Manual of
DERMATOLOGY
in General Practice

Manual of DERMATOLOGY in General Practice

2ND EDITION

Prof Dr Md Rokon Uddin
MBBS (DMC) DDV (BSMMU)
Consultant
Department of Dermatology and Laser Unit
Bangladesh Specialized Hospital
Dhaka, Bangladesh

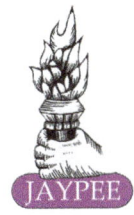

JAYPEE BROTHERS MEDICAL PUBLISHERS
The Health Sciences Publisher
New Delhi | London

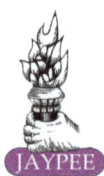 **Jaypee Brothers Medical Publishers (P) Ltd**

Headquarters
EMCA House
23/23-B, Ansari Road, Daryaganj
New Delhi 110 002, India
Landline: +91-11-23272143, +91-11-23272703
+91-11-23282021, +91-11-23245672
E-mail: jaypee@jaypeebrothers.com

Overseas Office
JP Medical Ltd.
83, Victoria Street, London
SW1H 0HW (UK)
Phone: +44-20 3170 8910
E-mail: info@jpmedpub.com

Corporate Office
Jaypee Brothers Medical Publishers (P) Ltd.
4838/24, Ansari Road, Daryaganj
New Delhi 110 002, India
Phone: +91-11-43574357
Fax: +91-11-43574314
E-mail: jaypee@jaypeebrothers.com

EU GPSR Authorised Representative
Logos Europe, 9 rue Nicolas Poussin
17000, La Rochelle, France
Phone: +33 (0) 6 67 93 73 78
E-mail: Contact@logoseurope.eu

Website: www.jaypeebrothers.com
Website: www.jaypeedigital.com

© 2024, Jaypee Brothers Medical Publishers

The views and opinions expressed in this book are solely those of the original contributor(s)/author(s) and do not necessarily represent those of editor(s) or publisher of the book.

All rights reserved. No part of this publication may be reproduced, stored or transmitted in any form or by any means, electronic, mechanical, photocopying, recording or otherwise, without the prior permission in writing of the publishers.

All brand names and product names used in this book are trade names, service marks, trademarks or registered trademarks of their respective owners. The publisher is not associated with any product or vendor mentioned in this book.

Medical knowledge and practice change constantly. This book is designed to provide accurate, authoritative information about the subject matter in question. However, readers are advised to check the most current information available on procedures included and check information from the manufacturer of each product to be administered, to verify the recommended dose, formula, method and duration of administration, adverse effects and contraindications. It is the responsibility of the practitioner to take all appropriate safety precautions. Neither the publisher nor the author(s)/editor(s) assume any liability for any injury and/or damage to persons or property arising from or related to use of material in this book.

This book is sold on the understanding that the publisher is not engaged in providing professional medical services. If such advice or services are required, the services of a competent medical professional should be sought.

Every effort has been made where necessary to contact holders of copyright to obtain permission to reproduce copyright material. If any have been inadvertently overlooked, the publisher will be pleased to make the necessary arrangements at the first opportunity.

Inquiries for bulk sales may be solicited at: jaypee@jaypeebrothers.com

Manual of Dermatology in General Practice / *Prof Dr Md Rokon Uddin*

First Edition: 2021

Second Edition: **2024**

ISBN: 978-93-5696-853-0

Dedication

This book is dedicated in loving memory of my father and to my mother.

Preface to the Second Edition

As a practicing dermatologist, I have had the privilege of witnessing remarkable advancements in my understanding and treatment options for various dermatological conditions throughout my career. It brings me immense pleasure to introduce the second edition of this comprehensive dermatology book.

This updated edition is tailored for both medical students and healthcare professionals, offering an in-depth exploration of dermatological conditions, their diagnoses, and a plethora of supporting illustrations. I am confident that this book will prove invaluable to readers seeking a profound grasp of dermatology, whether they are embarking on their journey in the field or are seasoned practitioners aiming to enrich their knowledge.

The second edition of this book presents a thorough overview of dermatological conditions, encompassing their symptoms and the latest advancements in diagnosis and treatment. It delves into a wide array of topics, ranging from common conditions to rare diseases and complex dermatological cases. Detailed descriptions, illustrations, and photographs of dermatological conditions are provided to empower professionals, enabling them to enhance their diagnostic skills with confidence. The book also offers guidance on distinguishing between similar-looking skin conditions by understanding their clinical presentations and utilizing appropriate diagnostic tools.

Dermatology is a continuously evolving field, and I firmly believe that by sharing our knowledge, experiences, and research, we can collectively work toward improving the care and well-being of our patients.

I genuinely hope that this book becomes a source of continual learning and innovation in the realm of dermatology. May it serve as an inspiration to the next generation of dermatologists, encouraging them to strive for excellence and contribute significantly to the overall well-being of the people they serve.

Prof Dr Md Rokon Uddin

Preface to the First Edition

The dream to compose the manual was set in my mind 20 years back while I had been undergoing training in the Department of Dermatology at Dhaka Medical College Hospital, Bangladesh where I found the entire academic and training environment made the learning difficult, complex and unenjoyable. So, the manual was structured to make the clinical dermatology fascinating and easily understandable to all the physicians requiring to diagnose and treat the dermatological problems of the patients.

The contents of the book were selected to cover the common clinical dermatological problems encountered by all the physicians spreading across the country.

All the segments of the book thoughtfully arranged here to fulfill the aim and satisfy the objectives of making the subject matter comprehensible to any medical graduate. For dermatologists as well as for postgraduate students and practitioners up-to-date clinical and surgical approaches of common skin disorders were special inclusions.

Clinical photographs were nominated keeping two objectives in mind. Firstly, to make the clinical aspects vivid and visible to the physicians; and secondly, to make the purpose of teaching easier and more attractive.

I hope this book should be a real help to generate interest among the physicians transforming clinical dermatology methodical, charming and easier.

Prof Dr Md Rokon Uddin

Acknowledgments

I would like to thank all my patients for being a part of my journey. It is because of them that I was able to acquire the knowledge, expertise, and photographs, shedding light on various diseases, necessary for the foundation of this book.

At the same time, I would like to extend my heartfelt gratitude to Shri Jitendar P Vij (Group Chairman), Mr Ankit Vij (Managing Director), Mr MS Mani (Group President), Ms Chetna Malhotra (Senior Director—Professional Publishing, Marketing, and Business Development), Ms Pooja Bhandari [Director—Production (Books and Journals)], Mr Sabyasachi Hazra, Associate Director (Publishing and Digital Sales), and Mr Akhilesh Saxena (Publishing Coordinator), M/s Jaypee Brothers Medical Publishers (P) Ltd, New Delhi, India, for constant encouragement and for publishing the *Manual of Dermatology in General Practice*.

Prof Dr Md Rokon Uddin

Contents

1. Basic Principles and Cutaneous Signs and Symptoms — 1
2. Pruritus and Dysesthesia — 11
3. Psoriasis and Related Disorders — 13
4. Dermatitis (Eczema) — 31
5. Psychoneurodermatitis — 45
6. Urticaria and Angioedema — 52
7. Erythema Multiforme, Stevens–Johnson Syndrome, Toxic Epidermal Necrolysis, and Fixed Drug Eruption — 55
8. Environmental and Occupational-related Dermatoses — 63
9. Endocrine, Metabolic, and Nutritional Diseases — 67
10. Genetic Diseases of Skin (Genodermatosis) — 83
11. Cutaneous Signs of Systemic Disease — 94
12. Cutaneous Manifestation of Bacterial, Viral, Protozoal, Worm, Fungal Infection, and Other Infections/Infestation — 96
13. Bullous Diseases (Genetic, Autoimmune and Acquired) — 161
14. Rheumatologic Dermatology — 171
15. Neutrophilic Dermatosis — 186
16. Disorders of Sebaceous, Eccrine, and Apocrine Glands — 190
17. Hair, Nail, and Mucous Membrane — 197

Index — 215

CHAPTER 1

Basic Principles and Cutaneous Signs and Symptoms

APPROACH TO DERMATOLOGICAL DIAGNOSIS

- *History taking*: Onset and course
  - *Constitutional symptoms*:
    - Exacerbating or relieving factors
    - History of skin disease, atopy, autoimmune disease, diabetes mellitus or any immunosuppressive conditions
    - Occupational, social history
    - Psychological history
    - Allergy history
    - *Drug history*: Both topical and systemic drugs including over-the-counter preparation.
- *Closer inspection*: Use magnifying lens or dermatoscope.
- Examination of skin, hair, nail, and mucous membrane
  - Type of lesion—Cutaneous signs
  - *Distribution pattern*:
    - Generalized or localized (Extensor surface, flexural areas, body folds, palm-sole)
    - Unilateral or bilateral—if bilateral symmetrical or asymmetric distribution.
    - Linear or random or grouped distribution—if grouped: Herpetiform or cluster.
    - Special pattern—if any-photodistribution, photoprotected, alone cleavage lines, contact area, and areas of occlusion.
  - Further characterization
    - *Color*—Pink, red, purple, white, tan, brown, black, blue, gray, and yellow.
    - Margination—Well- and ill-defined.
    - Shape—Round, oval, polygonal, polycyclic, annular (ring-shaped), iris, serpiginous (snakelike), umbilicated.
    - Palpation—Have to consider consistency (soft, firm, hard, fluctuant, boardlike); temperature (hot and cold); mobility; tenderness; depth of lesion (dermal or subcutaneous)
  - Morphology pattern.
- *General examination*: Includes lymph node examination.
  - Skin findings for systemic disease.

CUTANEOUS SIGNS

■ Primary Lesions

Initial lesions those are not altered by natural evolution, infection, trauma, or manipulations.

Macules: They are ≤1 cm sized flat, nonpalpable skin lesions with color change., e.g., freckle, lentigo, idiopathic guttate melanosis, etc. **(Figs. 1 and 2)**.

Patches: Flat skin lesions with color change >1 cm, e.g., vitiligo, melasma, dermal melanogenesis, café-au-lait spot, nevus depigmentosus, etc. **(Figs. 3 and 4)**.

Papules: They are circumscribed, discrete, solid, epidermal elevation varying in size from a pinhead to 1 cm (0.5 mm to 1 cm) **(Figs. 5 to 8)**.

Plaques: They are circumscribed, elevated solid lesion due to increased thickness of epidermis and/or cells or deposits within the dermis >1 cm in diameter. May be distinct lesion or formed by a confluence of papules **(Figs. 9 and 10)**.

Nodules: Dome-shaped, elevated, circumscribed lesions involving dermis and may extent to the subcutis; diameter >1 cm and on palpation can be compressible, soft, rubbery, or firm **(Figs. 11 to 14)**.

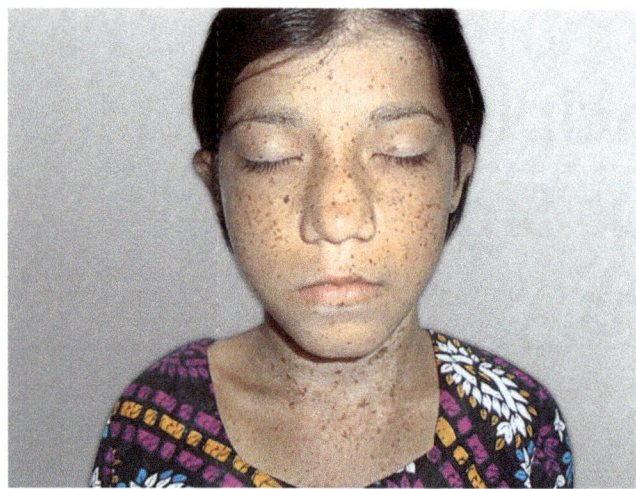

FIG. 1: Freckles-hyperpigmented flat lesions ≤1 cm.

FIG. 2: Rain drop hypopigmentation in chronic arsenicosis.

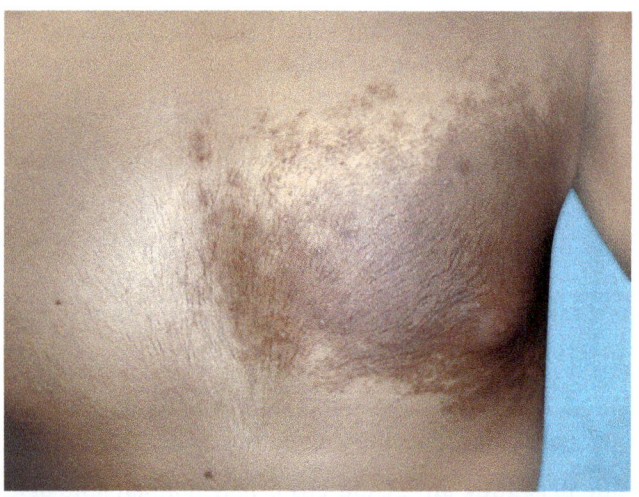

FIG. 3: Becker's nevus. Usually, unilateral tan to brown pigmentation ≥1 cm.

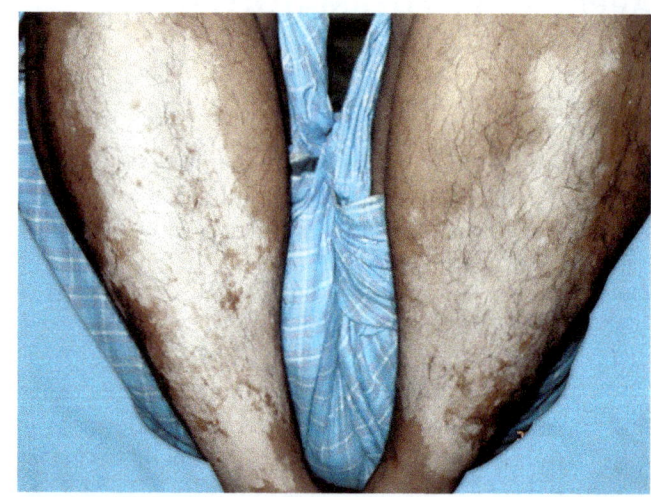

FIG. 4: Vitiligo—white flat area ≥1 cm.

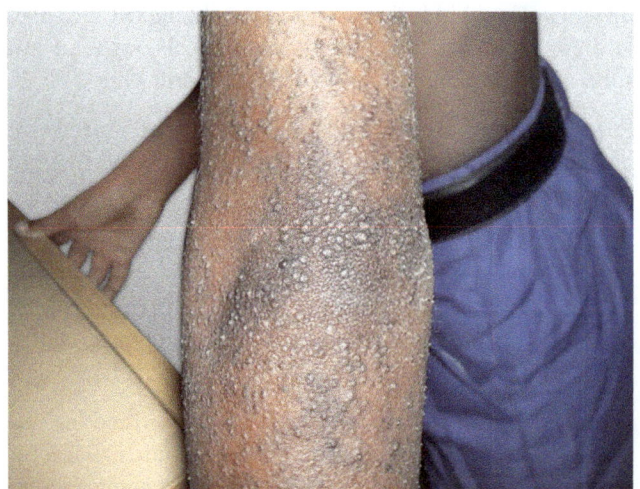

FIG. 5: Keratosis pilaris.

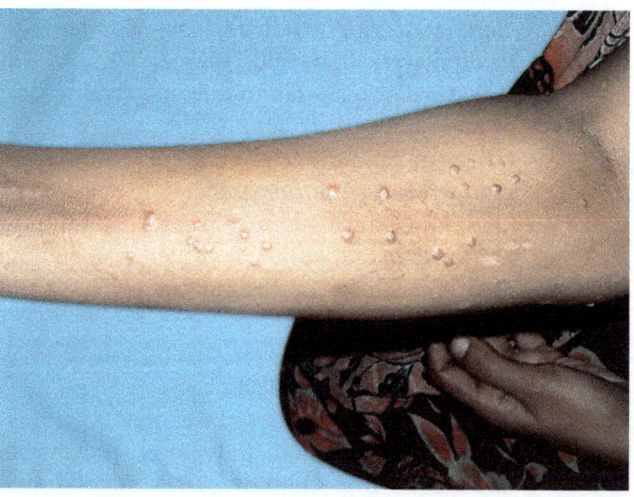

FIG. 6: Flat top papules in lichen planus.

CHAPTER 1 Basic Principles and Cutaneous Signs and Symptoms

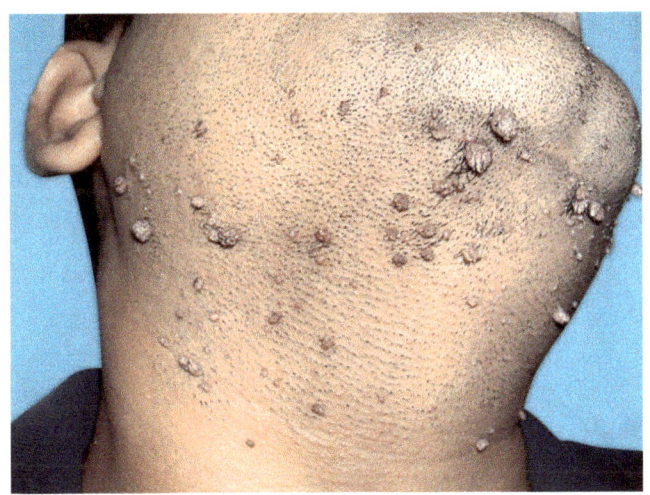

FIG. 7: Verrucous papules in viral warts.

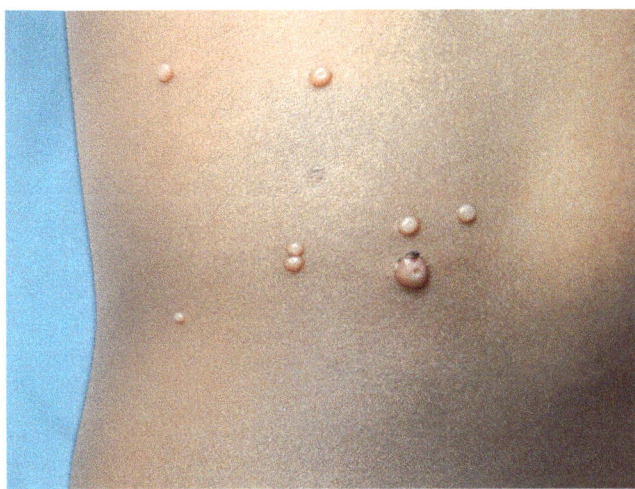

FIG. 8: Umbilicated papule in molluscum contagiosum.

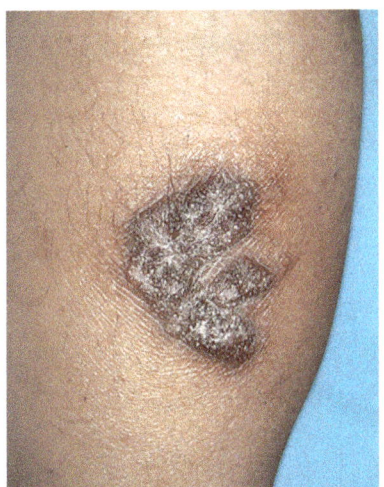

FIG. 9: Hypertrophic lichen planus. Solid elevated lesion >1 cm.

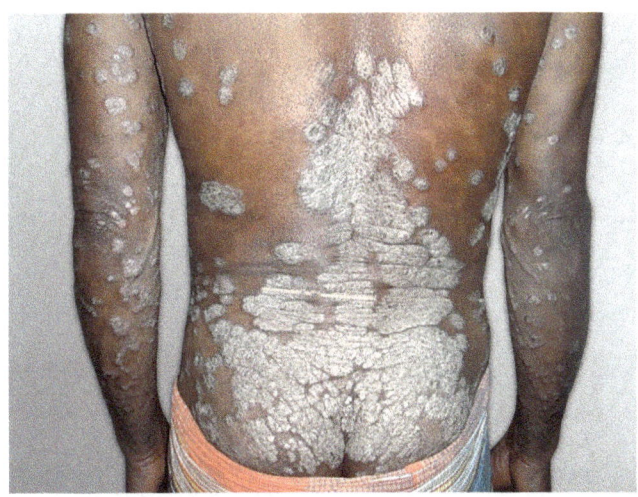

FIG. 10: Psoriasis. Soild elevated lesions ≥1 cm.

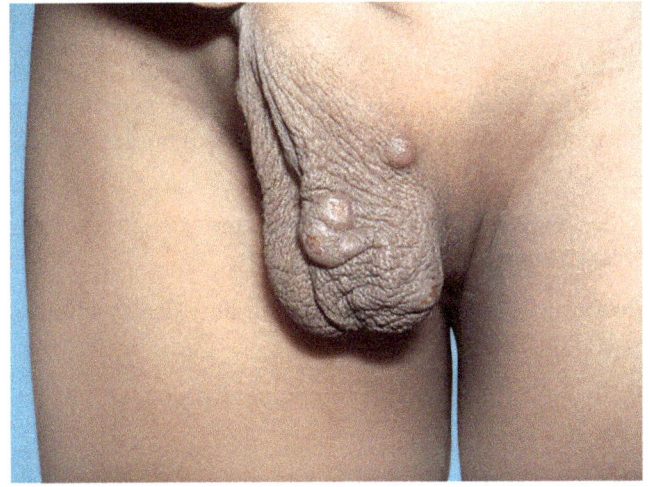

FIG. 11: Scabies: Dome-shaped lesion >1 cm.

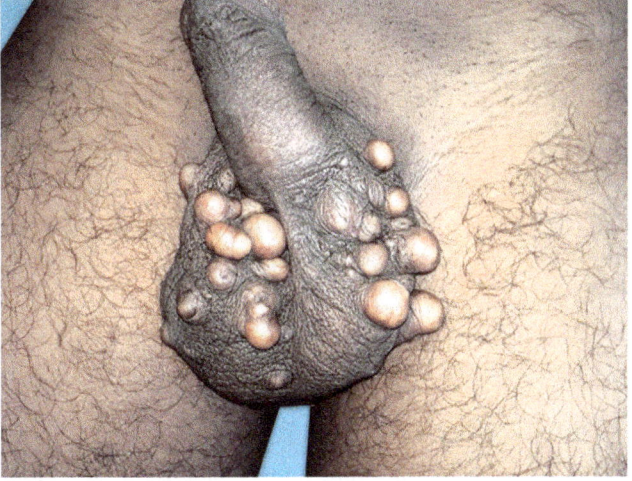

FIG. 12: Steatocystoma multiplex: Multiple cystic lesions on scrotum.

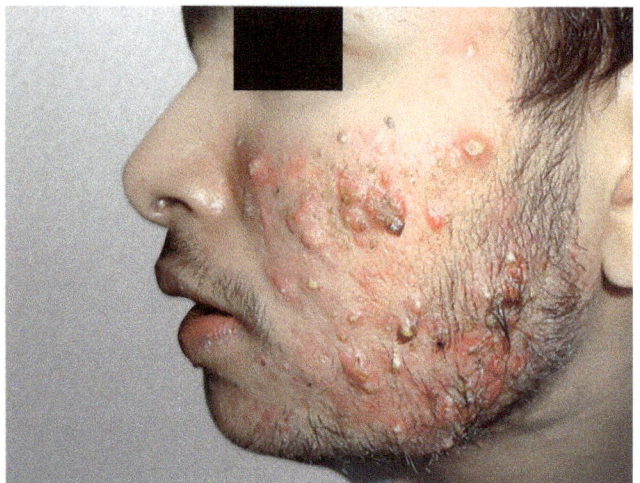

FIG. 13: Nodulocystic acne.

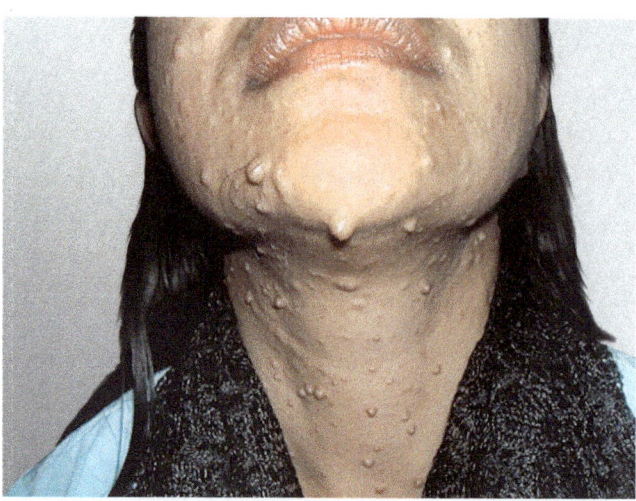

FIG. 14: Nodule in neurofibromatosis.

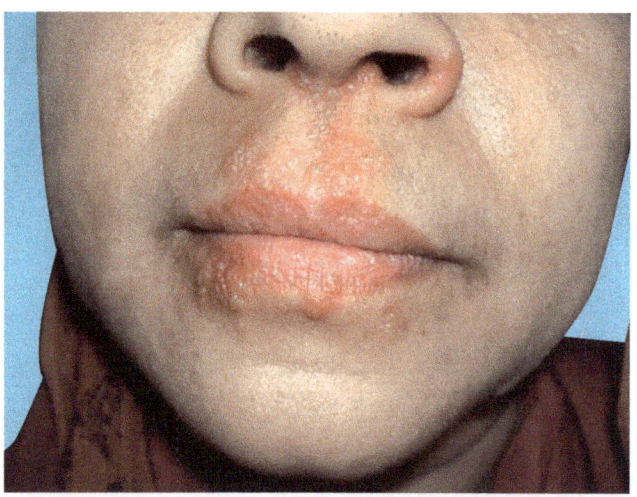

FIG. 15: Herpes simplex. Grouped vesicles on mucocutaneous area.

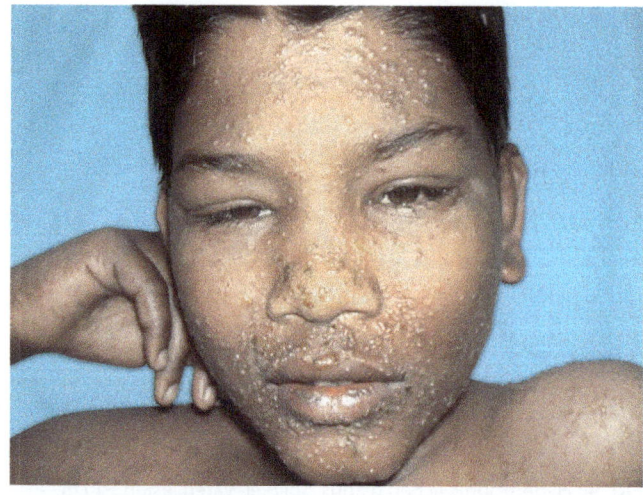

FIG. 16: Varicella. Discrete same stage vesicular lesions in an immunocompromised boy.

Vesicle: Elevated, circumscribed fluid containing lesion <1 cm diameter **(Figs. 15 and 16)**.

Bulla: Elevated, circumscribed fluid containing lesion >1 cm diameter **(Figs. 17 and 18)**.

Pustule: Elevated, circumscribed pus (infectious neutrophil or sterile) containing lesion <1 cm diameter **(Figs. 19 and 20)**.

Wheals: Evanescent, edematous, pruritic elevated lesion of various sizes **(Fig. 21)**.

■ Secondary Lesions

Lesions those are altered by natural evolution, infection, trauma, or manipulations.

Crust: Dried serum, pus, blood mixed with epithelial and sometimes bacterial debris. When crusts become detached, the base may be dry or red and moist **(Figs. 22 and 23)**.

Scale: They are dry or greasy, laminated masses of keratin **(Figs. 24 and 25)**.

Erosion: Partial or full loss of epidermis. Heals without a scar **(Fig. 26)**.

Excoriation: Linear or punctuate abrasion by trauma **(Fig. 27)**.

Fissures: Vertical loss of epidermis and partial or full thickness of dermis **(Fig. 28)**.

CHAPTER 1 Basic Principles and Cutaneous Signs and Symptoms

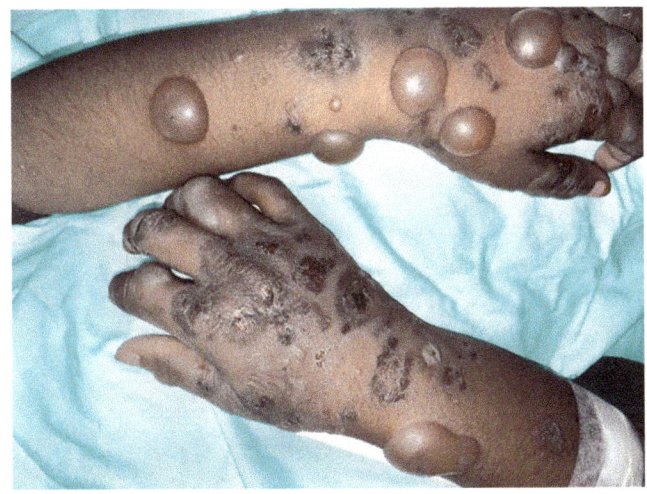

FIG. 17: Bullous pemphigoid. Classic presentation with multiple tense bullae arising on normal skin, some bullae have ruptured, leaving circular crusting and erosions.

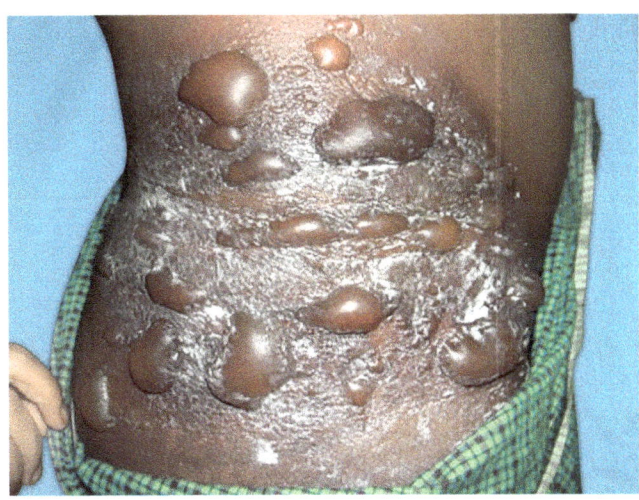

FIG. 18: Burn.

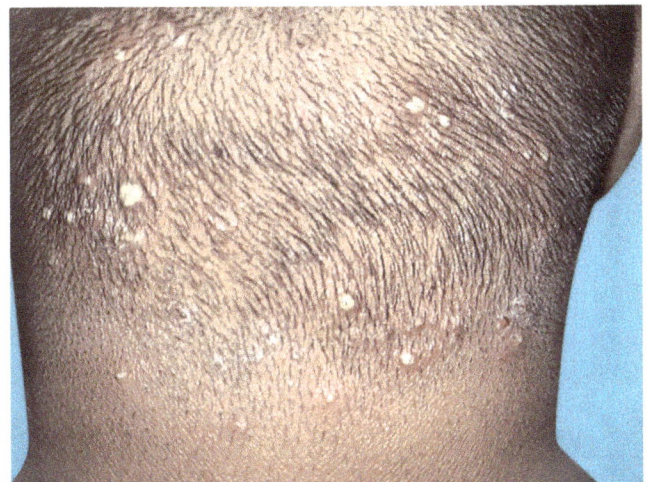

FIG. 19: Infectious–boil.

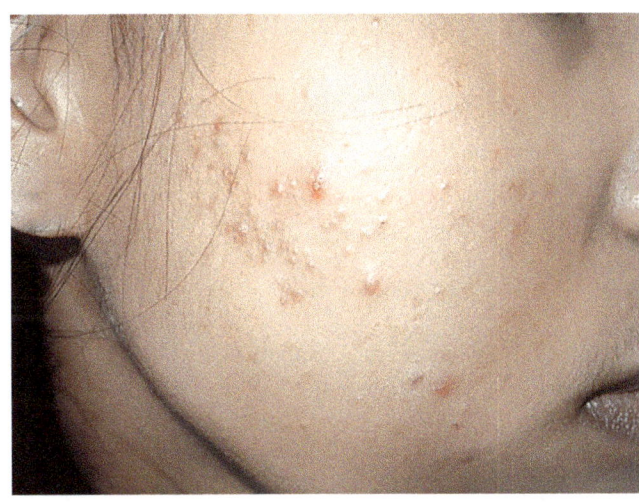

FIG. 20: Sterile pus formation in acne.

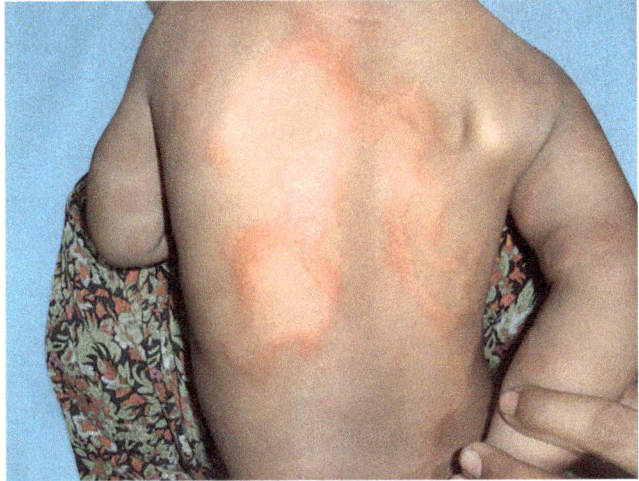

FIG. 21: Acute or chronic urticarial: Pruritic evanescent plaque.

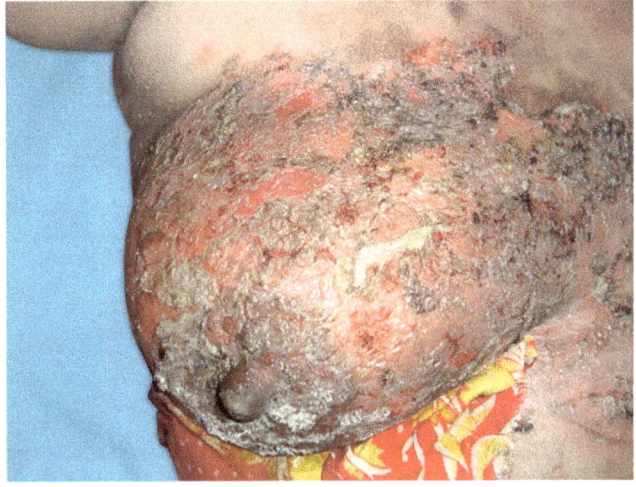

FIG. 22: Pemphigus vulgaris. Crusted lesions.

CHAPTER 1 Basic Principles and Cutaneous Signs and Symptoms

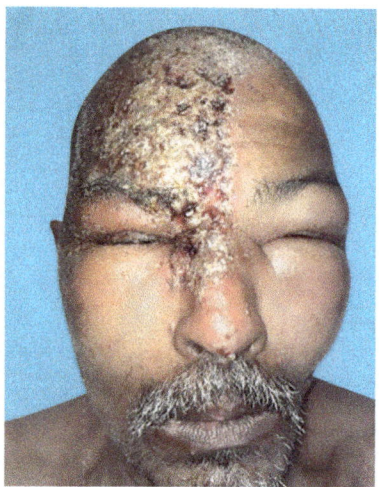

FIG. 23: Herpes zoster. Unilateral crusted lesions.

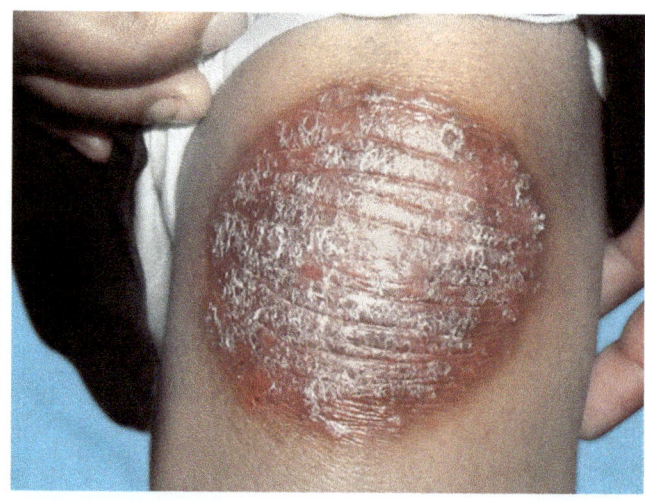

FIG. 24: Psoriasis. Silvery white scales.

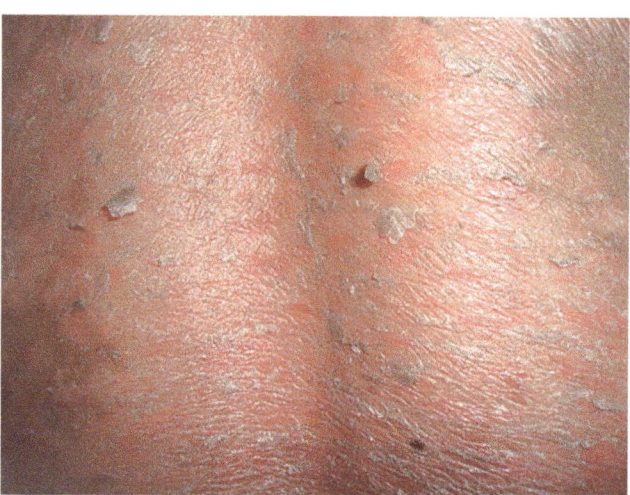

FIG. 25: Erythroderma.

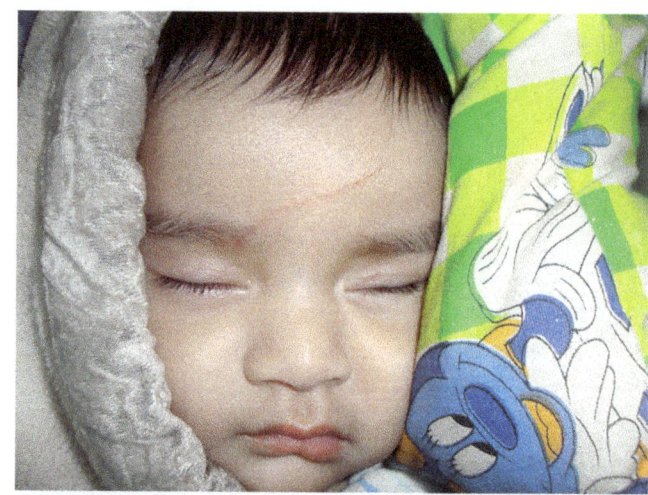

FIG. 26: Erosion.

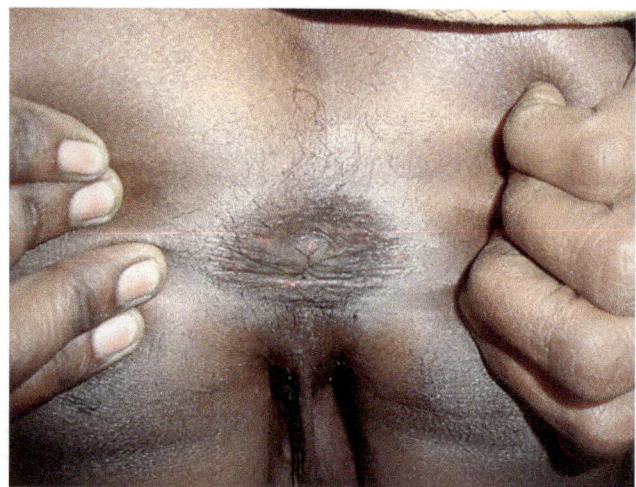

FIG. 27: Excoriation–punctate erosion.

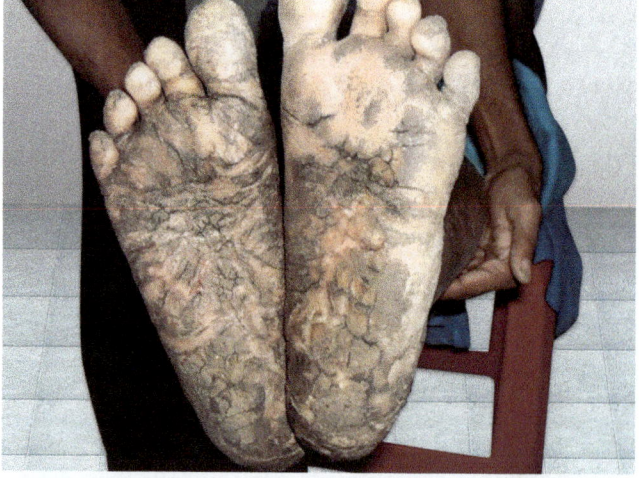

FIG. 28: Fissures.

Ulcers: Rounded or irregularly shaped complete loss of epidermis plus partial or complete loss of dermis **(Fig. 29)**.

Atrophy: Diminution of some or all layers of skin **(Figs. 30A and B)**.

Hypertrophy: Deposition of excessive amounts of collagen which are confined in wound area **(Figs. 31A and B)**.

Keloid: Deposition of excessive amounts of collagen which are not confined in wound area and are extended in normal surrounding area in claw-like fashion **(Figs. 32 and 33)**.

Petechiae

Pinpoint spots that appear on the skin due to extravasation of RBC.
- ≤3 mm diameter.
- Occurs in significant thrombocytopenia <20,000–40,000/mm^3 **(Figs. 34 and 35)**.

Purpura

Nonpalpable purpura are extravasation of blood in skin and mucous membrane <1 cm in diameter **(Figs. 35 and 36)**.

Palpable purpura occur due to vasculitis **(Figs. 37A and B)** and this is a common presentation of vasculitis.

Ecchymoses: Extravasation of blood usually >1 cm **(Figs. 38 to 41)**.

Causes are:
- *Defective coagulation*: Anticoagulant use, hepatic insufficiency and vitamin K deficiency.
- Poor dermal support of blood vessels.
- Platelet dysfunction.

Telangiectasis: Permanent dilatation of cutaneous blood vessels **(Figs. 42A and B)**.

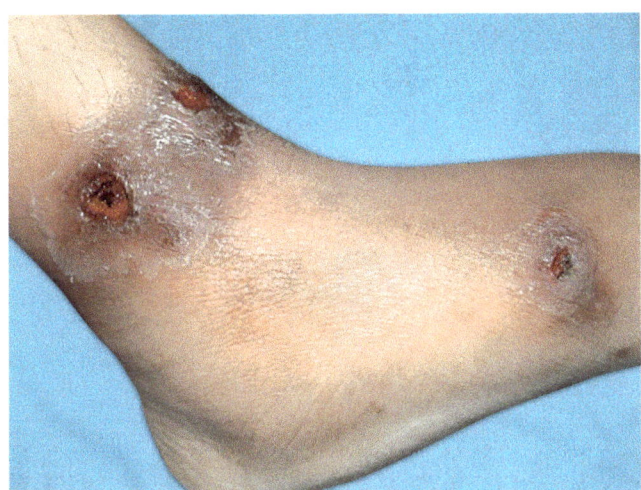

FIG. 29: Ulcers.

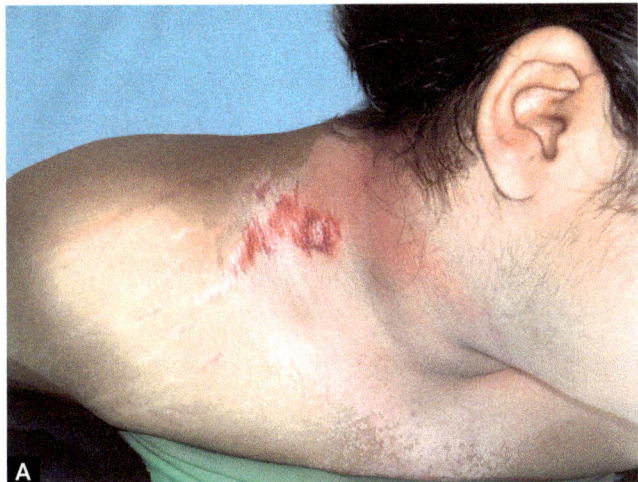
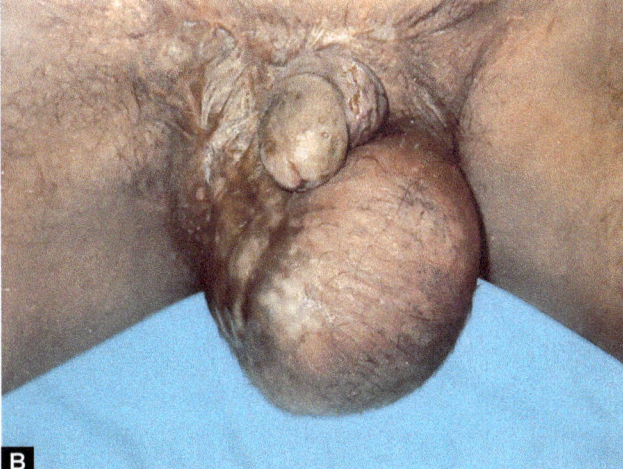

FIGS. 30A AND B: Atrophic scar. (A) Due to topical steroid. (B) Due to burn.

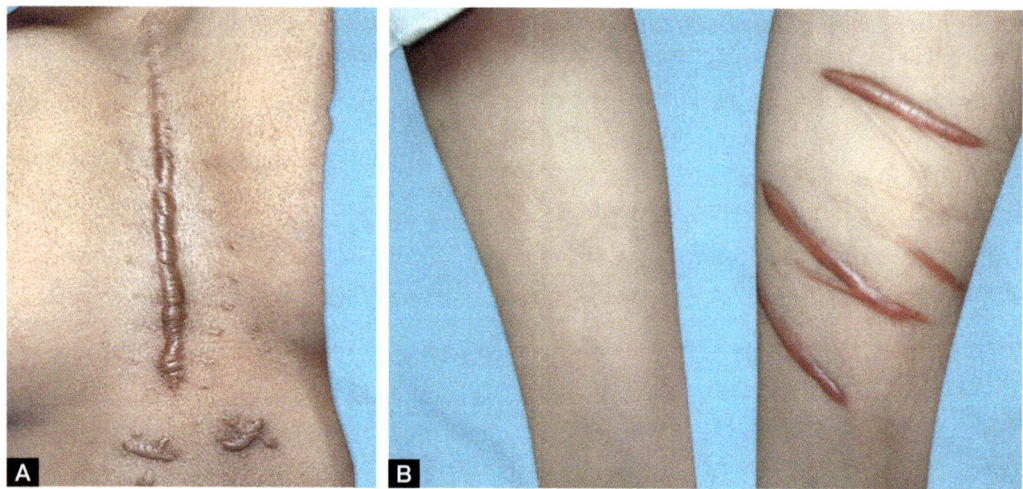

FIGS. 31A AND B: Hypertrophy—confined in wound area.

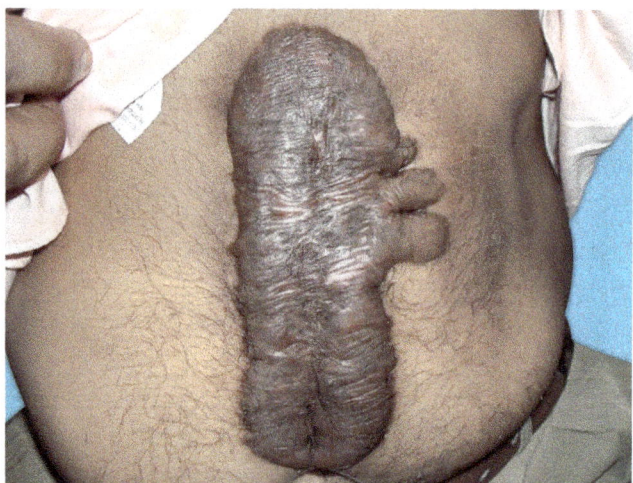

FIG. 32: Keloid at the site of incision—not confined in wound area and are extended in normal surrounding area.

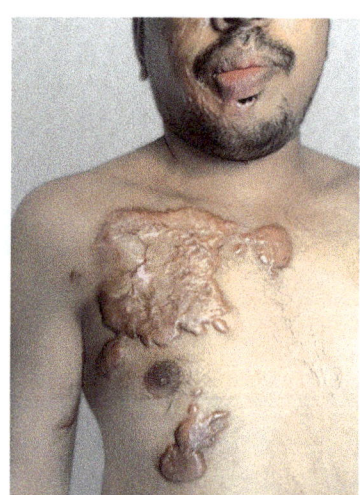

FIG. 33: Keloid on burns.

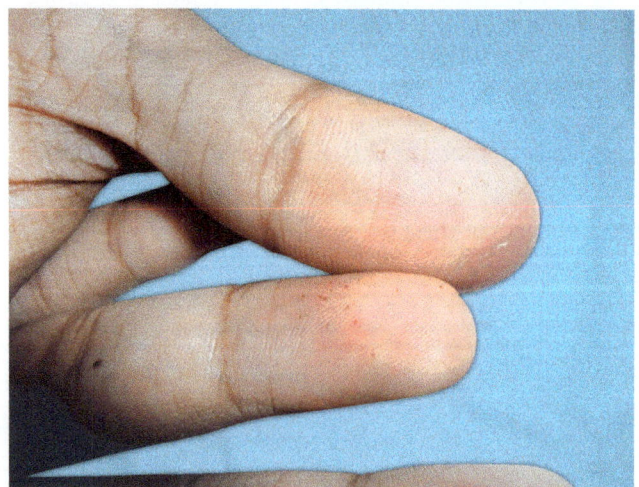

FIG. 34: Petechiae.

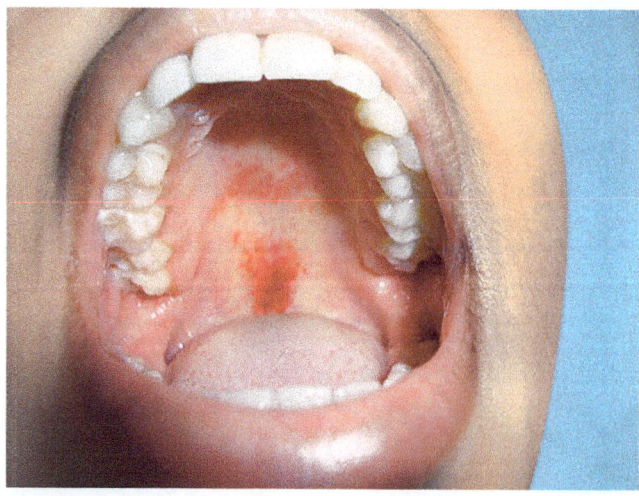

FIG. 35: Petechial hemorrhage.

CHAPTER 1 Basic Principles and Cutaneous Signs and Symptoms

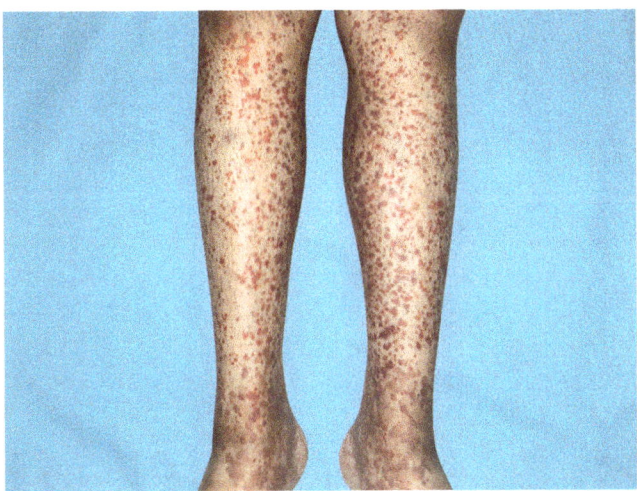

FIG. 36: Nonpalpable purpura.

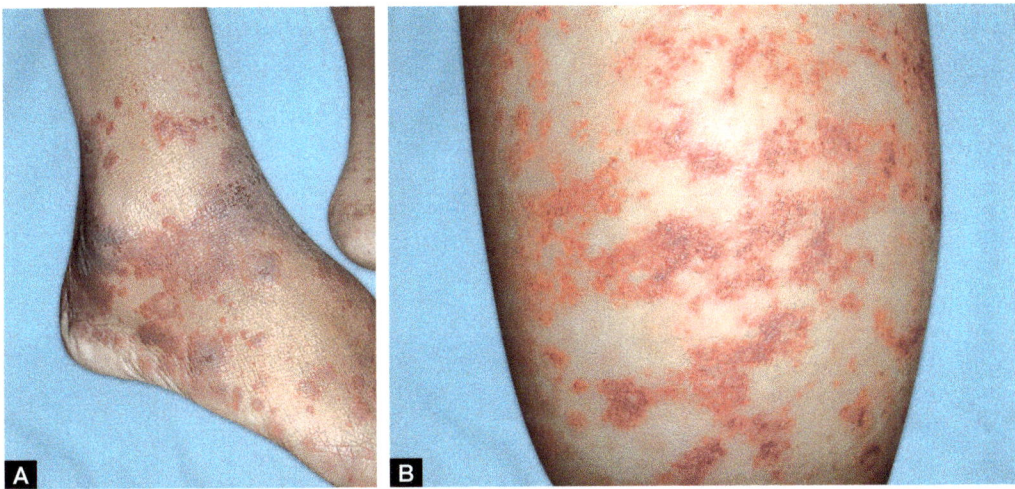

FIGS. 37 AND B: Red purple papule with a blanching erythema.

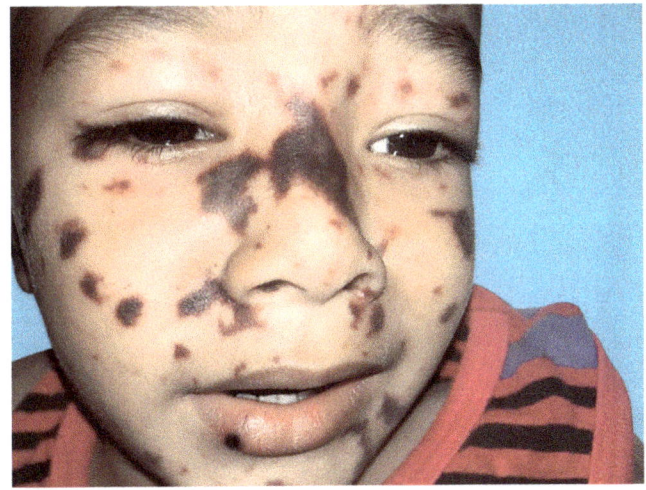

FIG. 38: Ecchymosis in disseminated intravascular coagulation.

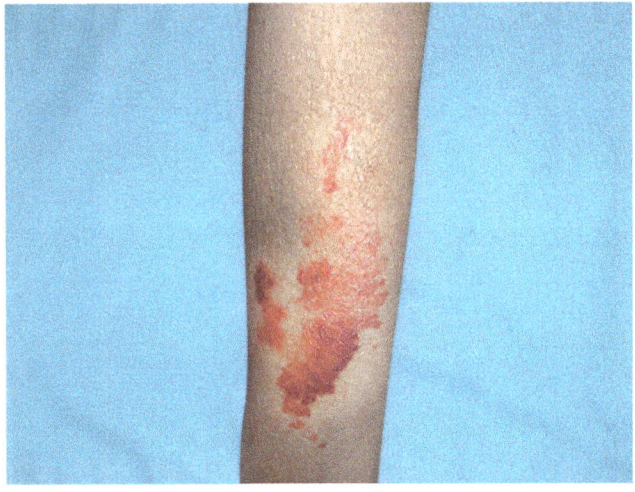

FIG. 39: Petechiae, purpura, ecchymosis in dengue hemorrhagic fever.

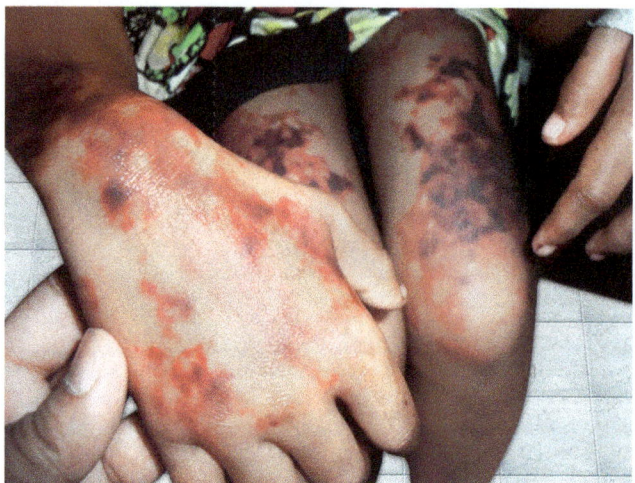

FIG. 40: Ecchymosis in meningococcal infection.

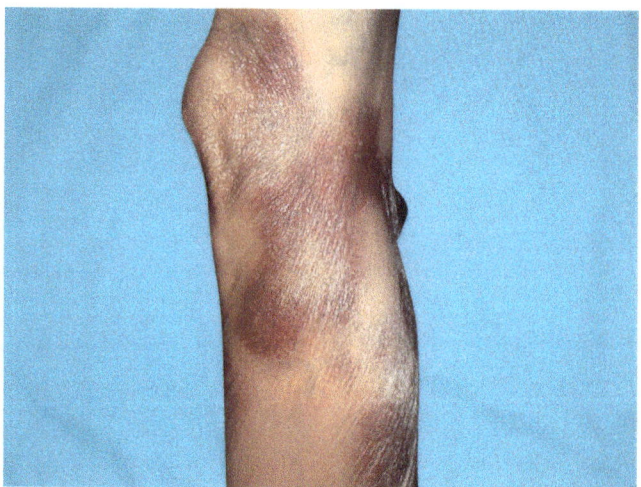

FIG. 41: Senile purpura and ecchymosis.

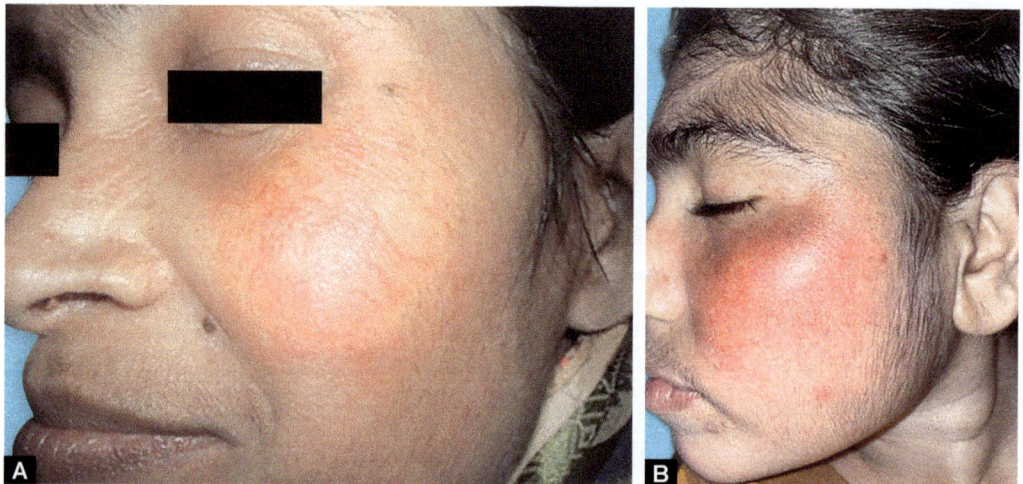

FIGS. 42A AND B: Permanent dilatation of cutaneous blood vessels due to topical steroid.

CHAPTER 2

Pruritus and Dysesthesia

PRURITUS

An unpleasant sensation of the skin that elicits a desire to scratch is known pruritus.

Causes of Pruritus

Dermatological Diseases

- Infestations/bites and stings—scabies, pediculosis, and arthropod bites
- Inflammation—atopic dermatitis, stasis dermatitis, allergic > irritant contact dermatitis, seborrheic dermatitis, psoriasis, lichen planus, urticaria, papular urticaria, drug eruption, mastocytosis, eosinophilic folliculitis, and pruritus associated with HIV
- Autoimmune connective tissue disease—lichen sclerosus, dermatomyositis, and lupus erythematosus
- Infections—bacterial, viral, fungal, and parasitic
- Neoplastic—cutaneous T-cell lymphoma
- Others—xerosis, scar associated, lichen simplex chronicus, prurigo nodularis, pregnancy dermatosis, neuropathic itch, and actinic pruritus.
- *Metabolic and endocrine conditions*:
  o Hyperthyroidism is probably due to increased blood flow.
  o Hypothyroidism is probably due to excessive dryness.
  o Pregnancy related
  o Diabetes mellitus
- *Malignant neoplasm*:
  o Lymphoma, myeloid and lymphocytic leukemia, myelodysplasia, multiple myeloma, and Hodgkin disease

- *Drug*: Aspirin, alcohol, dextran, polymyxin B, morphine, codeine, and scopolamine
- *Renal*: Due to dryness and deposition of excretory materials
- *Hematological*: 50% polycythemia vera patient experience aquagenic pruritus, paraproteinemia, and iron deficiency
- *Hepatic disease*: Obstructive biliary disease (starts acrally and then disseminates) and pregnancy (intrahepatic cholestasis)
- *Neurological*: Peripheral nerve damage and spinal nerve damage
- *Psychological states*: During periods of emotional stress, delusions of parasitosis, psychogenic pruritus, neurotic excoriation, and anorexia nervosa

Treatment of Pruritus

General Measures

- Use mild soap
- Use moisturizer
- Avoid woolens and harsh fabrics
- Avoid fabric softeners
- Keep nails short

Pruritus Secondary to a Specific Dermatological Condition

- Treat underlying skin disease
- Oral antihistamine
- *Thalidomide*: Consider for refractory prurigo nodularis, actinic prurigo, and chronic lupus erythematosus.

Primary Generalized Pruritus with No Identifiable Specific Skin Disease

- *Topical*:
  - Low-potency topical corticosteroids
  - Topical calcineurin inhibitors
  - Cooling agents (e.g., menthol and camphor)
- *Systemic*:
  - *Antihistamines*:
    - Nonsedative antihistamine in morning, plus
    - Sedating antihistamine at evening, plus
    - Oral doxepin 10–25 mg at bedtime
  - *Antipruritic anticonvulsants*:
    - Gabapentin ± mirtazapine
    - Pregabalin ± mirtazapine

Antipruritic antidepressants: Consider in underlying depression with paraneoplastic condition or polycythemia vera.

Selective serotonin reuptake inhibitors (SSRIs) and serotonin-norepinephrine reuptake inhibitors (SNRIs): Fluoxetine, paroxetine, sertraline, and venlafaxine.

Tricyclic antidepressants (TCAs): Amitriptyline and doxepin.

Opioid antagonists and agonists: Consider in underlying hepatic or renal disease.
- Naltrexone
- Nalfurafine (renal itch)
- Thalidomide

Physical Treatment

- *Ultraviolet (UV) therapy*: Ultraviolet B rays (UVB), and psoralen and ultraviolet A (PUVA)
- Acupuncture

DYSESTHESIA

An unpleasant, abnormal sensation that can be either spontaneous or evoked; abnormal, unpleasant sensations that may include pain, pruritus (neuropathic itch), tingling, burning, and "pins and needles".

CHAPTER 3
Psoriasis and Related Disorders

INTRODUCTION

- Psoriasis is a common skin disease. It affects up to 2% of the populations.
- Chronic inflammatory disease of skin, mucous membrane, nails, and joints with polygenic predisposing and triggering factors such as infections [especially streptococcal pharyngitis and human immunodeficiency virus (HIV) infection], minor trauma, anxiety, or drugs [beta-blockers, lithium, antimalarial drugs, interferon, systemic corticosteroids (rebound), etc.]. Alcohol ingestion is a putative trigger factor.
- Well-demarcated, erythematous papules and plaques with silvery white scale are most common presentation **(Figs. 1 to 17)**. Common sites are scalp, extensor elbow and knee, palm sole, back of trunk (intergluteal folds), and nails **(Fig. 18)**.
- Other lesions are sterile pustule, and glistening plaque in intertriginous areas **(Figs. 19 to 22)**.
- Major systemic association is psoriatic arthritis. Psoriatic arthritis occurs in 5–30% of patients.
- *Koebner phenomenon*: Isomorphic new lesions at the site of trivial injury.

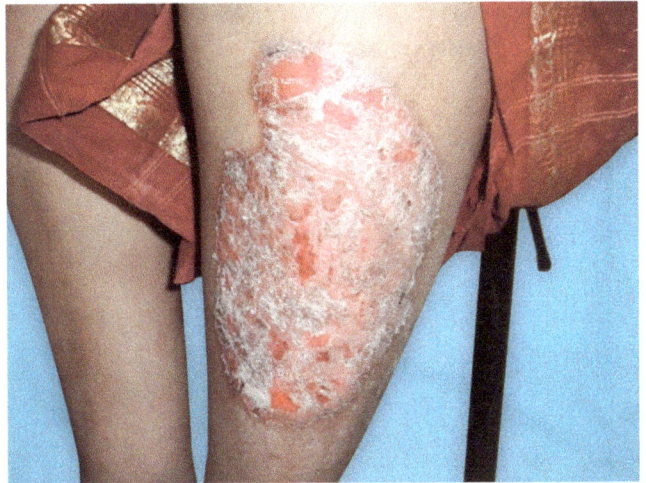

FIG. 1: Erythematous plaques with thick scale and desquamation on left shin.

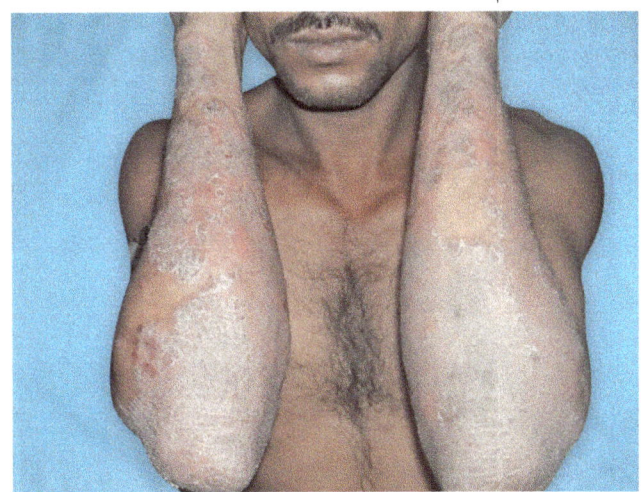

FIG. 2: Bilateral symmetrical erythematous papule-plaque with silvery white scale over both extensor forearms.

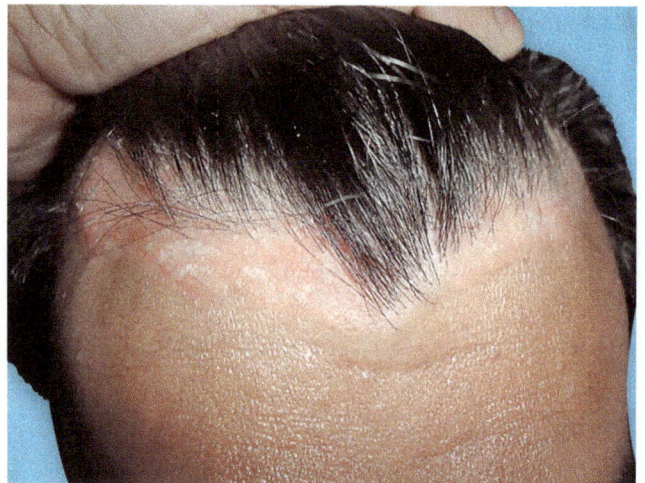

FIG. 3: Well-defined psoriatic plaque not crossing hair line.

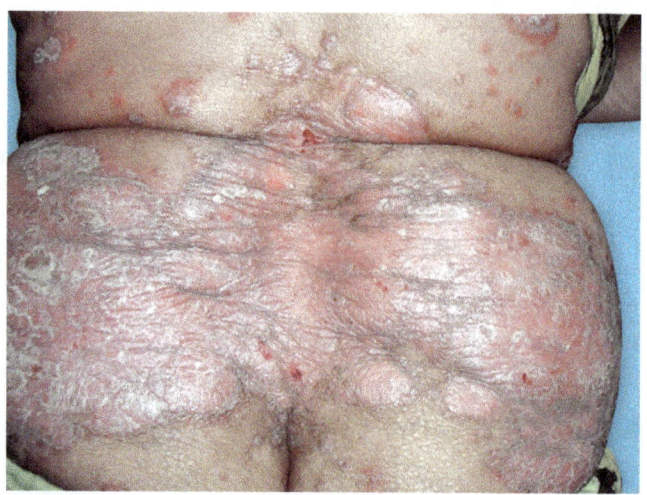

FIG. 4: Symmetric distribution of psoriatic plaque.

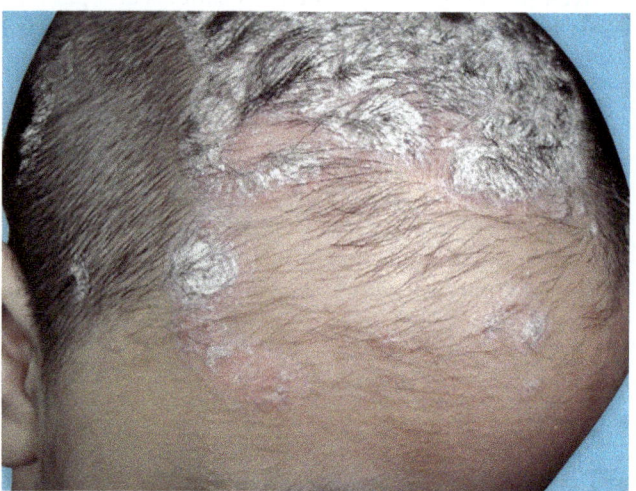

FIG. 5: Erythematous plaques with thick asbestos like scales over scalp of a 3-year-old child.

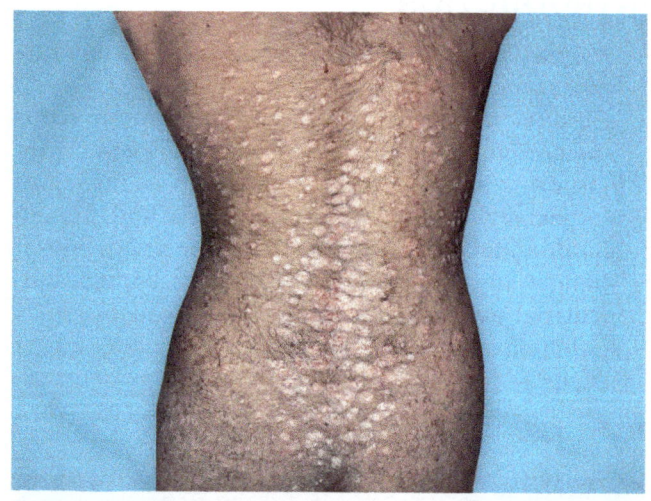

FIG. 6: Guttate psoriasis on back of trunk.

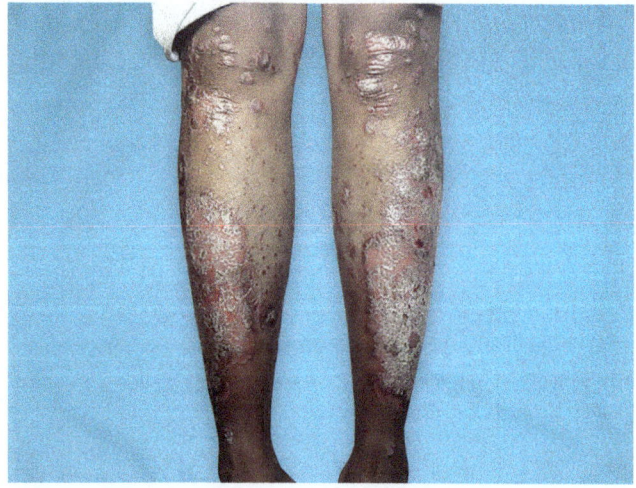

FIG. 7: Widespread chronic plaque psoriasis.

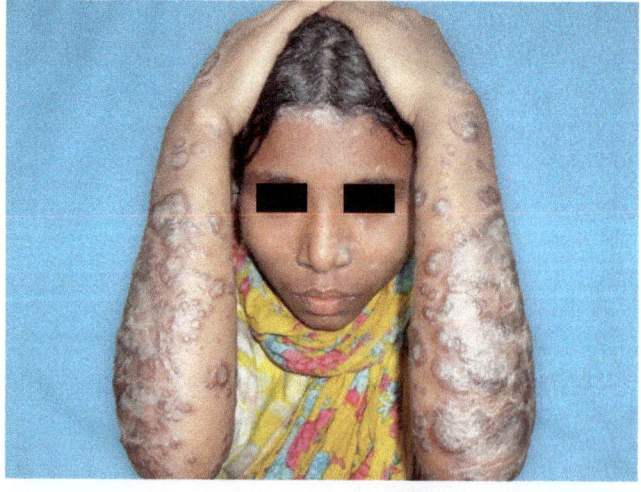

FIG. 8: Chronic stable plaque psoriasis on both extensor forearm.

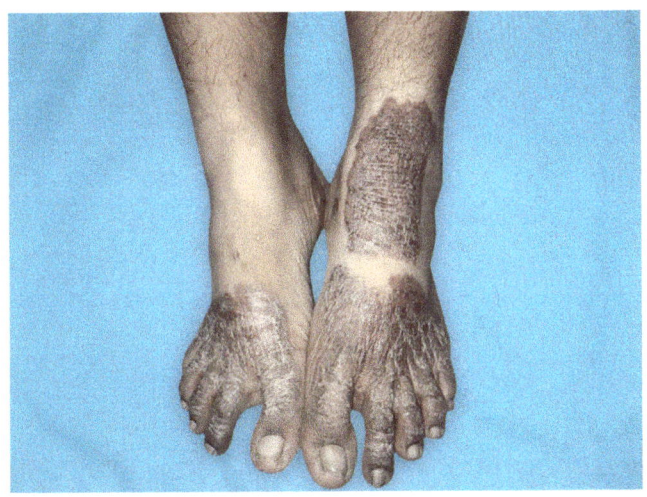

FIG. 9: Thick plaque on dorsum of foot easily confused with chronic eczema [lichen simplex chronicus (LSC)].

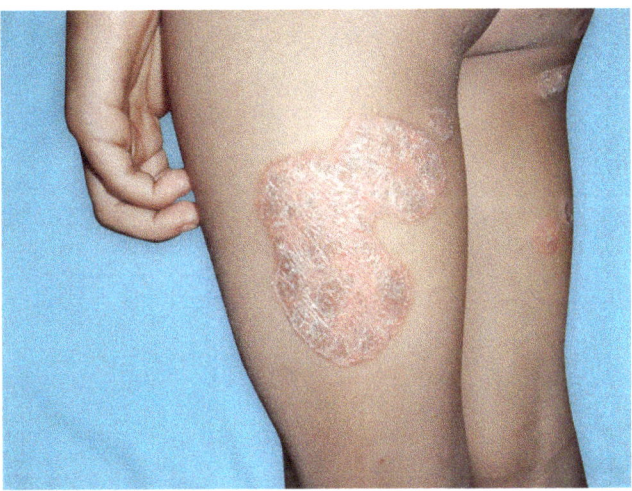

FIG. 10: Large scaling plaque on left thigh. Lesions are polycyclic and confluent forming geographic pattern.

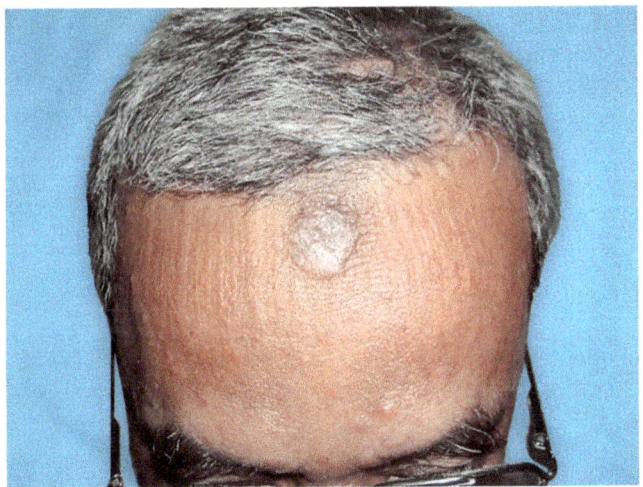

FIG. 11: Repeated trauma resultant psoriatic plaque on forehead.

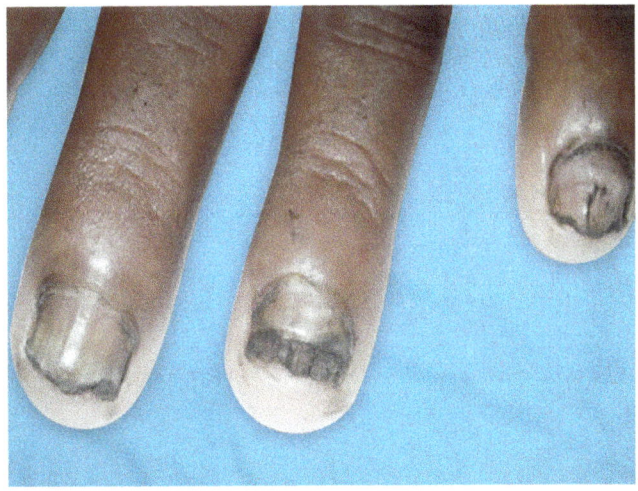

FIG. 12: Psoriatic nail change (thick nail plate).

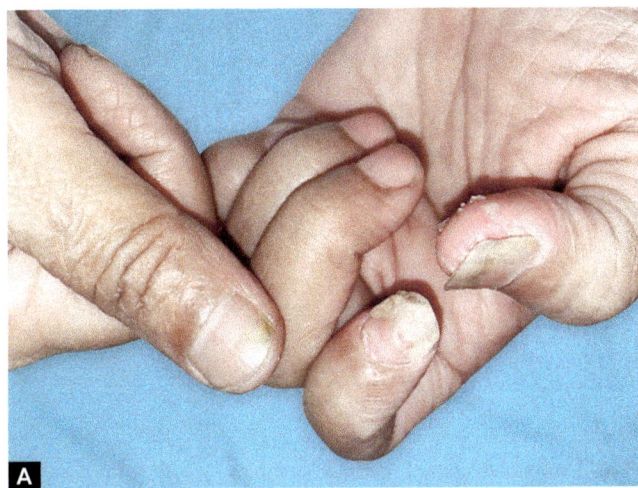

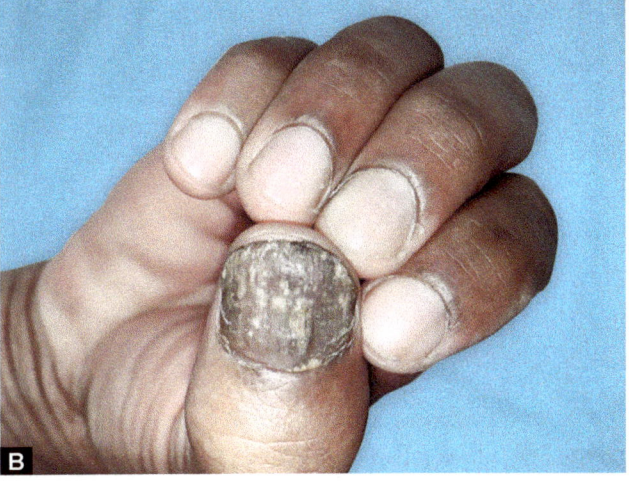

FIGS. 13A AND B: Pitting, onycholysis, thickening of nail plate on a psoriasis patient.

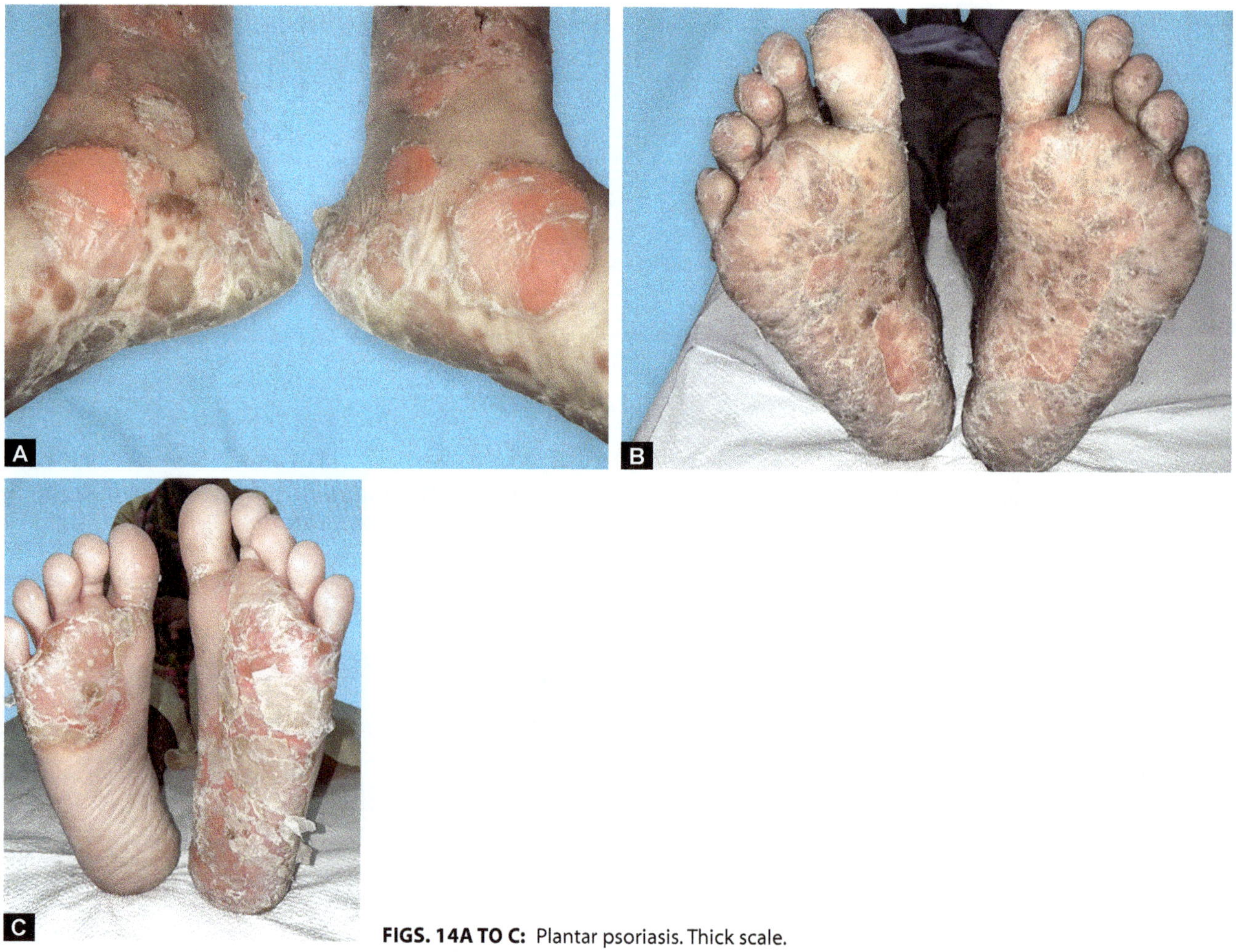

FIGS. 14A TO C: Plantar psoriasis. Thick scale.

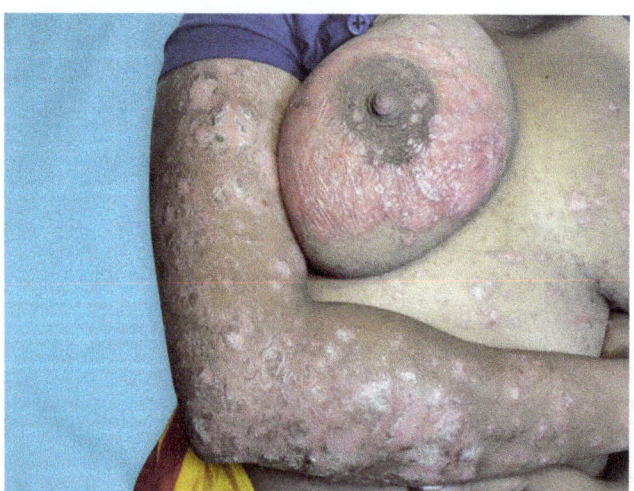

FIG. 15: Erythematous plaque with silvery white scale involving extensor upper extremity and right periareolar region.

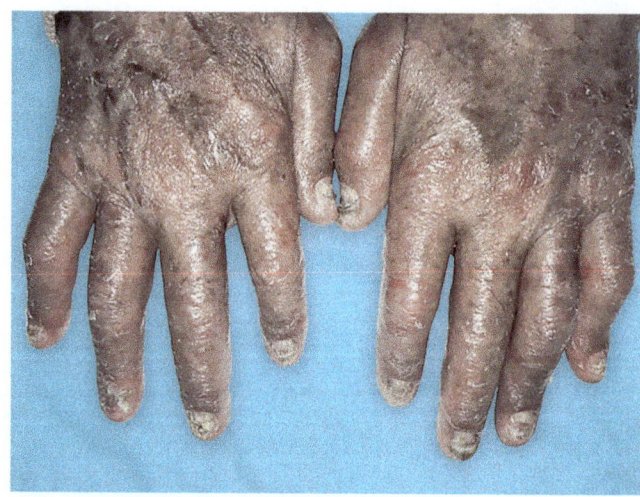

FIG. 16: Involvement of skin, nail, and joint.

CHAPTER 3 Psoriasis and Related Disorders

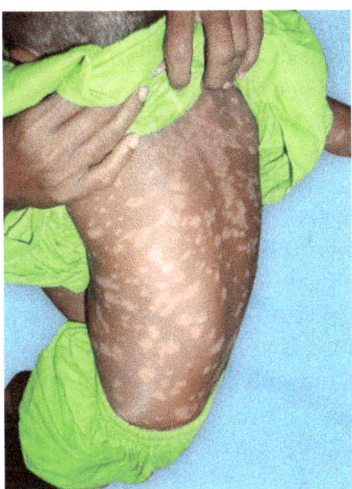

FIG. 17: Treated case: Hypopigmented patches just like pityriasis alba.

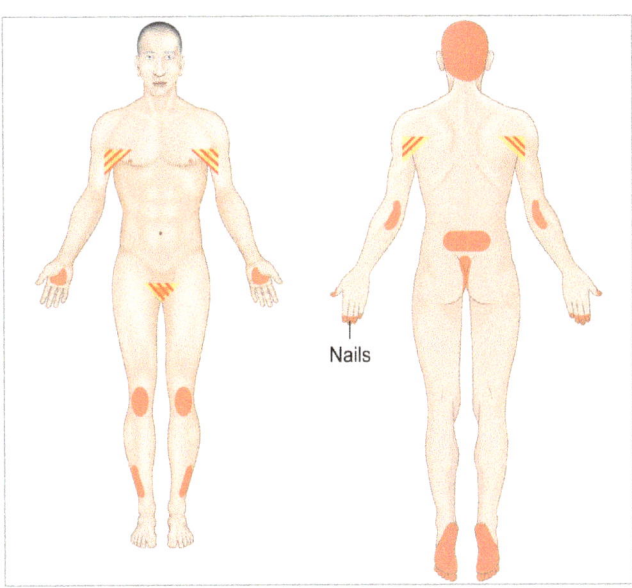

FIG. 18: Common sites where psoriasis occur.

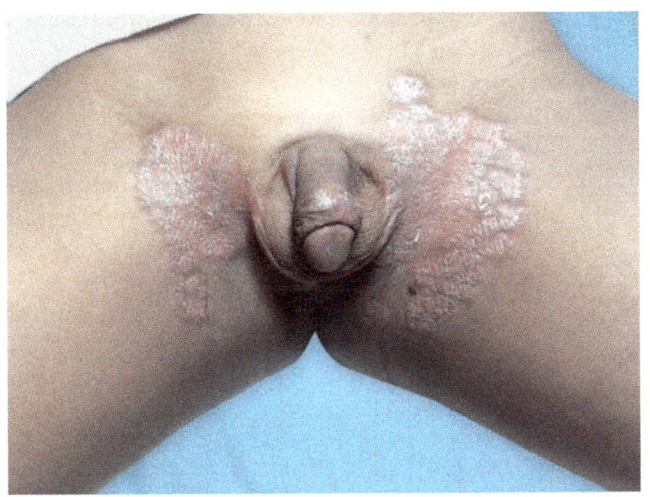

FIG. 19: Glistening plaque (inverse pattern psoriatic) on groin that mimic tinea cruris.

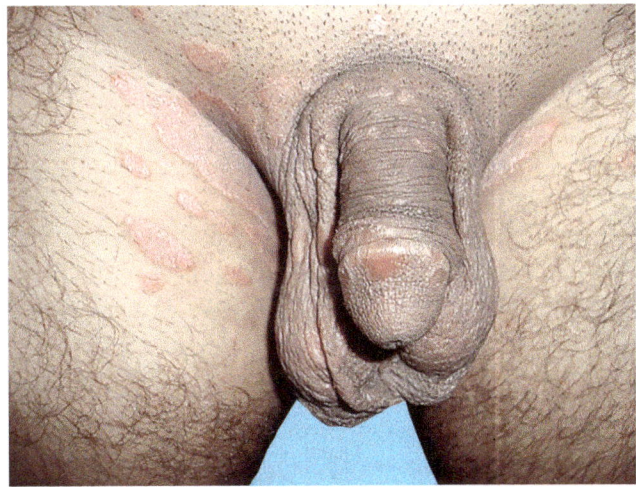

FIG. 20: Erythematous papule plaque on groin, glans penis in inverse pattern.

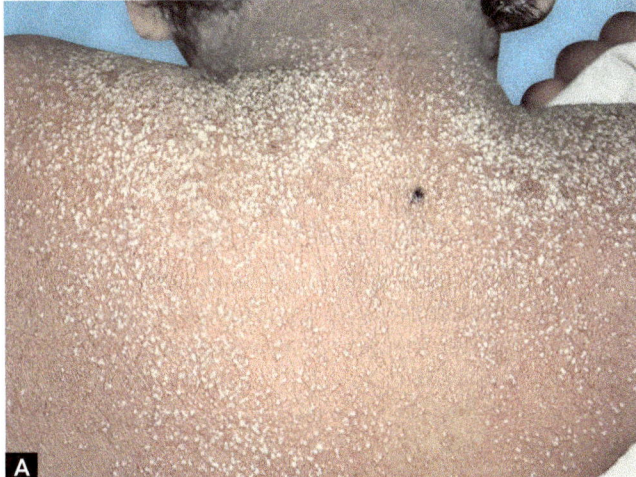

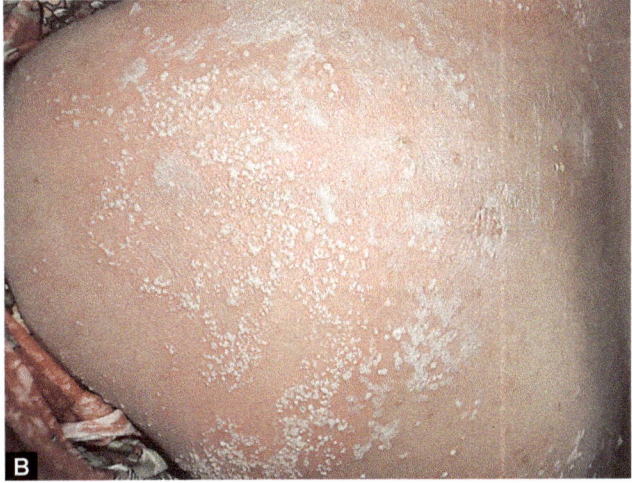

FIGS. 21A AND B: Creamy-yellow pustule that are confluent in some areas. Pustules are sterile and pruritic and when get larger, become painful.

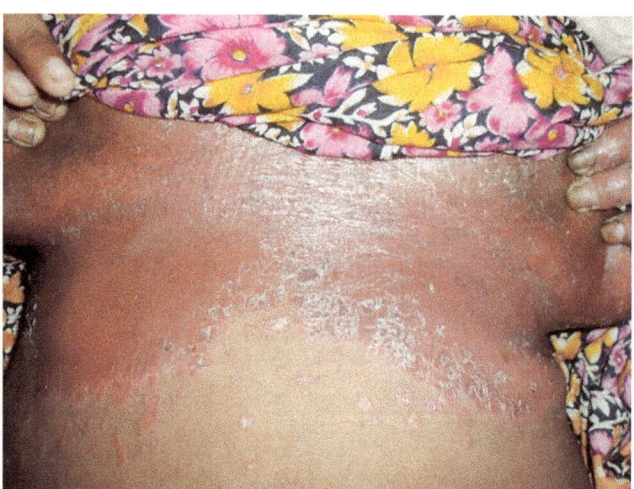

FIG. 22: Inverse pattern psoriatic plaque on submammary region.

COMMON SITES OF PSORIASIS

Common sites of psoriasis are shown in **Figure 18**.

■ Variants

- **Chronic plaque psoriasis:**
  - Typical lesion—well-demarcated, erythematous plaque with silvery scale
  - Often symmetrical lesions on the elbows and knees **(Figs. 2, 7, and 8)**, additional sites includes the scalp **(Figs. 3 and 5)**, presacral **(Fig. 4)**, hands **(Fig. 16)**, feet **(Figs. 9 and 14)**, intergluteal fold **(Figs. 19 and 20)** and umbilicus
  - It may be generalized.
- **Guttate psoriasis:**
  - Typical lesion—small papules or plaque (3 mm to 1.5 cm) with adherent scale **(Fig. 6)**
  - It affects children more than adults.
  - Usually, it is preceded by an upper respiratory tract infection.
  - In children, it may have spontaneous remission but often responds well to ultraviolet B (UVB).
- **Linear psoriasis:** Linear, erythematous, and scaly lesions that often follow the lines of Blaschko.
- **Erythrodermic psoriasis:**
  - Generalized erythema, plaques with scaling
  - Gradual or acute onset
  - Nail changes, facial sparing, and a history of typical plaque type psoriasis may be helpful clues.
  - It may be seen after abrupt tapering of medication, especially CS.
- **Pustular psoriasis:**
  - Generalized pustular psoriasis (von Zumbusch pattern)
    - Erythema and sterile pustules arising within erythematous, painful skin; lakes of pus characteristic **(Figs. 21A and B)**
    - Often associated with fever
    - Triggering factors—pregnancy (termed impetigo herpetiformis), rapid tapering of corticosteroids (CS), hypocalcemia, and infections.
- **Palmoplantar pustulosis:**
  - Sterile pustules on palms/soles
  - It may have no evidence of psoriasis elsewhere
  - Triggering factors—infections, stress, and smoking
  - Associated with inflammatory bone lesions

■ Special Sites

- Scalp psoriasis:
  - Well-demarcated, erythematous plaques with silvery scale
  - Scales may be attached for some distance onto scalp hairs, giving an asbestos like appearance.
  - Occasionally, alopecia may be seen within lesions **(Figs. 3 and 5)**.
- Inverse psoriasis:
  - Shiny, pink, well-demarcated thin plaques with minimal scale
  - Common sites include the axilla, inguinal crease, intergluteal cleft, and inframammary are and retroauricular fold.
  - Mucous membrane:
    - Migratory, annular lesions with central denuded areas and white borders
    - Similar to geographic tongue clinically and histopathologically
- **Nail changes:**
  - Fingernails are more affected than toenails.
  - It is associated with psoriatic arthritis.
  - Findings—nail pitting, oil spots (salmon patch), onycholysis with proximal red rim, splinter hemorrhages, and subungual debris

INVESTIGATIONS

Skin biopsy for histopathological examinations confirmation.

■ Psoriatic Arthropathy (Figs. 23A to C)

- It occurs in about 5–30% of patients with psoriasis.
- Most commonly as an asymptomatic oligoarthritis affecting the distal interphalangeal joints
- More rarely but classically is arthritis of all the interphalangeal joints.
- Occasionally presented as rheumatoid arthritis like, affecting small and medium-sized joints symmetrically.

CHAPTER 3 Psoriasis and Related Disorders

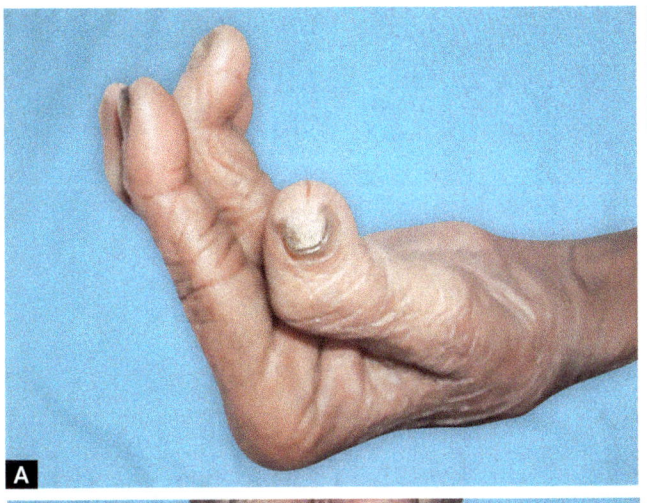
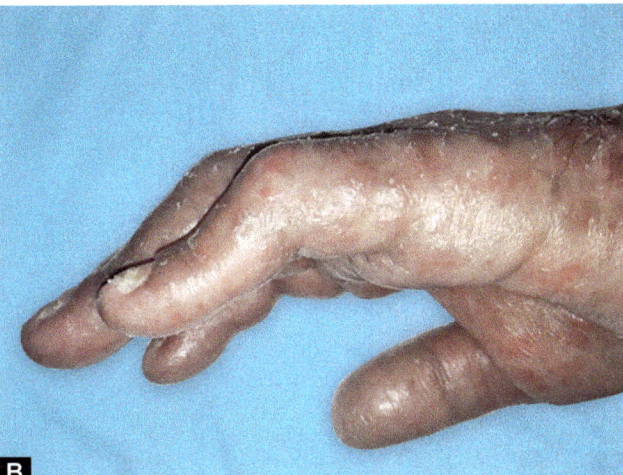
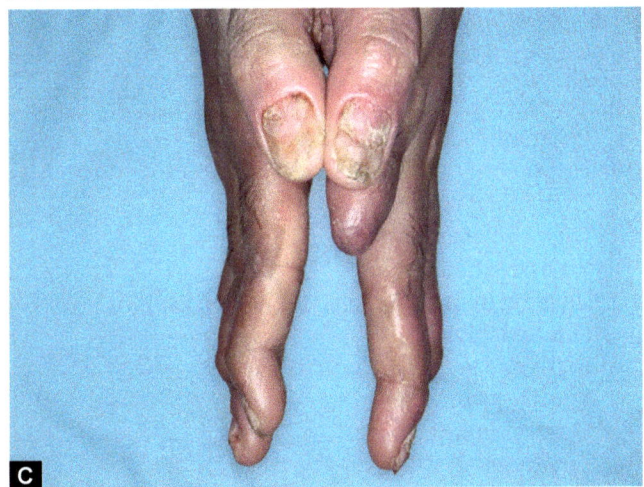

FIGS. 23A TO C: Psoriatic arthropathy changes.

Reactive Arthritis (Previously Referred to as Reiter's Disease)

- Urethritis, arthritis, ocular findings (conjunctivitis), and oral ulcers in addition to psoriasiform lesions especially on the sole [keratoderma blennorrhagicum **(Figs. 24A and B)**] or genital (balanitis circinata).
- This disease occurs chiefly in young men of HLA-B27 genotypes, generally following a bouts of urethritis or diarrheal diseases.
- Course is often self-limited.

TREATMENT

Topical Agents

- *First line*:
  - Topical corticosteroid (e.g., clobetasol propionate)
  - Vitamin D3 analog (calcipotriene and calcitriol)
- *Second line*:
  - Calcineurin inhibitor (tacrolimus may be first line for sensitive areas)
  - Tars
  - Anthralin
  - Tazarotene

Systemic Agents

- *First line*:
  - Phototherapy: UVB and psoralen plus ultraviolet A (PUVA)
  - Methotrexate (MTX)
  - Oral retinoids (e.g., acitretin and isotretinoin)
- *Second line*:
  - Targeted immunomodulators (biological agents)
  - Cyclosporine

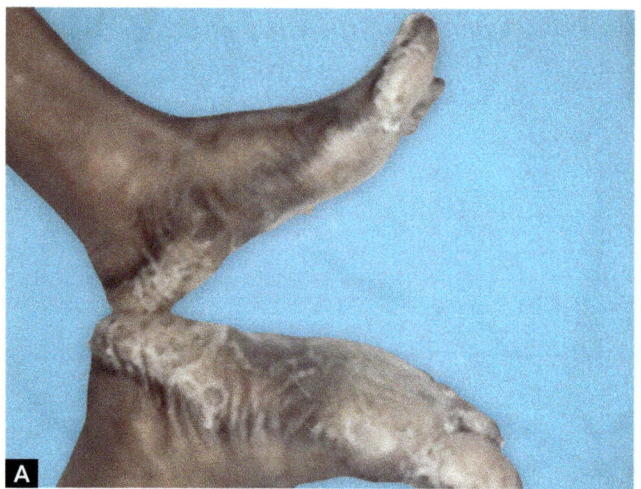
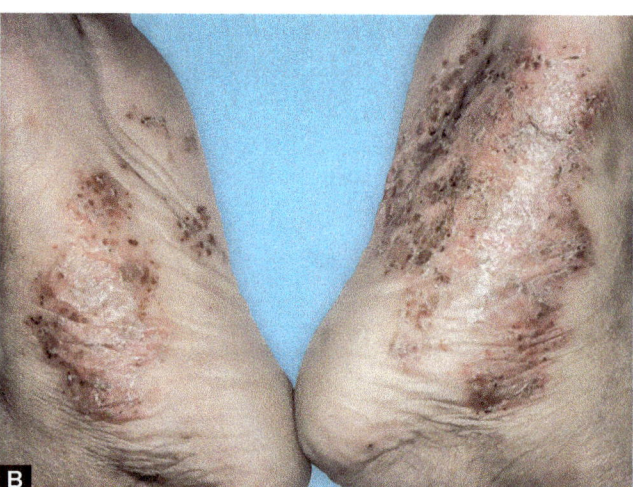

FIGS. 24A AND B: Plantar lesions of keratoderma blennorrhagicum.

Adalimumab

Adalimumab is a recombinant human immunoglobulin G1 (IgG1) monoclonal antibody specific for tumor necrosis factor (TNF). It binds specifically to TNF-α and blocks its interaction with the p55 and p75 cell surface TNF receptors. TNF is a naturally occurring cytokines that is involved in normal inflammation and immune responses. In psoriatic arthritis, nail psoriasis and plaque type psoriasis adalimumab bring excellent outcome.

Secukinumab

Secukinumab works by selectively binding to interleukin-17A (IL-17A) which is main proinflammatory cytokines produced by T-helper cells. IL-17A mediates innate immunity to infecting substances and it can also contribute to the development of chronic disease characterized by inflammation.

Cyclosporine

Cyclosporine is most often used for recalcitrant psoriasis that does not respond to other systemic treatments.

Cyclosporine can provide rapid relief from symptoms. Some improvement symptoms after two weeks of treatment, particularly with stronger doses. However, it may take from three to four months to reach optimal control. Cyclosporin is usually used for the induction of psoriasis remission at a daily dose included in the range of 2.5–5 mg/kg and with intermittent short-term regimens, lasting on average 3–6 months. The magnitude and rapidity of response are dose dependent, as well as the risk of development of adverse events. Therefore, the dose should be tailored to patient's needs and general characteristics and adjusted during the treatment course according to both the efficacy and tolerability.

Adverse effects:
- Decreased kidney function
- Headache
- High blood pressure
- High cholesterol
- Excessive hair growth
- Tingling or burning sensation in the arms or legs
- Skin sensitivity
- Increased growth of gum tissues
- Flu-like symptoms
- Upset stomach
- Tiredness

Contraindication:
- A compromised immune system
- Abnormal kidney function
- High blood pressure
- Cancer, or a history of cancer (other than basal or squamous cell skin cancers)
- Severe gout
- Pregnant or breastfeeding
- Undergoing radiation treatment

Individuals previously treated with methotrexate or other immunosuppressive agents, PUVA, UVB, coal tar, or radiation therapy are at an increased risk of developing skin cancer when taking cyclosporine. Additional risks with cyclosporine include kidney damage.

Methotrexate

Indication:
- Chronic plaque psoriasis [>10% bovine serum albumin (BSA) or interference with employment or social functioning]
- Pustular psoriasis
- Erythrodermic psoriasis
- Psoriasis arthritis

- Severe nail psoriasis
- Psoriasis is not responding to topical tacrolimus, photo therapy, and/or systemic retinoids.

Contraindication:
- *Absolute*:
  - Severe anemia, leukopenia, and/or thrombocytopenia
  - Significant liver function test (LFT) abnormalities
  - Concomitant medications that increased MTX level, e.g., trimethoprim/sulfamethoxazole.
  - Significant reduced pulmonary fibrosis
  - Pregnancy or lactation
  - Severe infections
  - Peptic ulcer (active)
  - Hypersensitivity of MTX
  - Unreliable patient
- *Relative*:
  - Impaired kidney infections (creatinine clearance <60 mL/min)
  - Concomitant hepatotoxic medications
  - Currently planning to have children (discontinue MTX 3 months prior to attempts to conceive)

PITYRIASIS ROSEA

- The etiology is unknown, but viral infections may serve as a trigger.
- It occurs most commonly in adolescents and young healthy adults.
- Pityriasis rosea is an acute erythematous eruption (pink to salmon-colored papules or plaque) with their long axis following Langer's lines of cleavage (**Figs. 25 and 26**), creating a "Christmas tree" pattern on the trunk.

Initially, a single (primary or herald) plaque lesion develops with a collarette scale on the trailing edge of the advancing border. Usually on the trunk, 1–2 weeks later, a generalized secondary eruption develops.

The average duration of illness is 6–8 weeks, while some cases last for months.

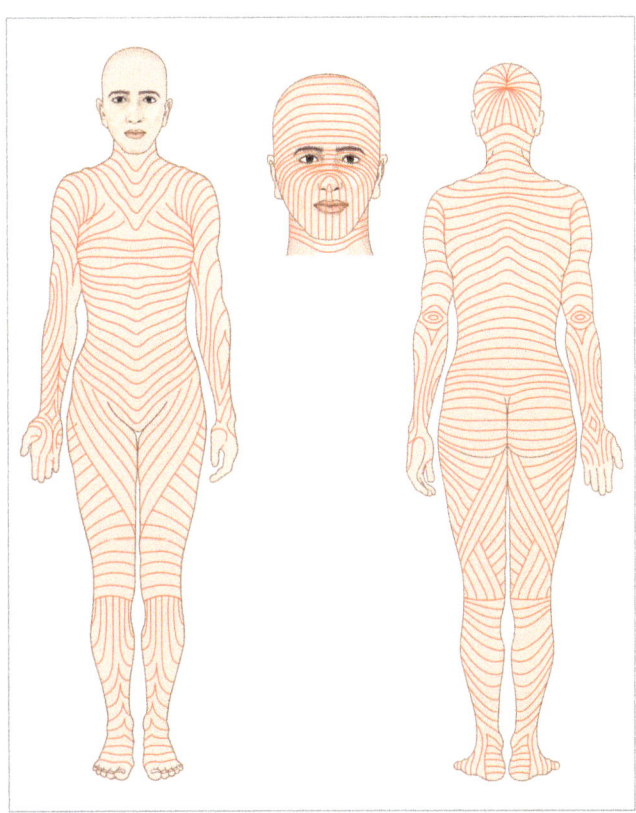

FIG. 25: Langer's lines of cleavage.

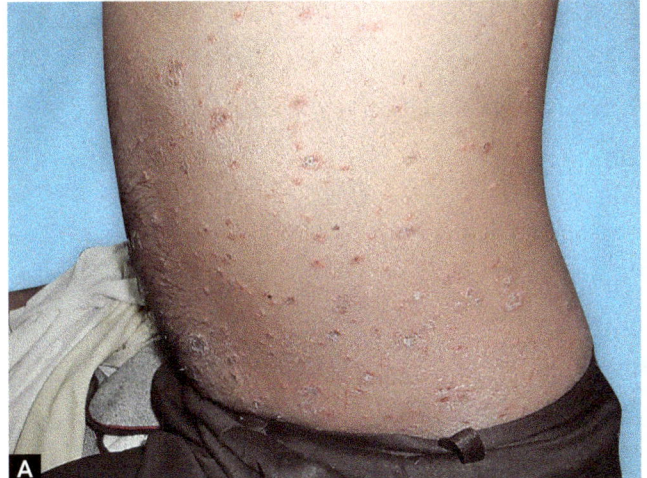
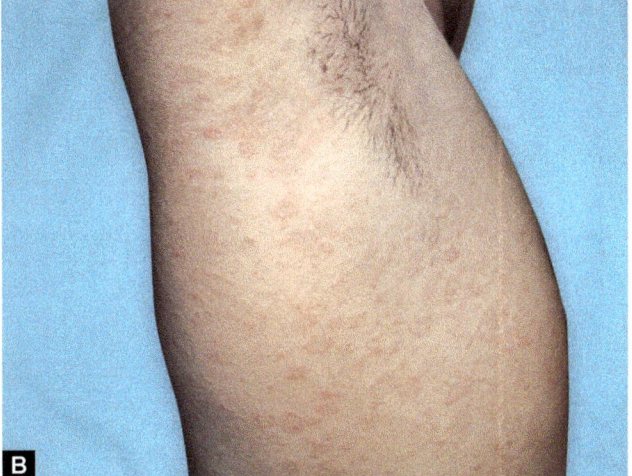

FIGS. 26A AND B: Papule and plaque with oval configurations that follow the lines of cleavage. Plaque has collarette scale in which scale attached at periphery and loose toward the center of lesion.

Diagnosis

Biopsy and histopathological examination.

Treatment

- Topical antipruritic lotion or corticosteroid
- Natural sunlight
- 14 days course of erythromycin or 10 days course of azithromycin

PITYRIASIS RUBRA PILARIS

- Rare, chronic, papulosquamous disorder often progressive to erythroderma of unknown etiology.
- Characterized by a salmon or orange red color **(Figs. 27 to 30)**, islands of sparing, follicular papules, and waxy keratoderma
- It may be exacerbated by exposure of UV light; classic form spontaneously resolves with 3–5 years.

Diagnosis

- Diagnosis is made on clinical grounds.
- Confirmation by biopsy and histopathology examination

Treatment

- Topical therapies consist of emollients, keratolytic agents, vitamin D3 (calcipotriol), glucocorticoids, and vitamin A analogue (tazarotene).
- Oral isotretinoin, acitretin, MTX, TNF-α inhibitors response within 6 months.

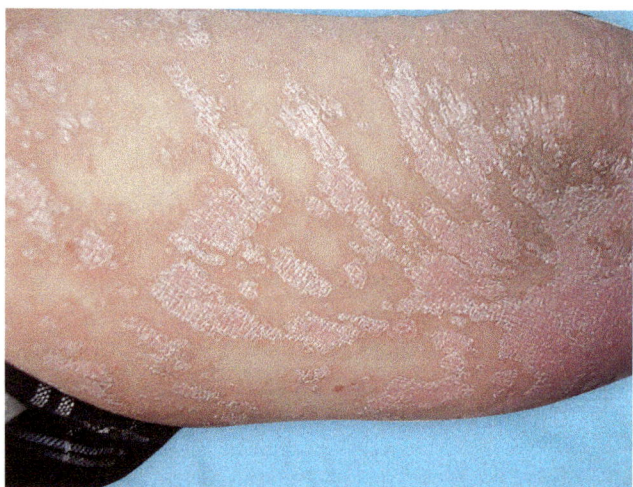

FIG. 27: Orange-red follicular papules. These are sharply demarcated islands of unaffected normal skin.

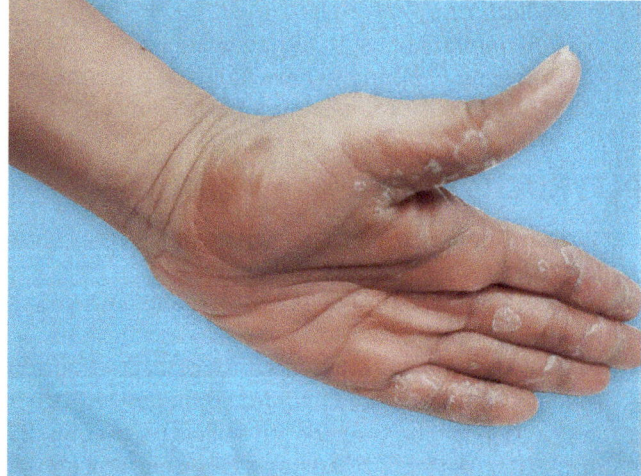

FIG. 28: Diffuse waxy hyperkeratosis of left palm with an orange hue.

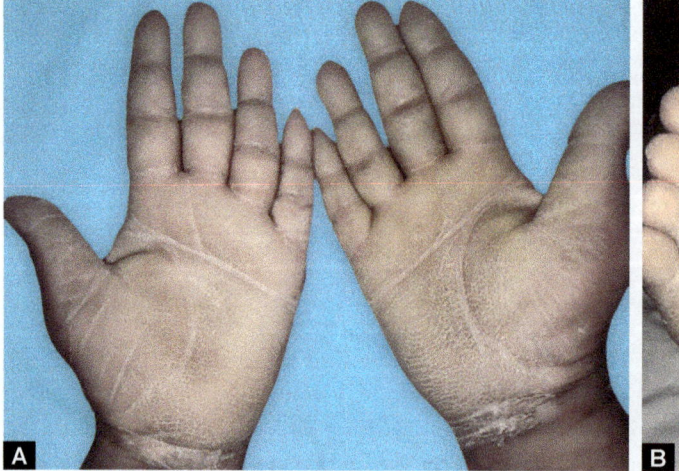
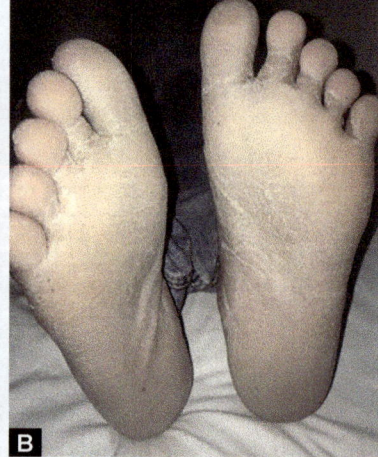

FIGS. 29A AND B: Diffuse, waxy hyperkeratosis of both palm and sole.

LICHEN PLANUS AND LICHENOID DERMATOSES

■ Lichen Planus

- Lichen planus (LP) is an acute or chronic inflammatory dermatosis involving skin, nail, and/or mucous membrane (oral, vulvovaginal) of unknown origin **(Figs. 31 to 41)**.
- Characterized by flat topped (lichenoid) papules; pink to violaceous, shiny, and pruritic polygonal papules **(Figs. 42 and 43)**.
- For easy remember 4P: Papule, purple, polygonal, and pruritic
- A characteristic finding is Wickham's striae, a network of fine white lines on the surface of papules and plaques **(Fig. 44)**.

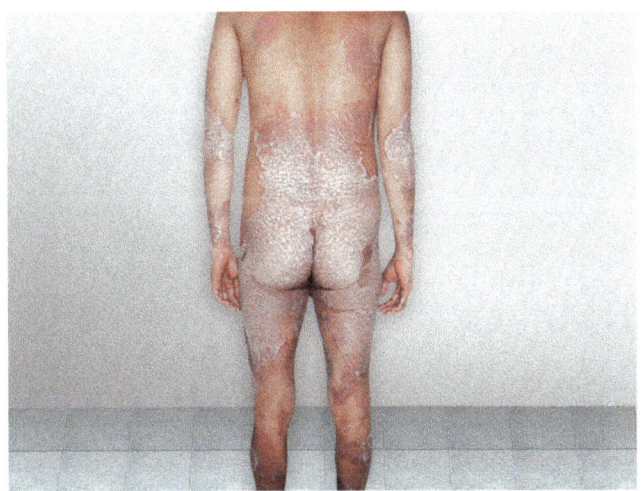

FIG. 30: Widespread involve—pityriasis rubra pilaris.

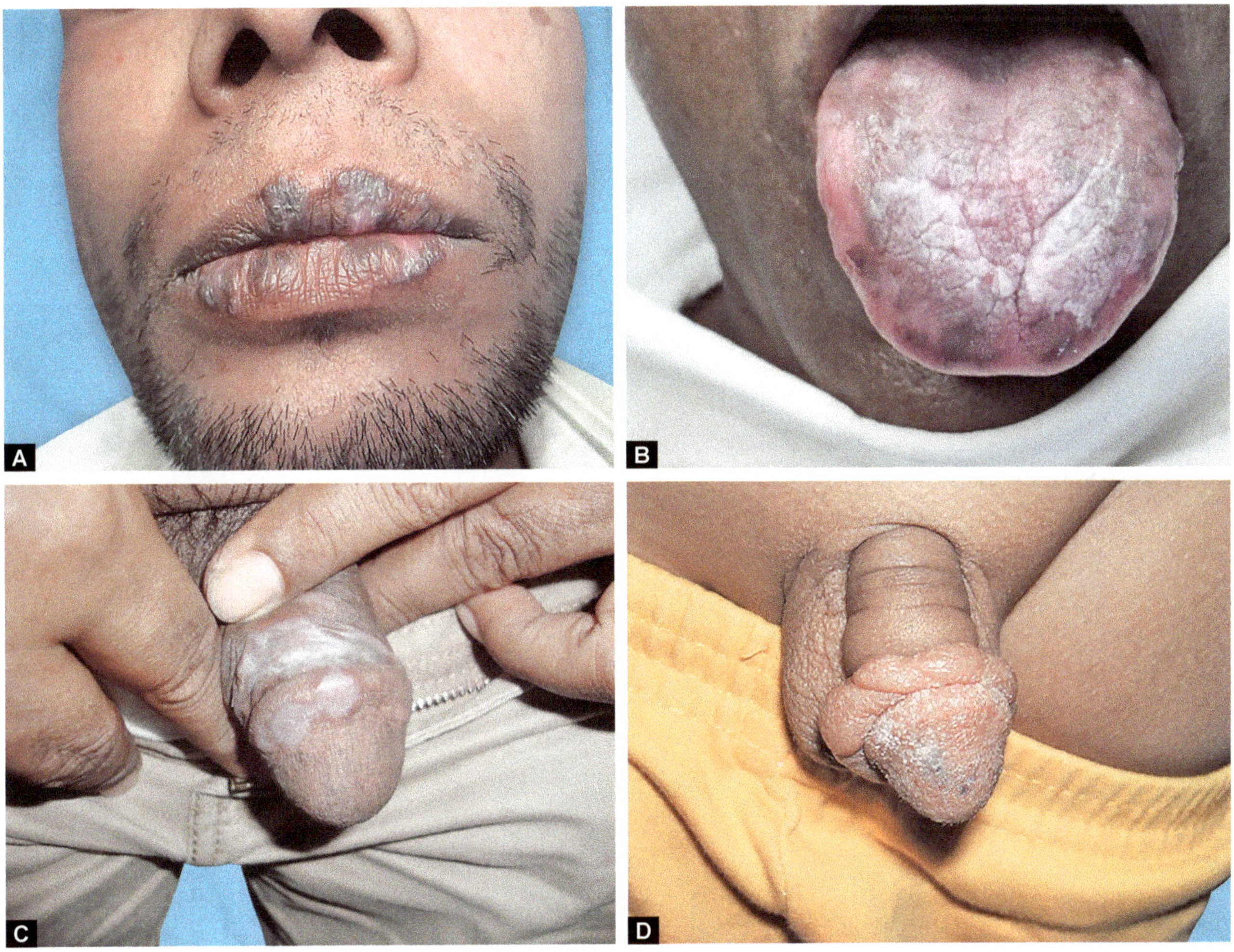

FIGS. 31A TO D: Violaceous papules and plaques on mucous membrane of different sites.

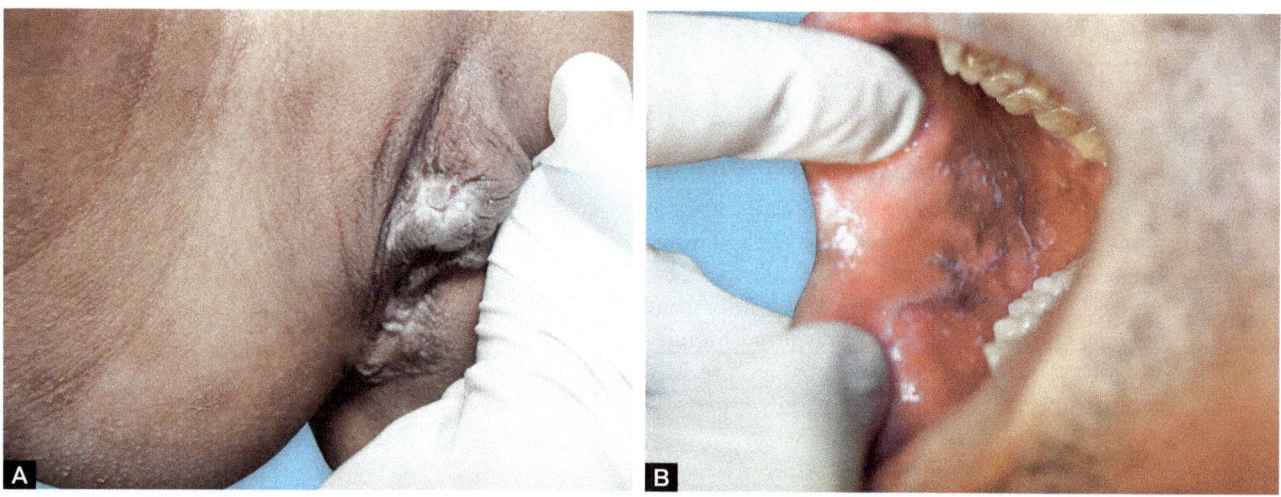

FIGS. 32A AND B: Hyperkeratotic papules plaque; reticular, lacy pattern on mucous membrane.

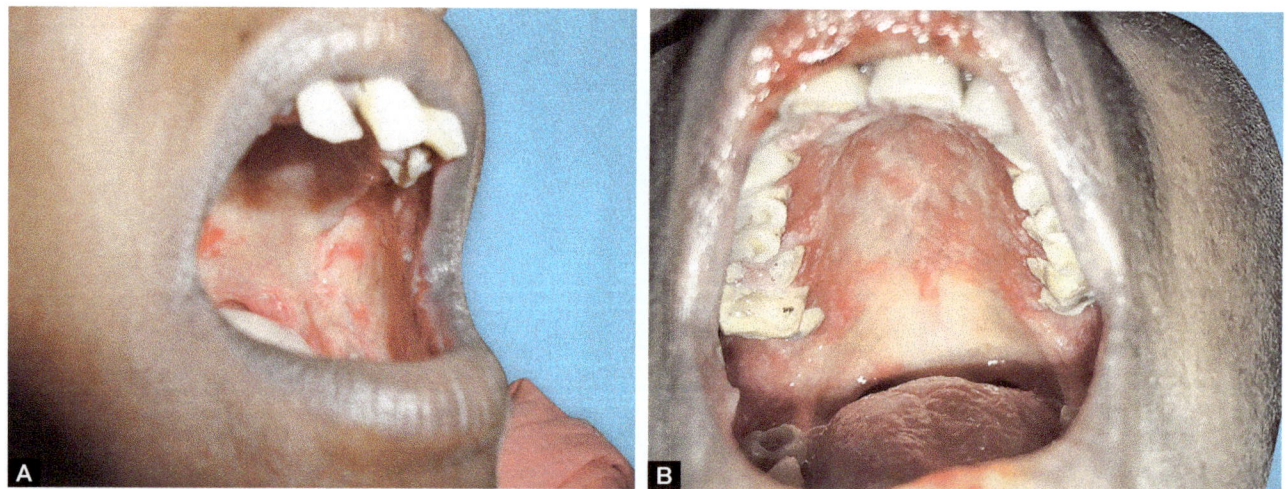

FIGS. 33A AND B: Erosive pattern on mucous membrane.

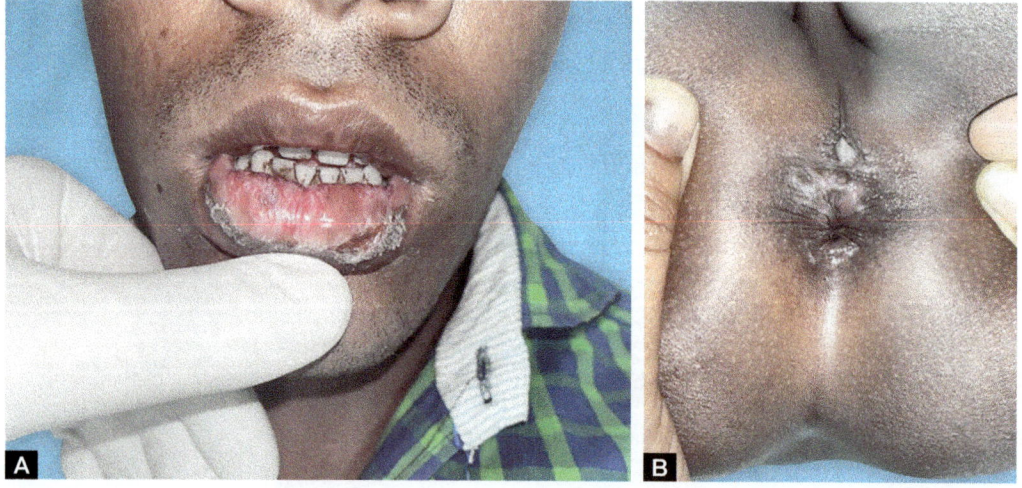

FIGS. 34A AND B: Erosive, ulcerative, and scarring of mucous membrane.

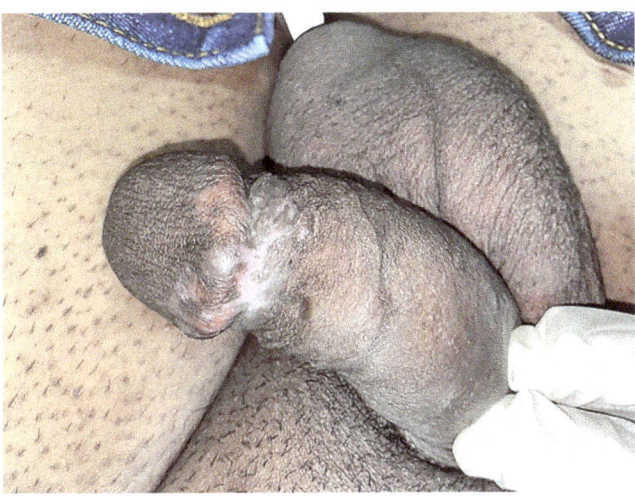

FIG. 35: Violaceous scarring on coronal sulcus.

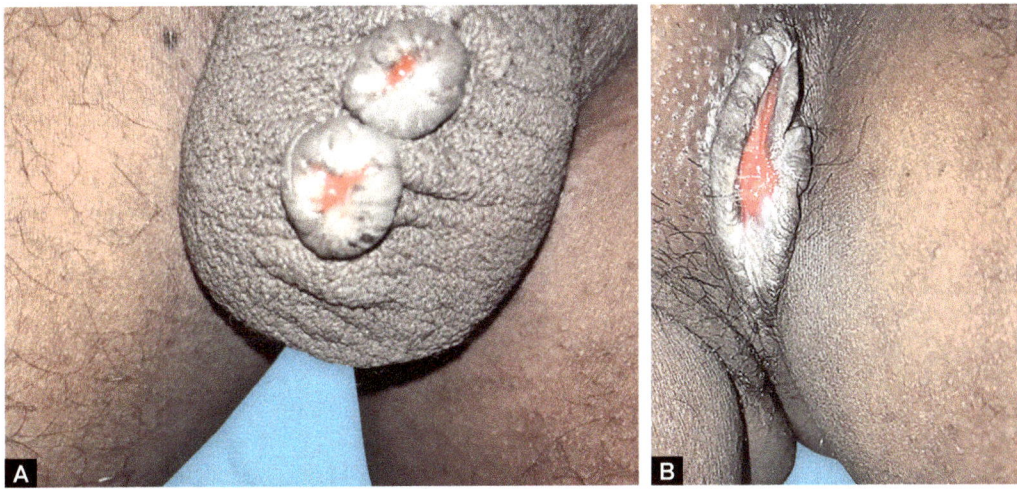

FIGS. 36A AND B: Hypertrophic lichen planus.

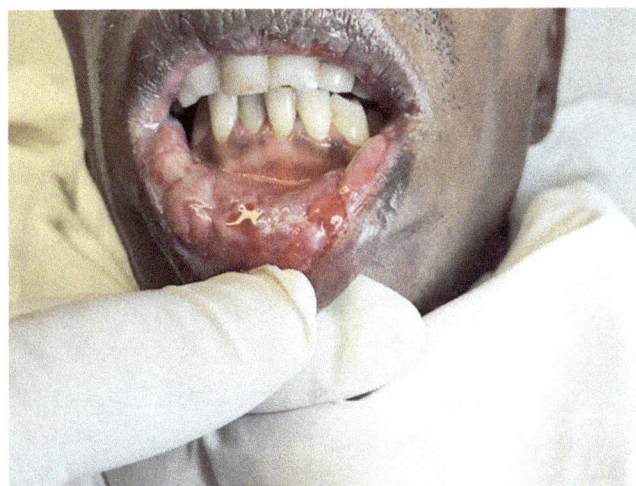

FIG. 37: Erosive, ulcerative lesion.

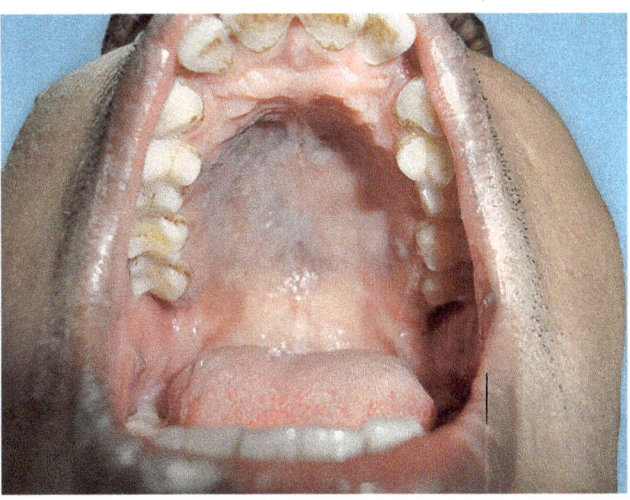

FIG. 38: Hard palate involvement.

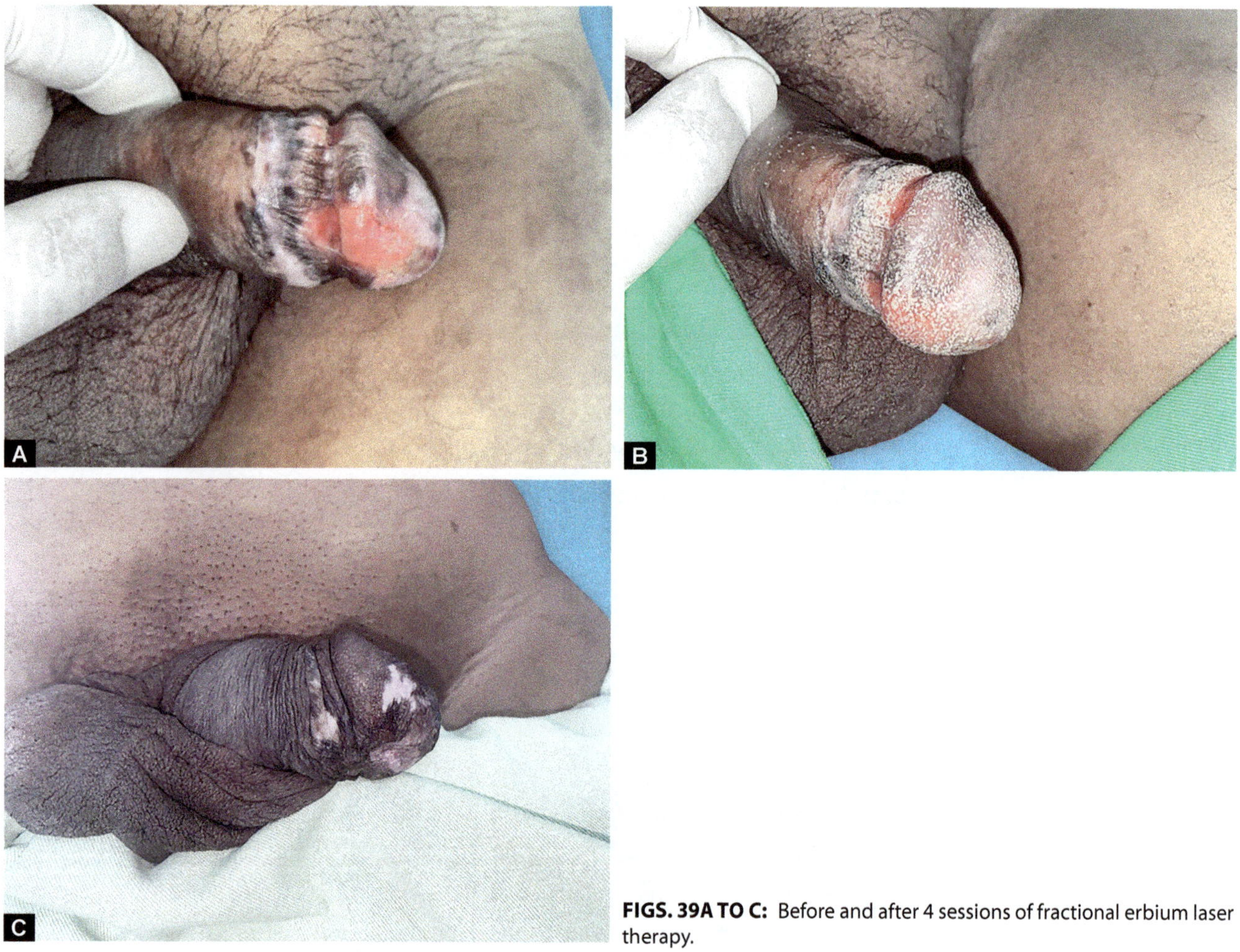

FIGS. 39A TO C: Before and after 4 sessions of fractional erbium laser therapy.

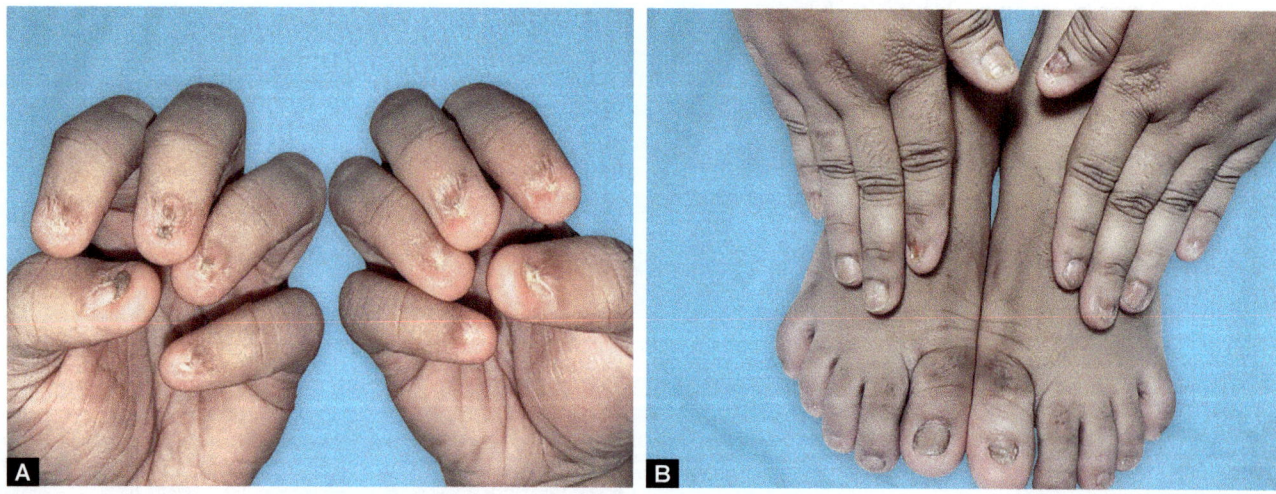

FIGS. 40A AND B: Twenty-nail dystrophy (5–10% lichen planus patients associated with nail involvement).

CHAPTER 3 Psoriasis and Related Disorders

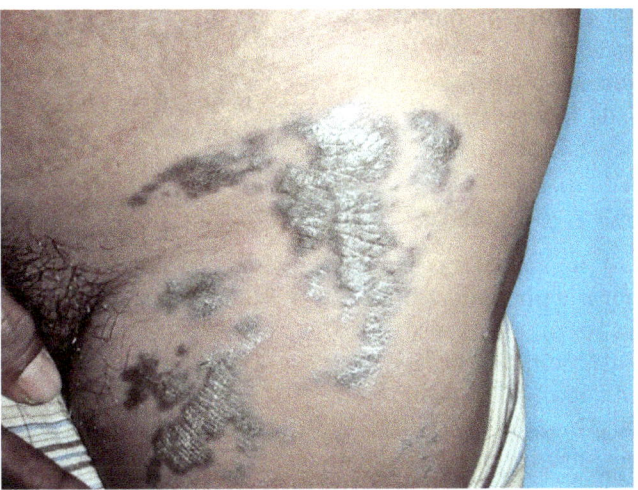

FIG. 41: Violaceous flat-topped papules and plaques–classic lesions.

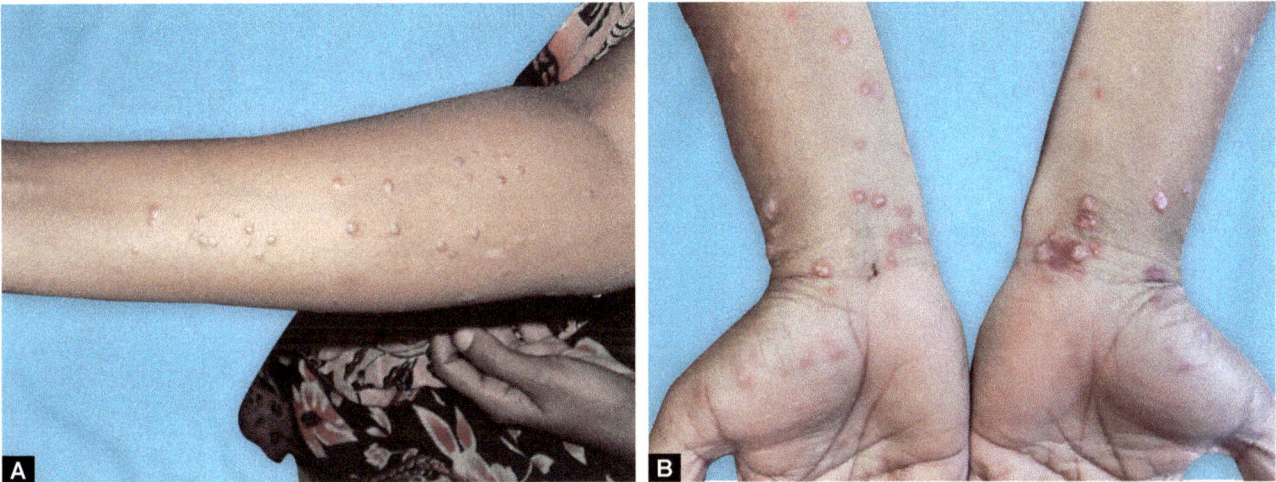

FIGS. 42A AND B: Flat-topped, polygonal, sharply defined papules of violaceous color, grouped and confluent. Surface is shiny and upon close inspection with a hand lens, fine white lens are revealed (Wickham's striae).

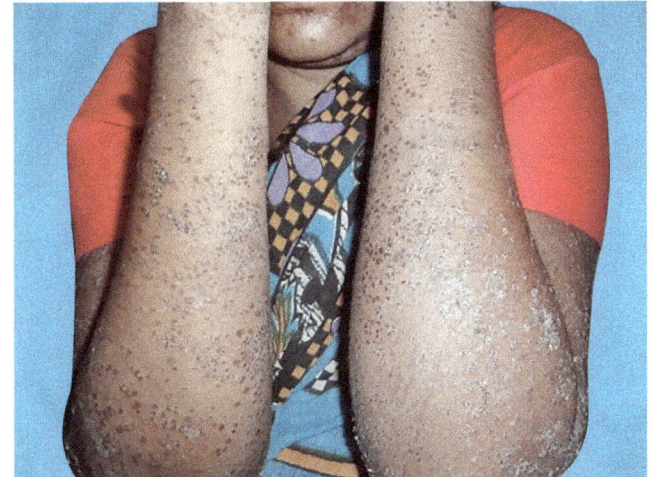

FIG. 43: Violaceous papules distributed on symmetrical fashion on both forearm.

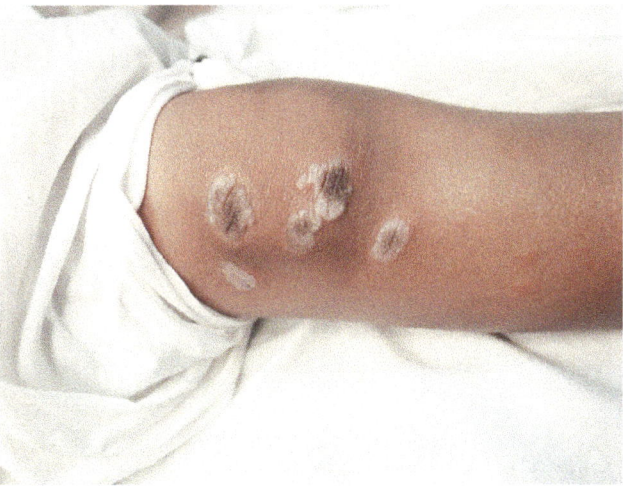

FIG. 44: Hypertrophic lesion—Wickham's striae.

- Squamous cell carcinoma arising in maltreated hypertrophic LP lesions **(Fig. 45)**.
- Common sites of involvement are, scalp, flexor wrists, forearm, genitalia, and distal lower extremities, in particularly on shin and presacral areas.

Lichenoid Drug Eruption (Fig. 46)

A drug-induced eruption that has an appearance similar to LP; often more generalized or is a photo distribution, more eczematous, psoriasiform, or pityriasis rosea like, often a latent period of months after initiating drug.

Angiotensin-converting enzyme (ACE) inhibitors, thiazide diuretics, antimalarials, beta-blockers, TNF-α inhibitors, and quinidine are most common culprit drugs.

Lichen Striatus

- Linear array of small 2–4 mm, flat topped (lichenoid) papules **(Fig. 47)** whose color ranges from skin colored to pink to tan (i.e., hypopigmented, especially in darkly pigmented patients).
- It favors children (median age 2–3 years), with a single streak along one extremity, spontaneously resolves over months to a few years.
- Acral streaks associated with nail dystrophy (e.g., onycholysis and splitting)
- Linear LP

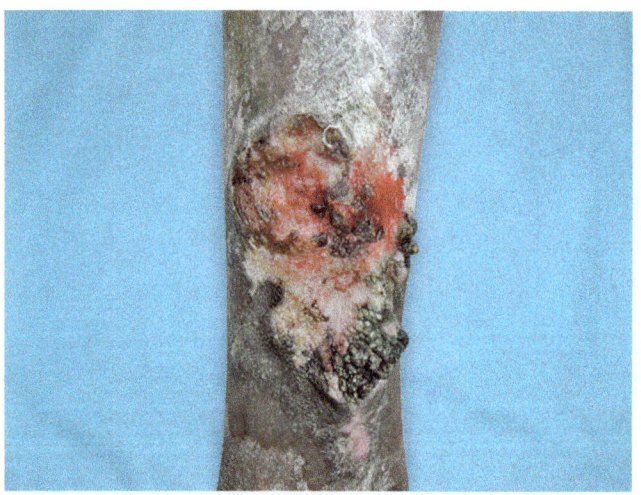

FIG. 45: Squamous cell carcinoma arising in maltreated hypertrophic lichen planus lesions.

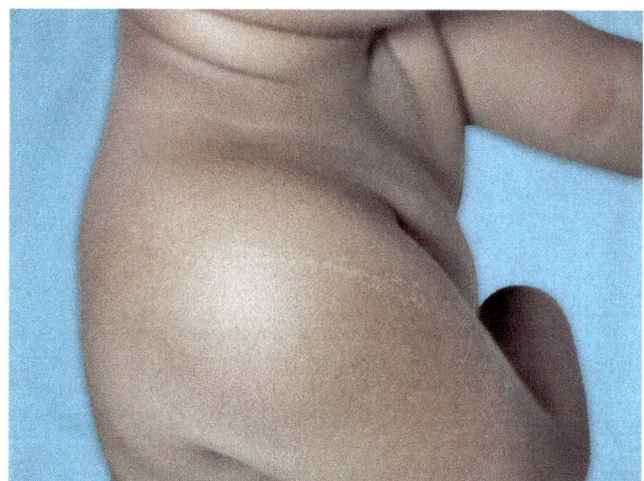

FIG. 47: Linear flat-topped papules.

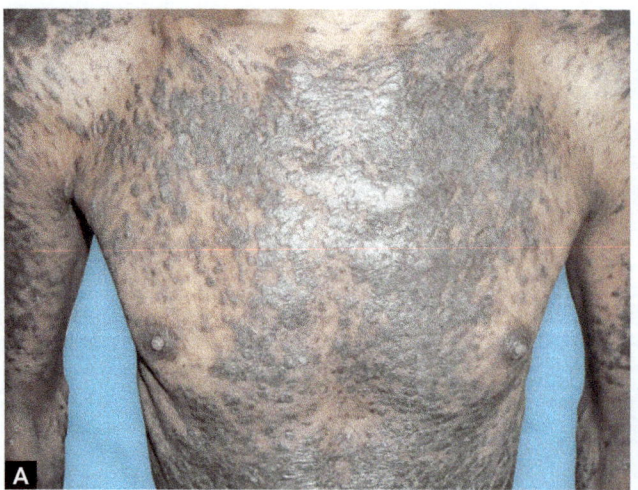

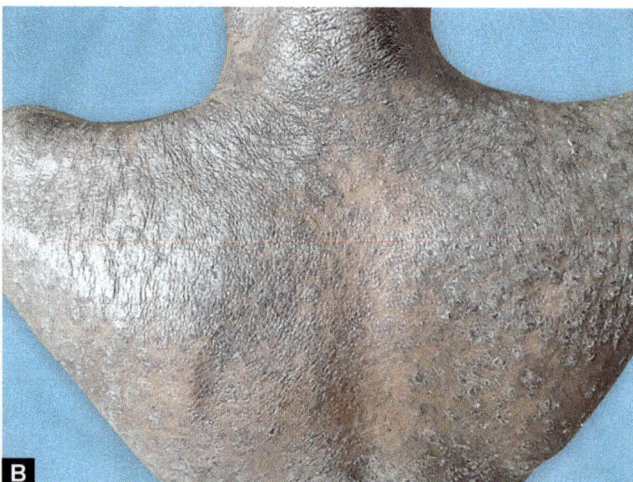

FIGS. 46A AND B: Lichenoid drug eruption, often more generalized.

Treatment
- No specific effective therapy
- Spontaneous resolution
- Topical corticosteroids, topical calcineurin inhibitors may be given.

Lichen Nitidus
- Multiple, tiny, discrete, flat-topped papules **(Figs. 48A to C)**
- Uniform in size and usually pink to brown in color or hypopigmented or shiny in darkly pigmented individuals
- *Site*: Anterior trunk, genitalia, and upper extremities
- A linear arrangement of papules may be seen (Koebner phenomenon) **(Fig. 49)**.
- It persists for months to year.
- *Differential diagnosis*: Flat warts, LP, popular eczema, and lichen nitidus

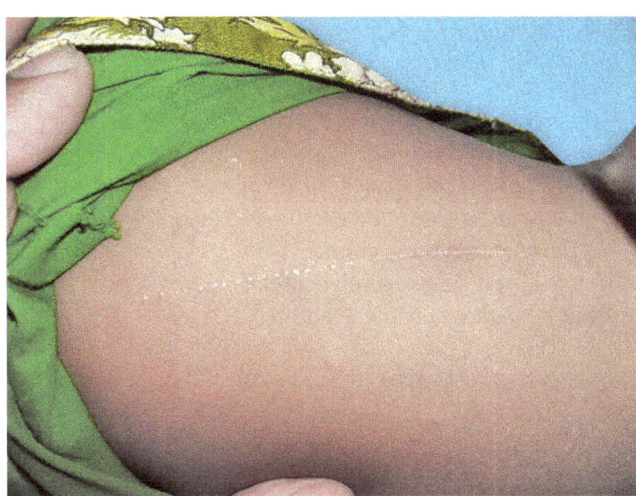

FIG. 49: Koebner phenomenon: Isomorphic new lesions at the side of minor trauma.

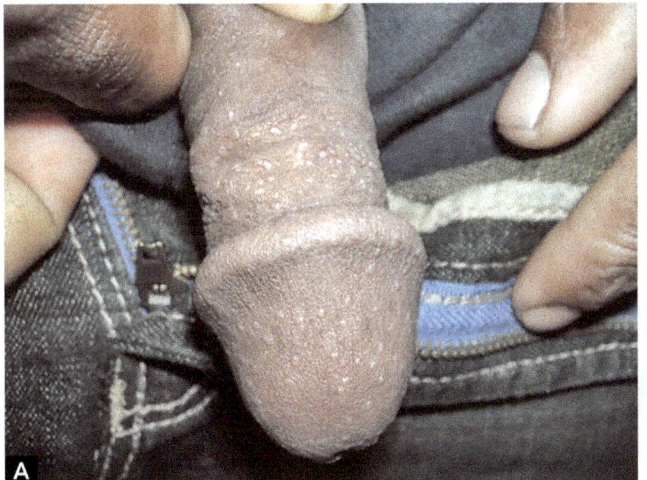

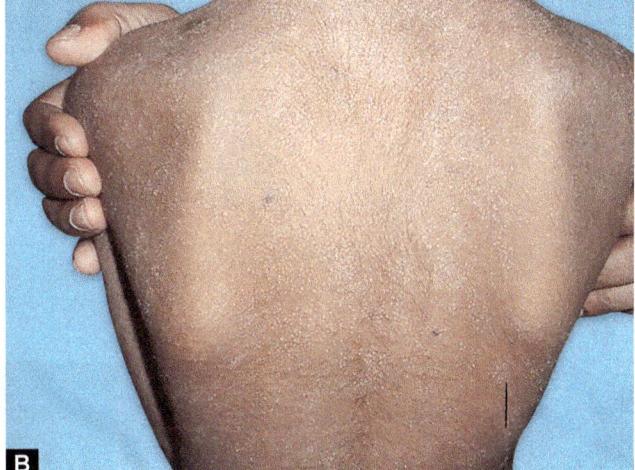

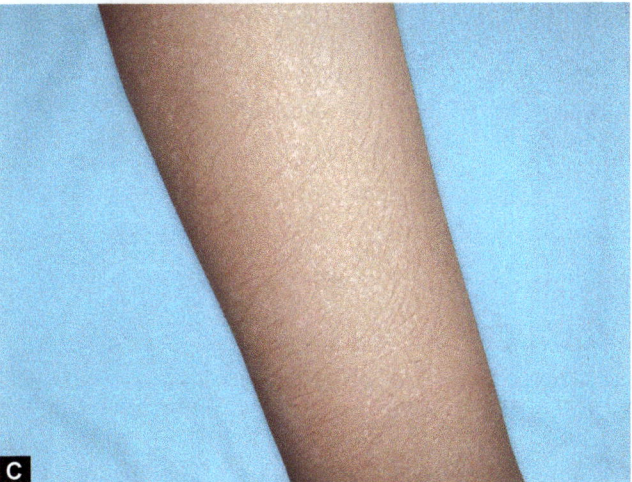

FIGS. 48A TO C: Numerous tiny flat-topped papules on the glans, hand, and back of trunk.

Erythema Dyschromicum Perstans (EDP, Ashy Dermatosis)

- Systemic distribution of multiple oval-shaped gray to gray-brown macules and patches **(Figs. 50A to E)**
- *Site*: Neck, trunk, and proximal upper extremities
- Slowly progressive, asymptomatic disorder that favors children and young adults
- In children, it may resolve after a few years (2–3 years), but it is more chronic in adults.

Differential Diagnosis

- Fixed drug eruption
- Post-inflammatory hyperpigmentation
- Lichen planus pigmentosus

Treatment

- No specific therapy
- Dapsone bring excellent outcome in some cases
- Fractional erbium laser followed by 10% trichloroacetic acid (TCA) and platelet-rich plasma (PRP) bring excellent outcome in recalcitrant cases.

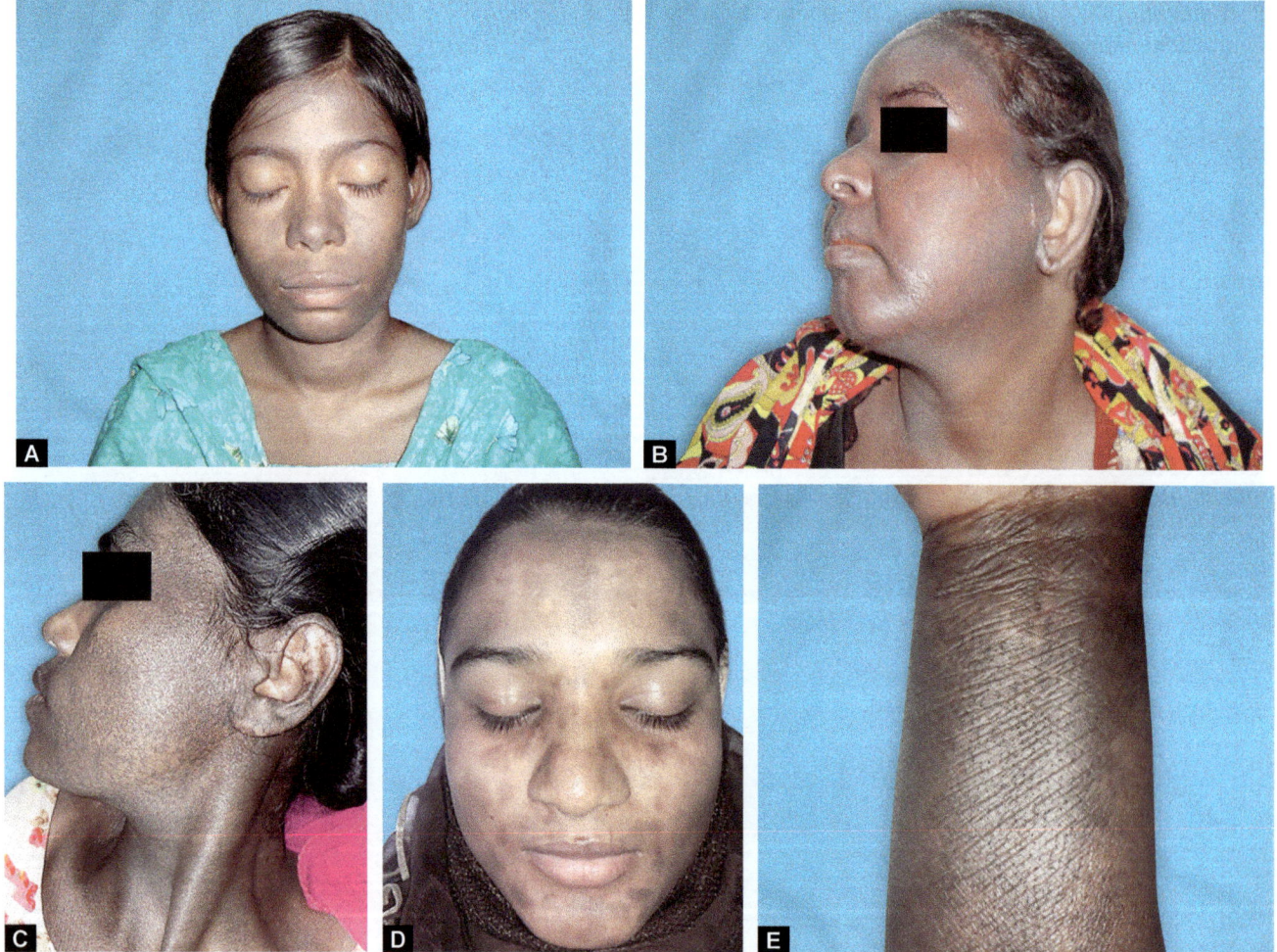

FIGS. 50A TO E: Numerous, oval to polygonal, diffuse macules, and patches distributed over face, neck, and forearm.

CHAPTER 4

Dermatitis (Eczema)

ATOPIC DERMATITIS (AD)

- Common inflammatory skin disease that affects 10–25% of children and 2–10% of adults.
- Atopic dermatitis is caused by both a defective barrier function of the skin and by an allergy to variety of environmental and dietary allergens.
- Onset usually in infancy or early childhood, with development in the 1st year of life in >50% and before 5 years of age in >85% of affected individuals.
- Sequalae often include—sleep disturbances, psychological distress, disrupted family dynamics, impaired functioning at school which leads to growth retardation and decreased intelligence.
- Often accompanied by other atopic disorders such as, asthma, allergic rhinoconjunctivitis.

■ Diagnostic Features and Triggers of Atopic Dermatitis (Figs. 1 to 4)

Essential features (must be present and are sufficient for diagnosis):
- Pruritus
- *Typical morphology and distributions*:
  - Facial and extensor involvement in infancy
  - Flexural lichenification in adults
  - Chronic or relapsing course

Important features (seen in most cases, support the diagnosis):
- Onset during infancy or early childhood
- Personal and/or family history of atopy

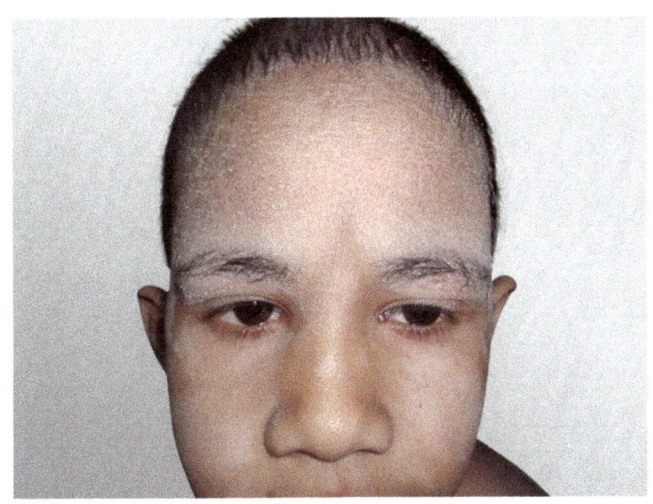

FIG. 1: Dry, scaly, and hypopigmented (pityriasis alba) face.

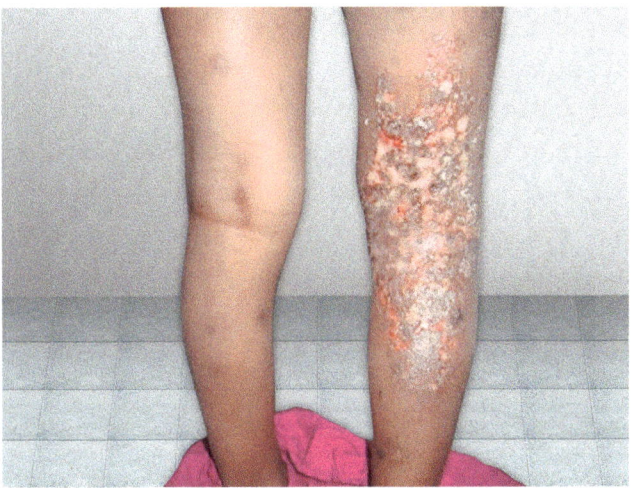

FIG. 2: Secondary bacterial infection on lichenification.

32 CHAPTER 4 Dermatitis (Eczema)

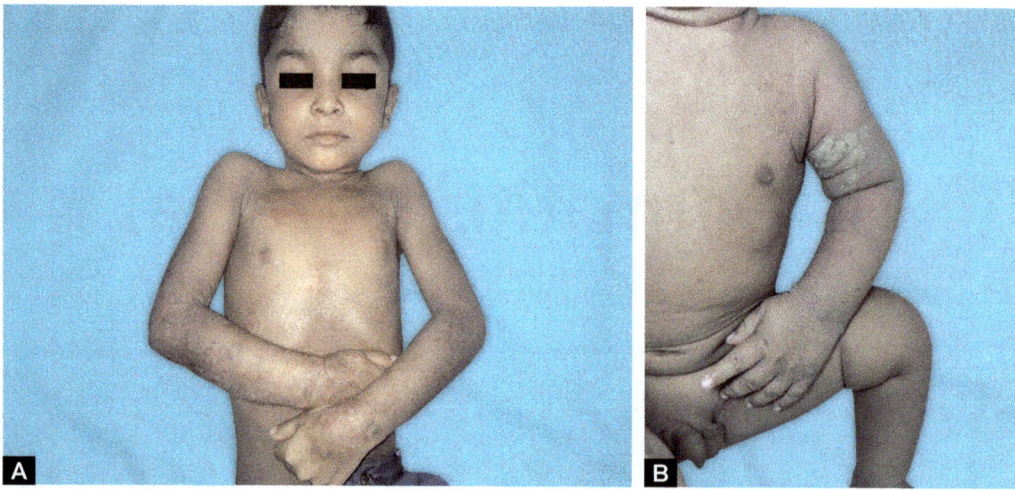

FIGS. 3A AND B: Dryness, erosions, and lichenification on whole body—related with food.

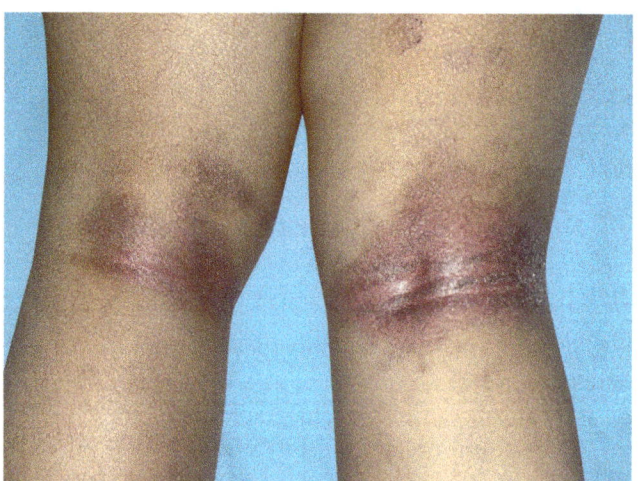

FIG. 3C: Dryness, erosions, lichenification on popliteal fossa.

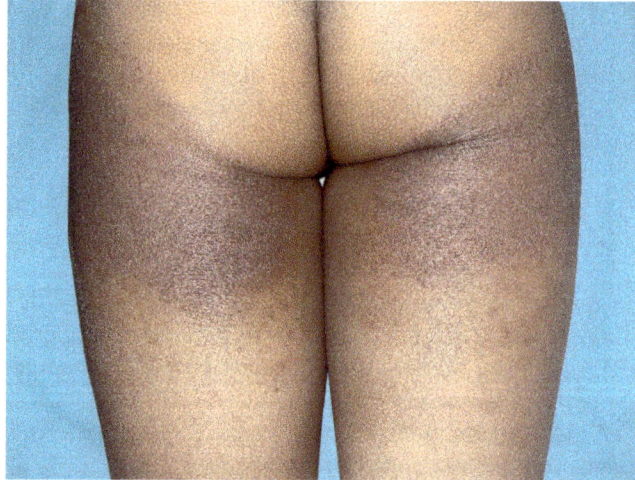

FIG. 3D: Dryness and hyperpigmentation on upper back of thigh due to contact (commode).

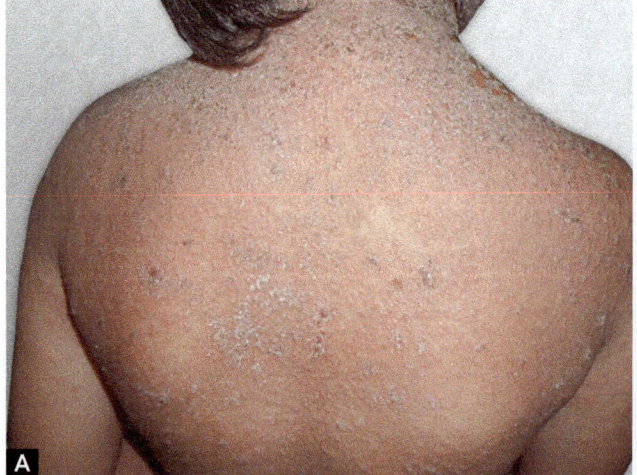

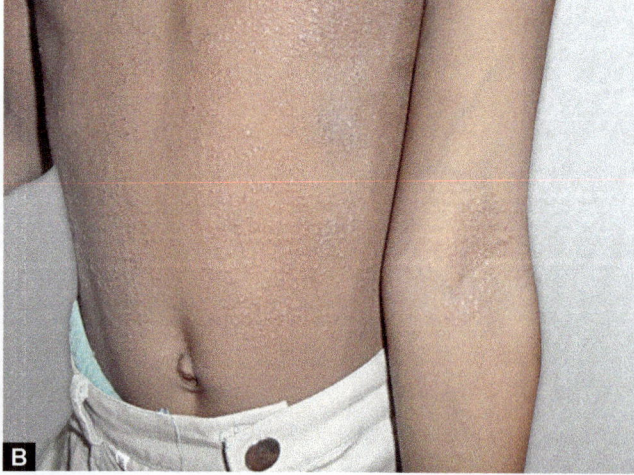

FIGS. 4A TO H: *Continued*

Continued

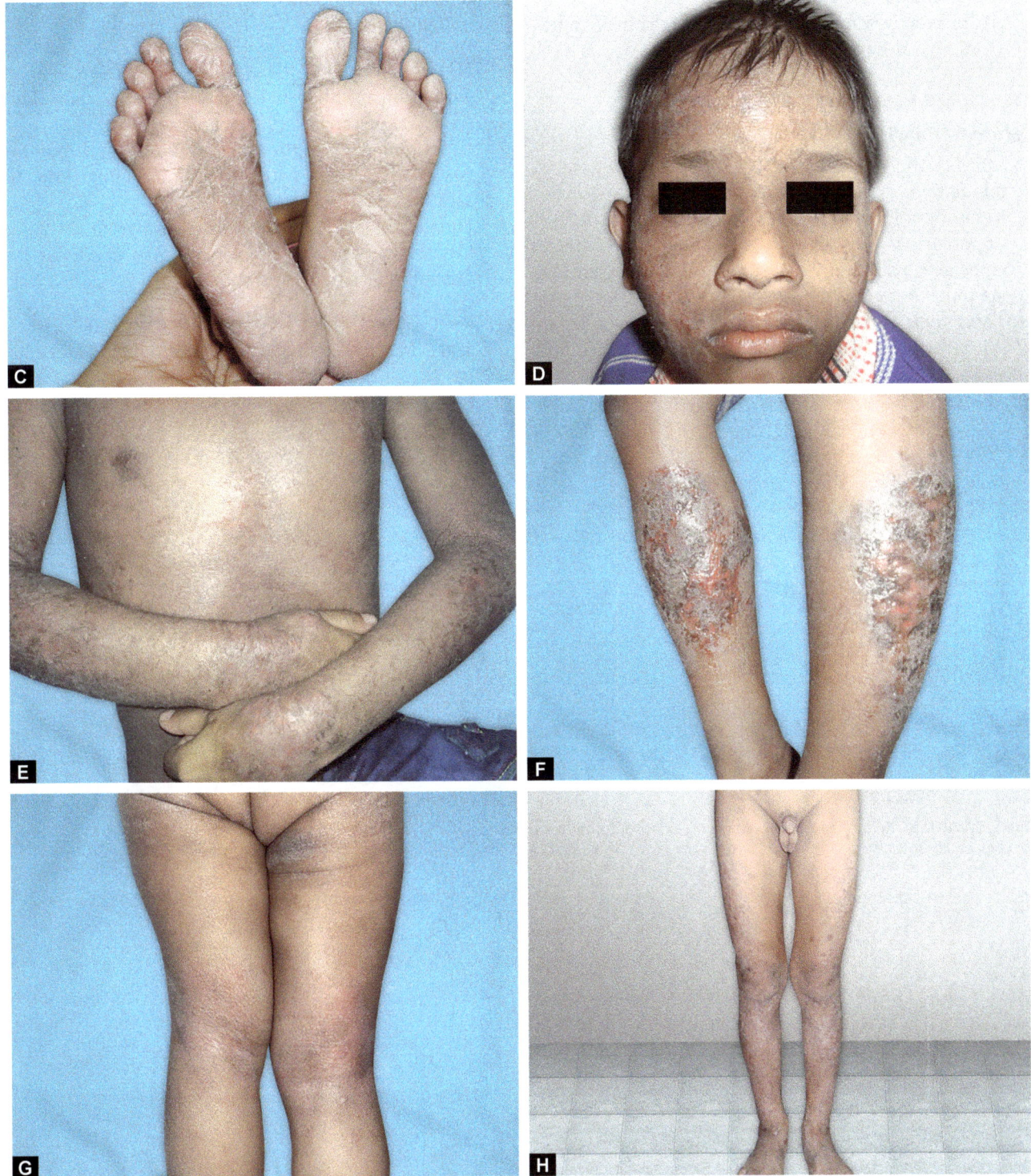

FIGS. 4A TO H: Xerosis, lichenification in different parts of body.

- *Xerosis*: Dry skin and fine scale.
  - Often leads to pruritus.
  - IgE reactivity [immediate skin test reactivity, radio-allergosorbent test (RAST) positive].

Associated Features of Atopic Dermatitis
Keratosis Pilaris
- Affects >40% of patient with AD and 15% of general population.
- Keratotic follicular papules on the lateral aspect of upper arms, buttocks, thighs, and lateral cheeks (specially in children); the trunk and distal extremities are much less common sites **(Figs. 5A and B)**.
- *Treatment*: Keratolytic agents—lactic, glycolic, or salicylic acid; topical retinoids may be used. But best one, use petroleum-based emollient without keratolytic agents because keratolytic agents may produce irritation on skin.

Pityriasis Alba
- Common in children/adolescents, especially those with AD and tan or darkly pigmented skin.
- Illdefined hypopigmented macules and patches (usually 0.5–3 cm) with subtle fine scaling **(Figs. 6A and B)**.
- Located on face, shoulders, trunk, and arms.
- *Treatment*: Regular use of sunscreens and emollients.
- Use full sleeve pants and shirt.

Typical Infraorbital Fold (Dennie–Morgan Sign)
Typical infraorbital fold has been described in **Figure 7**.

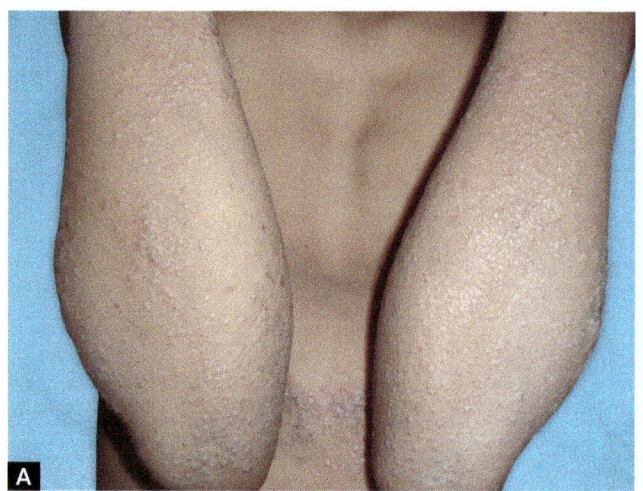
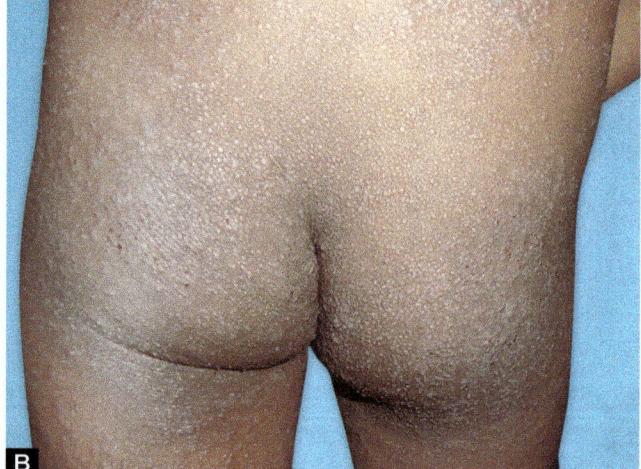

FIGS. 5A AND B: Keratotic follicular papule on extensor forearm and buttock.

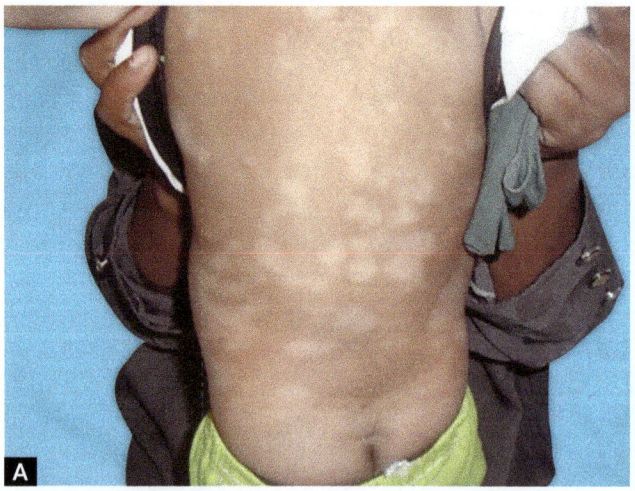
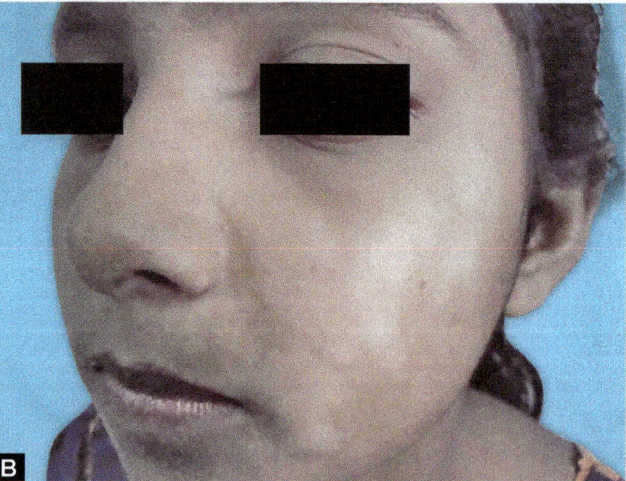

FIGS. 6A AND B: Hypopigmented macules and patches over back of trunk and face.

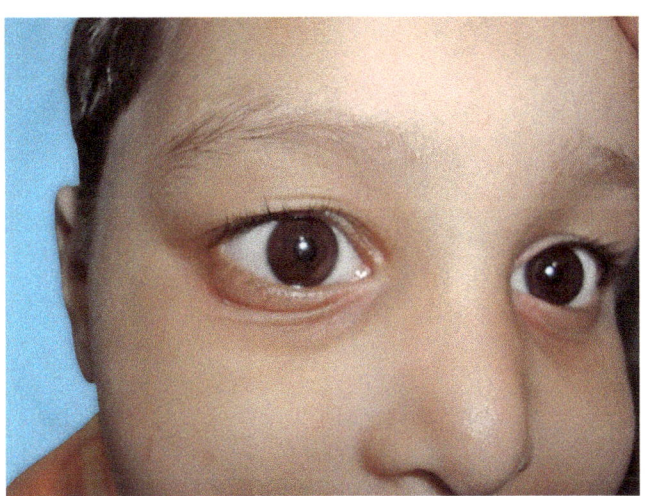

FIG. 7: Typical infraorbital fold (Dennie–Morgan sign).

Triggering Factors of Atopic Dermatitis

Multiple environmental and psychological factors can trigger or exacerbate AD.
- House dust mite, dermatophagoides pteronyssinus.
- *Food*: Eggs, peanuts, milk, fish, soybeans, wheat.
- Contact allergens
- Wool or other rough cloth
- Premenstrual flaring is common in pregnancy, parturition or menopause
- Stress
- Sweating
- Animal exposure during first few months of life, viral infections and maternal cigarette smoke.

■ Treatment

Following a growth chart is one of the simplest and best ways to detect any major impact on child growth and health.
- *Basic skin care*:
  - Daily bath, not >5 minutes, use mild soap during bath, topical emollients within 3 minutes after bath.
  - Use full sleeve pant and shirt.
  - Use covered shoes.
  - Use umbrella or sunscreen for photo protection.
- *Antihistamine*:
  - Hydroxyzine (e.g., 2 mg/kg/day every 6 hours).
- *Topical anti-inflammatory agents*:
  - 1st line topical corticosteroids
  - 2nd line topical calcineurin inhibitors (e.g., tacrolimus)
- *Phototherapy and systemic anti-inflammatory agents*:
  - Narrow band ultraviolet B (UVB)
  - Oral cyclosporine
  - Systemic corticosteroid (CS)

SEBORRHEIC DERMATITIS (SD) (FIGS. 8A TO D)

- Chronic, superficial, inflammatory disease characterized by redness and scaling, which occurs in sebaceous glands bearing skin.
- Common disorder with both as infantile and an adult form; unusual in children.
- Possible related to components of sebum and *Malassezia* species.
- This is probably the single most common scalp problem for which a patient seeks medical attention.
- The scalp is scaly and mildly erythematous.
- Seborrheic dermatitis is also common on the oily areas of the face (e.g., nasolabial folds, eyebrows), intrascapular region, presternal area, and in body folds.

■ Diagnosis

Dermatopathology.

■ Course and Prognosis

Recurrence and remissions, especially on scalp related with seasons, age, sunlight, dust, etc.

■ Treatment

- Topical antifungal creams.
- Daily shampoo (e.g., ketoconazole, ciclopirox, selenium sulfide, or zinc containing shampoo alternating with a gentle shampoo).
- Mild corticosteroids
- Topical calcineurin inhibitors (e.g., tacrolimus ointment)

ASTEATOTIC DERMATITIS (XEROTIC ECZEMA, FIG. 9)

- Arises in areas of dry skin, especially during winter months, in dry climate, in old adults and associated with diabetes mellitus (DM), chronic kidney disease, hypothyroidism, hot shower, etc.
- The areas of dermatitis resemble a dried riverbed or "crazyparing" with superficial cracking of skin.
- Favors the shin, mouth, lower flanks, and posterior axillaries line; may become more widespread but with sparing of the face, palms, and soles.
- Should exclude stasis dermatitis, ichthyosis vulgaris, adult atopic dermatitis, allergic or irritant contact dermatitis (ICD).
- Decrease frequency of bathing
- Apply mild CS

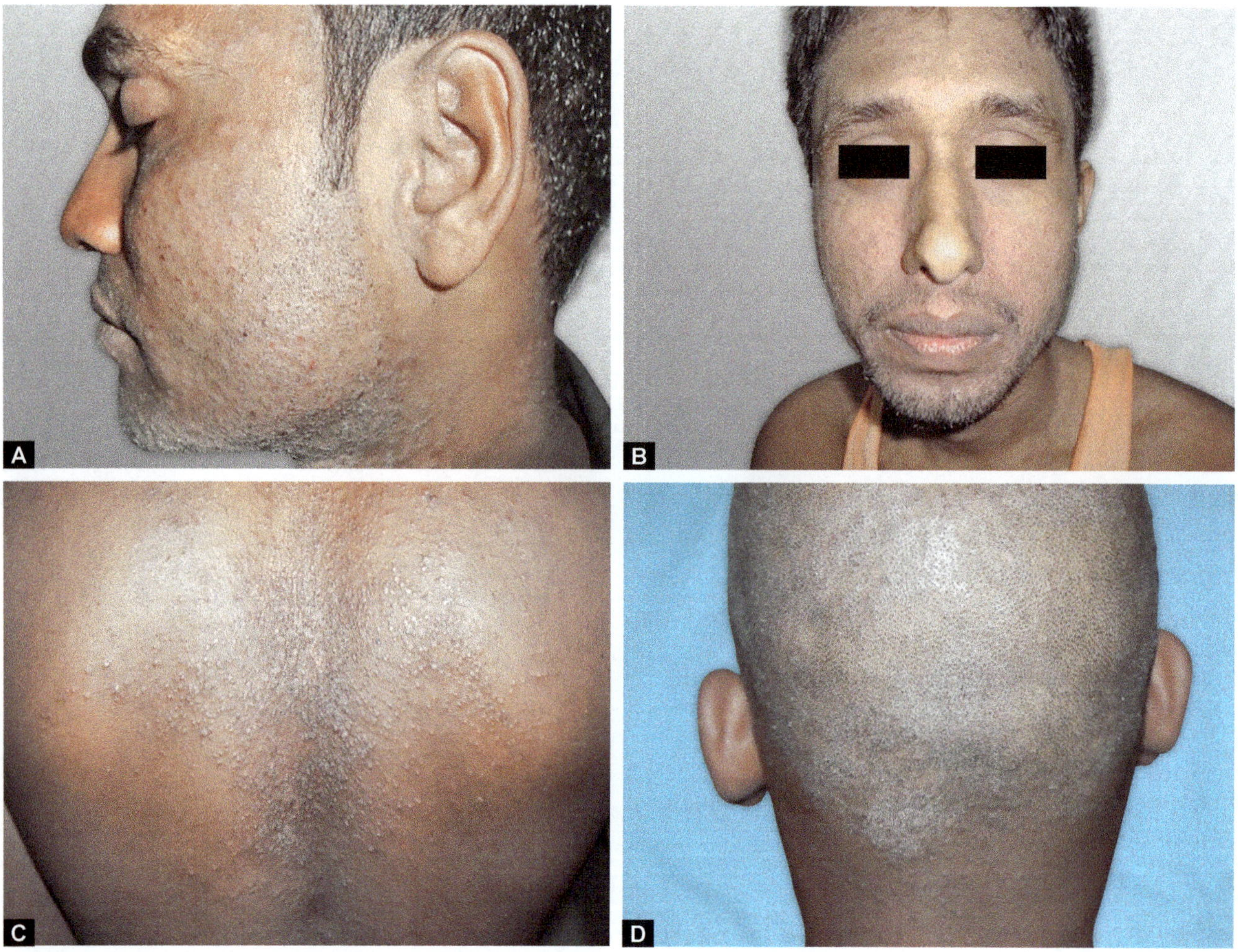

FIGS. 8A TO D: Erythema and yellow-orange scaling of face, scalp, and intrascapular region.

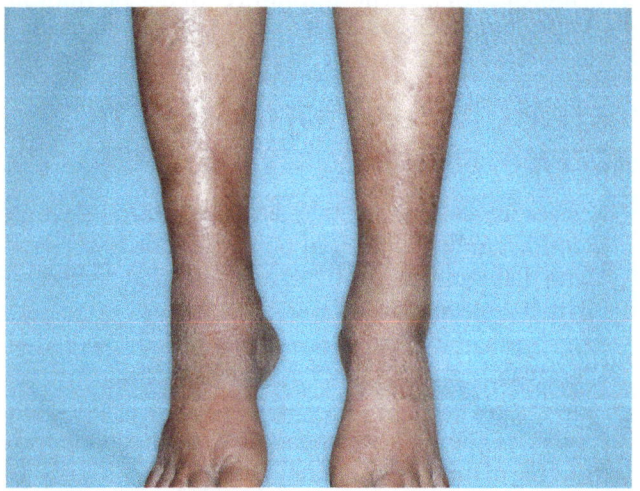

FIG. 9: Xerosis and dermatitis.

STASIS DERMATITIS (FIGS. 10 TO 12)

Pruritic dermatitis with scalecrust and sometimes oozing that favors the shins and calves, historically often begins near the medial malleolus.

Cutaneous signs of chronic venous hypertension include:
- Edema, often tender.
- Varicosities
- Stasis dermatitis.
- Stasis purpurapetechiae on yellow brown discoloration due to hemosiderin deposits.
- Lipodermatosclerosis
- Patients often have a history of chronic lower extremely edema and may have a history of deep vein thrombosis and/or recurrent cellulitis.

CHAPTER 4 Dermatitis (Eczema)

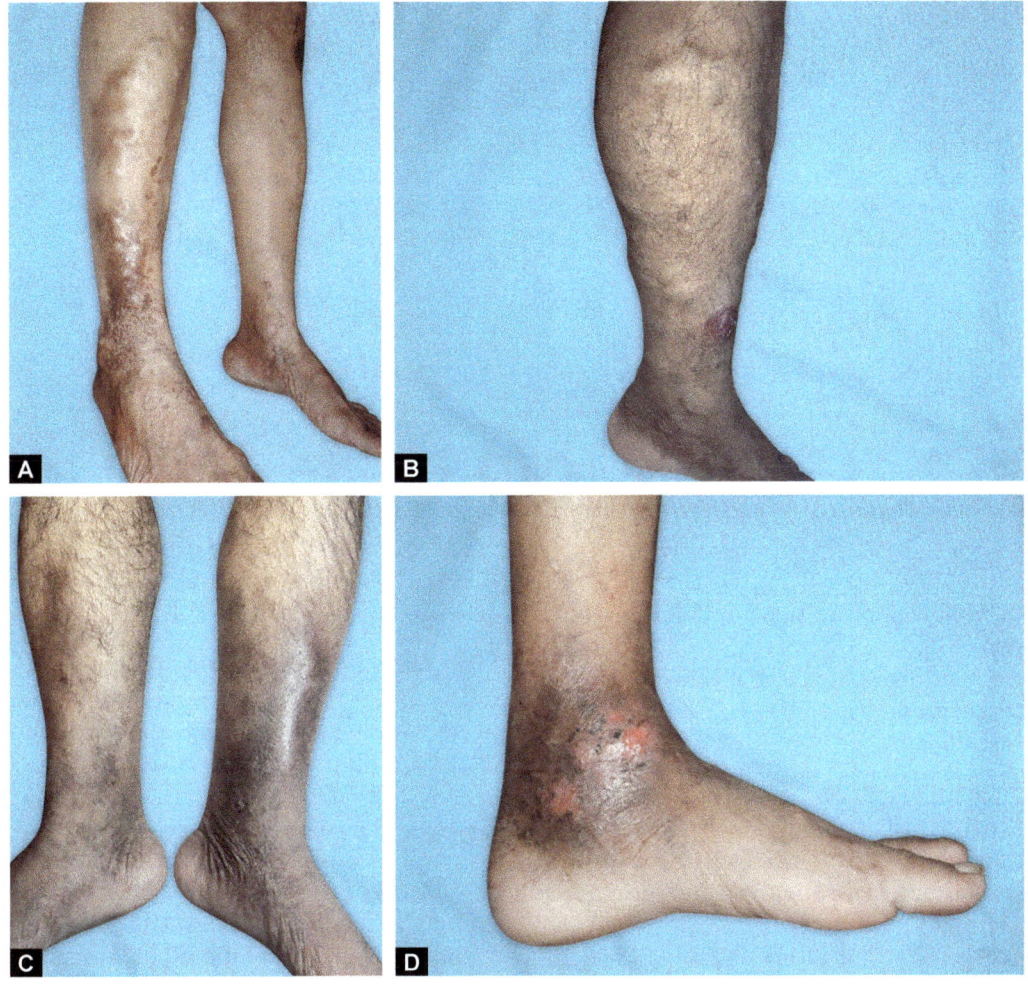

FIGS. 10A TO D: Engorged leg veins with sign of chronic eczema.

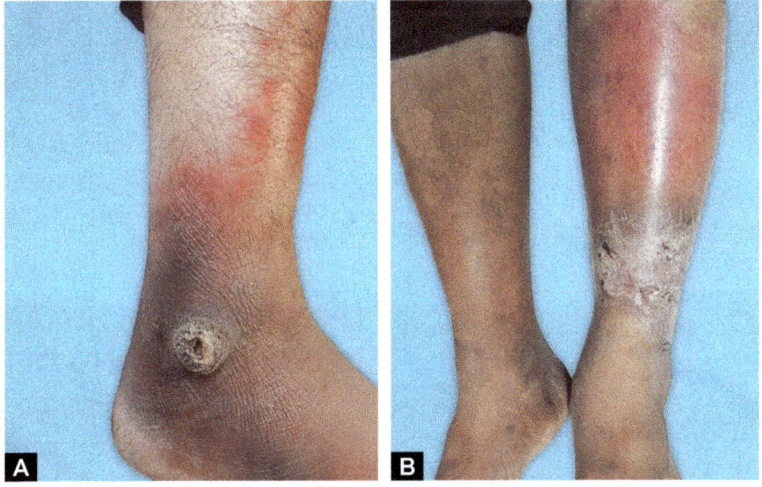

FIGS. 11A AND B: Erythema, edema with ulceration and crusting present.

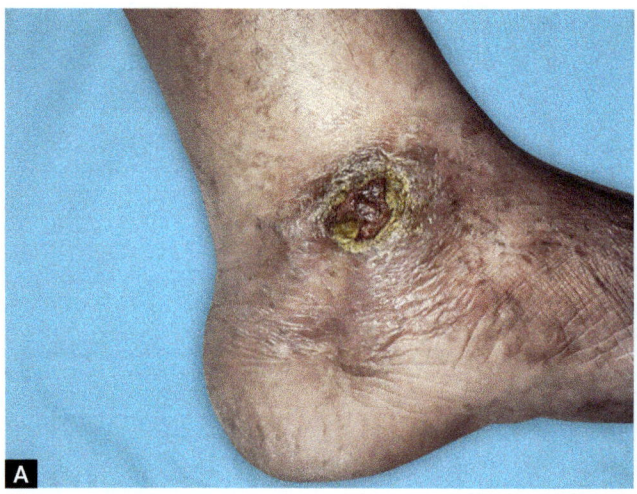
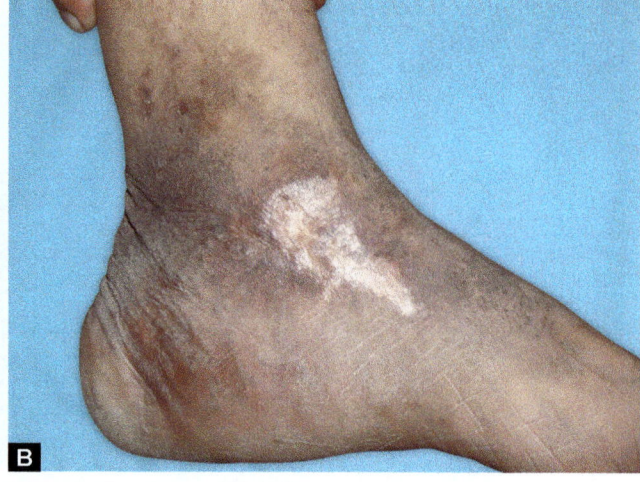

FIGS. 12A AND B: Stasis ulcer healed with conservative treatment.

- Often associated with other signs of chronic venous hypertension.
- Stasis ulcerations (above medial malleolus).
- Acroangiodermatitis.
- Livedoid vasculopathy.

■ Differential Diagnosis

Allergic contact dermatitis (ACD), ICD, asteatotic eczema, nummular eczema, cellulitis, acute or chronic lipodermatosclerosis.

■ Treatment

- Mild topical corticosteroid
- Leg elevation
- Pressure stocking
- Endovascular ablation of large varicosities

NUMMULAR ECZEMA

- Very pruritic, coin-shaped lesions of chronic dermatitis, usually measuring 2 or 3 cm in diameter.
- Occurs primarily on the extremities, classically the legs in men and the arms in women.
- A chronic relapsing course is common.
- *Synonyms*: Discoid eczema, microbial eczema (**Figs. 13A to C**).

■ Differential Diagnosis

Atopic dermatitis, stasis dermatitis, contact dermatitis, tinea corporis, vesicular pityriasis rosea, mycosis fungoides.

■ Treatment

Main aim of treatment is hydration of skin with moisturizer.

In addition to topical CS and calcineurin inhibitors, often requires phototherapy to clear.

BREAST ECZEMA (NIPPLE ECZEMA)

- Eczema of the breasts usually affects the areolar and may extend onto the surrounding skin. The area around the base of the nipple is usually spread, and the nipple is usually spared, and the nipple itself is less frequently affected (**Figs. 14A and B**).
- Painful fissuring is frequently seen in nursing mothers.
- Nipple eczema may be the sole manifestation of adult variant AD.
- Nipple eczema in the breast feeding women is a therapeutic challenge and can form AD, ACD, irritant dermatitis, infection, or food allergy. Poor positioning during breast feeding is a common cofactor in the development of nipple eczema. The role of secondary bacterial infection and *Candida* should be considered in breast feeding women.

DYSHIDROTIC ECZEMA (ACUTE AND RECURRENT HAND DERMATITIS)

- Firm, pruritic vesicles of the palms, soles as well as the lateral and medial aspect of the digits.
- A chronic and relapsing course is common.
- Intact vesicles within the epidermis are more longlived because of thick stratum corneum in acral sites.

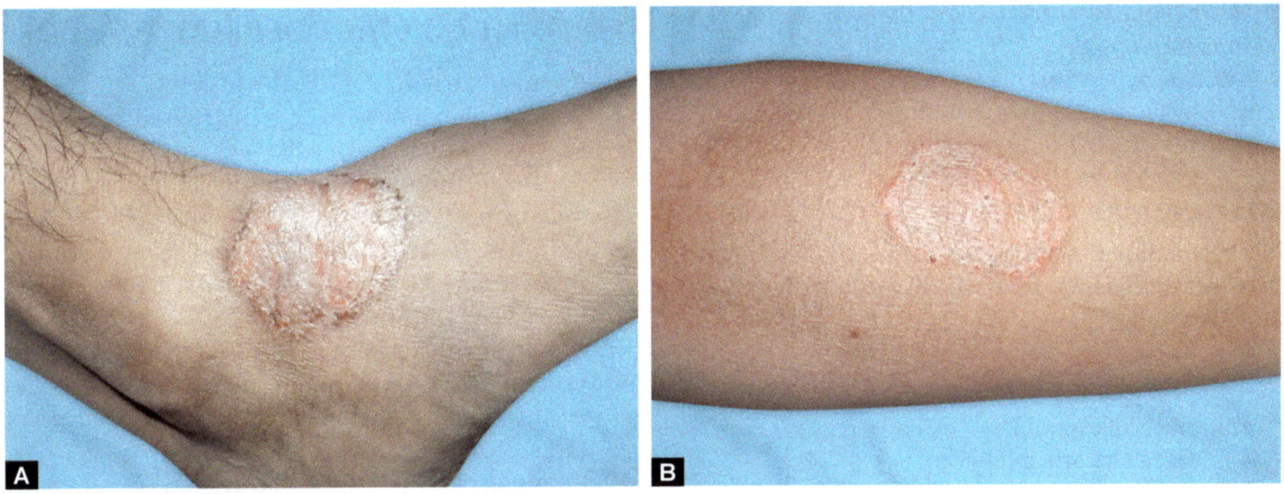

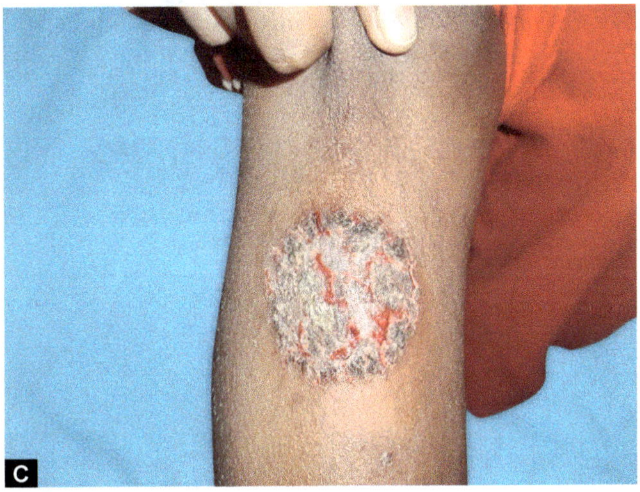

CHAPTER 4 Dermatitis (Eczema)

FIGS. 13A TO C: Coin-shaped lesion composed of small papules, vesicles, erosions, fissuring, and crust.

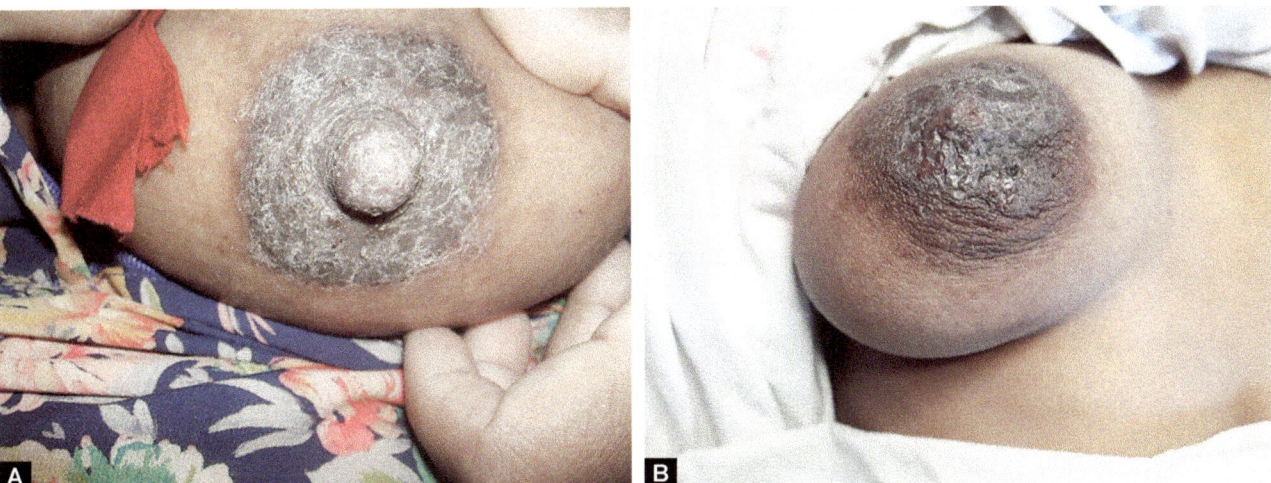

FIGS. 14A AND B: Lichenification and scaling of areola and periareolar skin.

- When longer vesicles develop, the term pompholyx is sometimes used.
- Can flare with stress, allergic or ICD and administration of intravenous immunoglobulin (IVIG), seen in patients with AD and hyperhidrosis.

Differential Diagnosis

Id reaction, inflammatory tinea pedis or mannum, ACD, scabies, palmoplantar psoriasis (if, secondarily infected), herpetic whitlow.

Treatment

- Topical corticosteroid
- Topical calcineurin inhibitors
- Bath PUVA (psoralen plus ultraviolet A)
- Systemic corticosteroid (when severe)

IRRITANT CONTACT DERMATITIS (ICD)

- Approximately 80% of all cases of CD.
- Secondary to a local toxic effect caused by a topical substance or physical insult.
- Localized, nonimmunologically mediated inflammatory reactions.
- *In chronic state*: Lichenification and pigmentation.
- *In acute state*: Erythema, edema, vesiculation followed by erosions and scaling.
- *In severe cases*: Epidermal necrosis (chemical burn).
- Commonly affects the hands. Search for any contact, occupational or environmental exposure, if suspected **(Figs. 15 to 17)**.
- Common cause of cheilitis (lip licking).
- *Common causes*: Soaps, cement, and cutting oils.

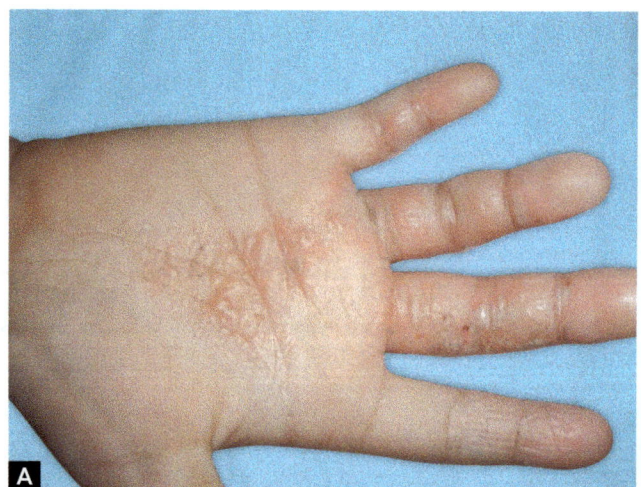
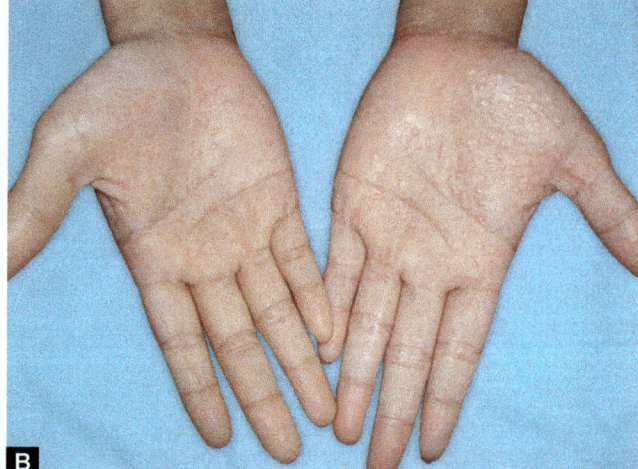

FIGS. 15A AND B: Clusters of firm vesicles along the lateral aspect of fingers, palms, and around wrist.

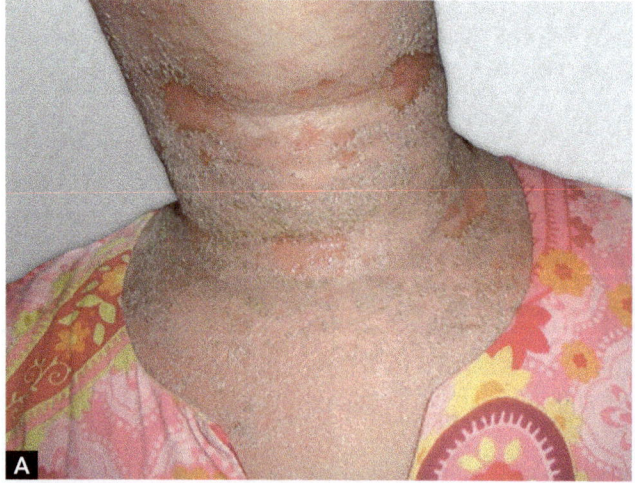
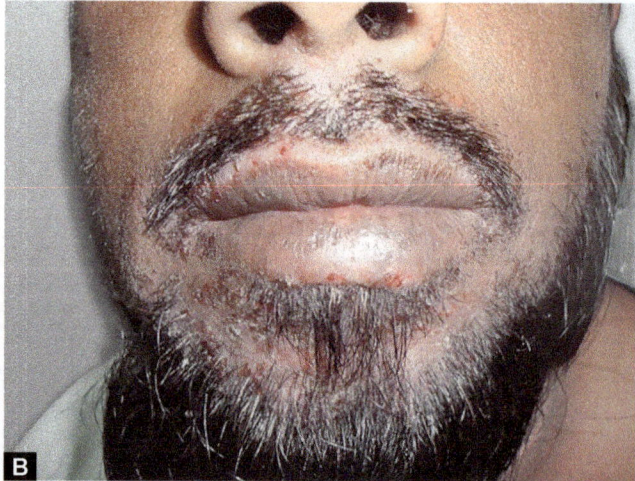

FIGS. 16A AND B: Irritant contact dermatitis involving neck and perioral area resulting vesiculation, exudation, and erosion.

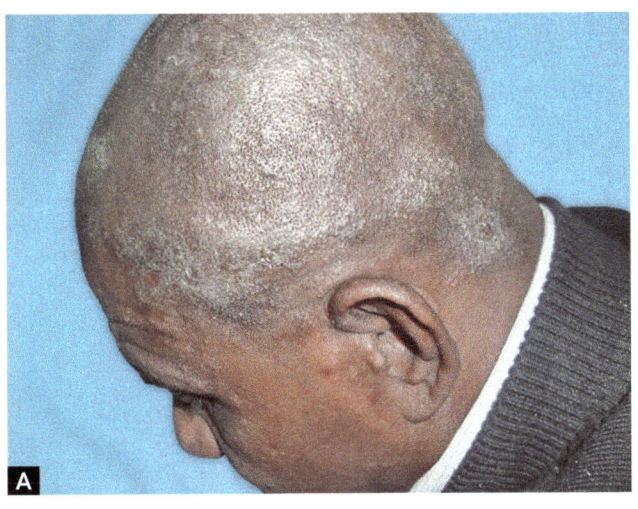 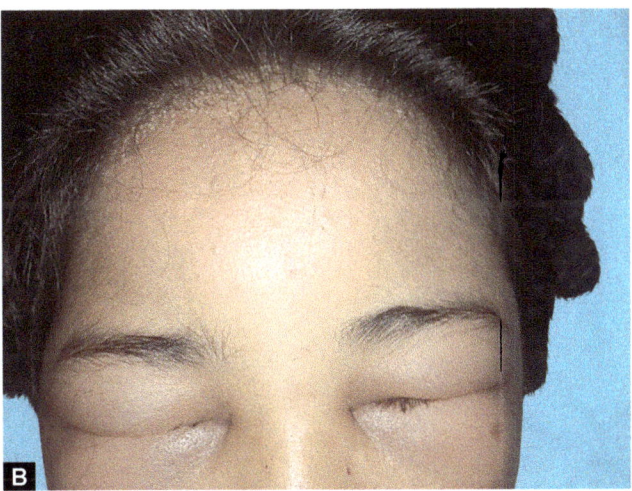

FIGS. 17A AND B: Vesiculation and edema due to hair dye.

■ Differential Diagnosis

Thermal burn, ICD, and ACD.

■ Treatment

Primarily avoidance of irritants.

ALLERGIC CONTACT DERMATITIS (ACD) (FIGS. 18 TO 20)

- Accounts for 20% of all causes of ACD.
- A delayed type of hypersensitivity reaction to a substance to which the individual has been previously sensitized.
- In contact to ICD, more commonly presents with pruritus during acute phase, the chronic phase has significant overlap with ICD.
- Initially, welllocalized to the site of contact.
- *In acute phase*: Erythema and edema, vesicobullous lesions and weeping develop **(Figs. 21 to 23)**.
- *In chronic phase*: Lichenification and scaling.
- Common allergens are metal, fragrances, preservatives, topical antibiotics, plants, and poison ivy.
- Occupational ACDs are rubber, nickel, epoxy resin, and aromatic amines.

■ Differential Diagnosis

- ICD
- AD
- Stasis dermatitis
- Seborrheic dermatitis

■ Common Allergens

- *Metals*: Nickel, chromate, cobalt, and gold.
- *Topical antibiotics*: Neomycin sulfate, bacitracin, and topical CS.
- *Fragrances*: Balsam of Peru.
- *Preservatives*: Formaldehyde, thimerosal, quaternium-15.

■ Treatment

- Short-term topical and systemic CS
- Avoidance of allergens

RADIODERMATITIS

Radiation dermatitis is an effect of external beam ionizing radiation resulting intense erythema and vesiculation of skin, may be observed in radiation ports **(Figs. 24A and B)**.

Administration of many chemotherapeutic agents, during or about the time of radiation therapy, may induce an enhanced radiation reaction **(Figs. 25A and B)**. In some cases, months to years after radiation treatment, the administration of a chemotherapeutic agent may induce a reaction within the prior radiation port, with features of radiation dermatitis. This phenomenon has been termed "radiation recall".

Besides the skin, internal structures such as gut may also affected.

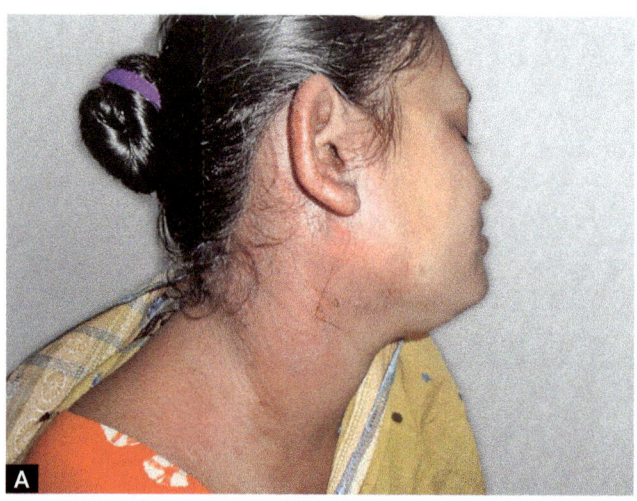
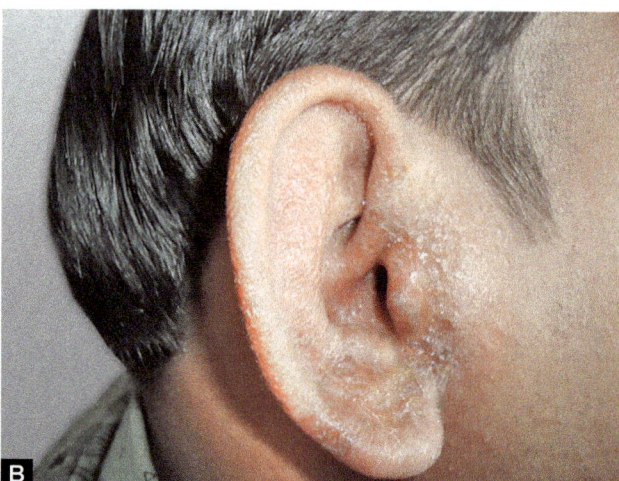

FIGS. 18A AND B: In acute phase erythema, vesiculation and exudation.

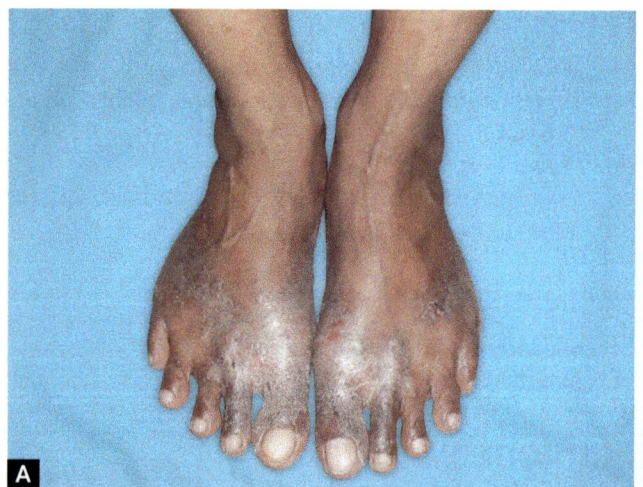
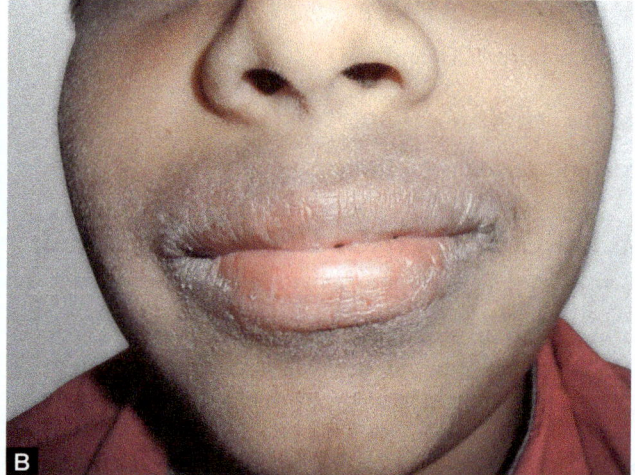

FIGS. 19A AND B: In chronic phase lichenification, pigmentary change occurs.

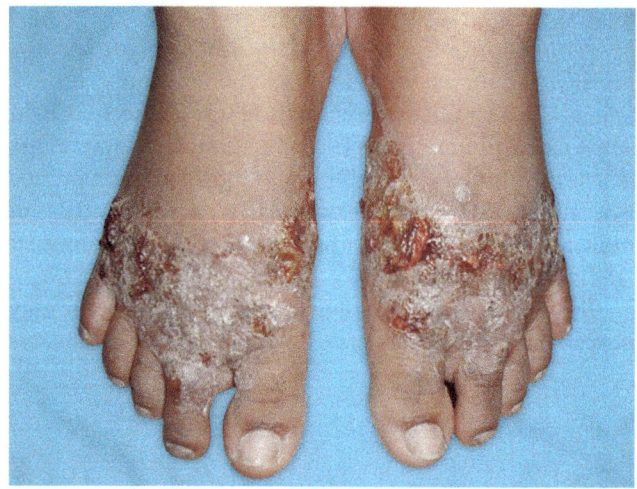

FIG. 20: Acute on chronic dermatitis.

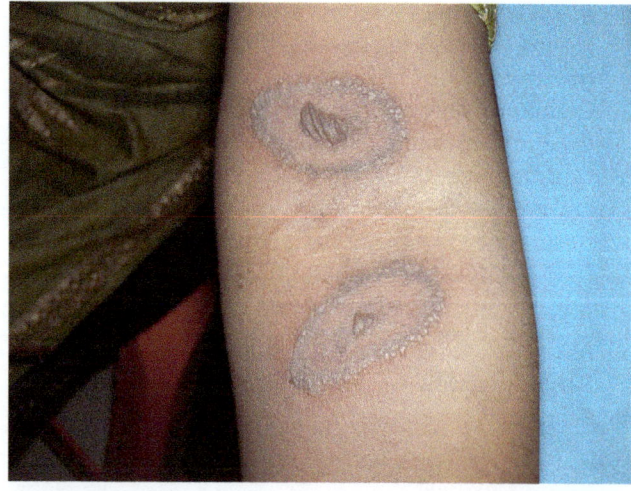

FIG. 21: Vesiculation and erythema, edema due to chemical component of insect.

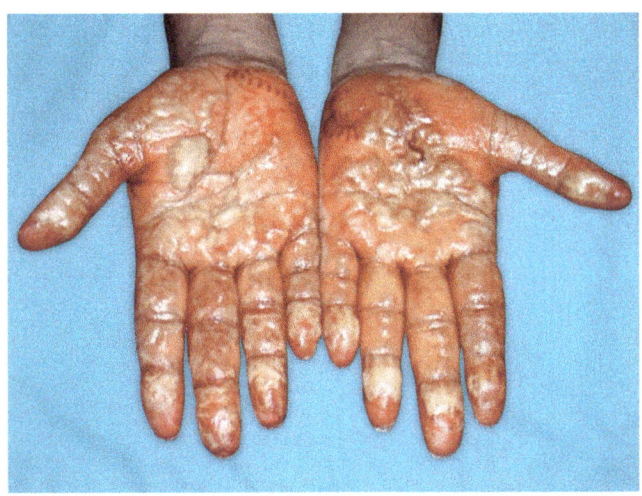

FIG. 22: Vesicles and bulla due to chemical component of Henna (*mehndi*).

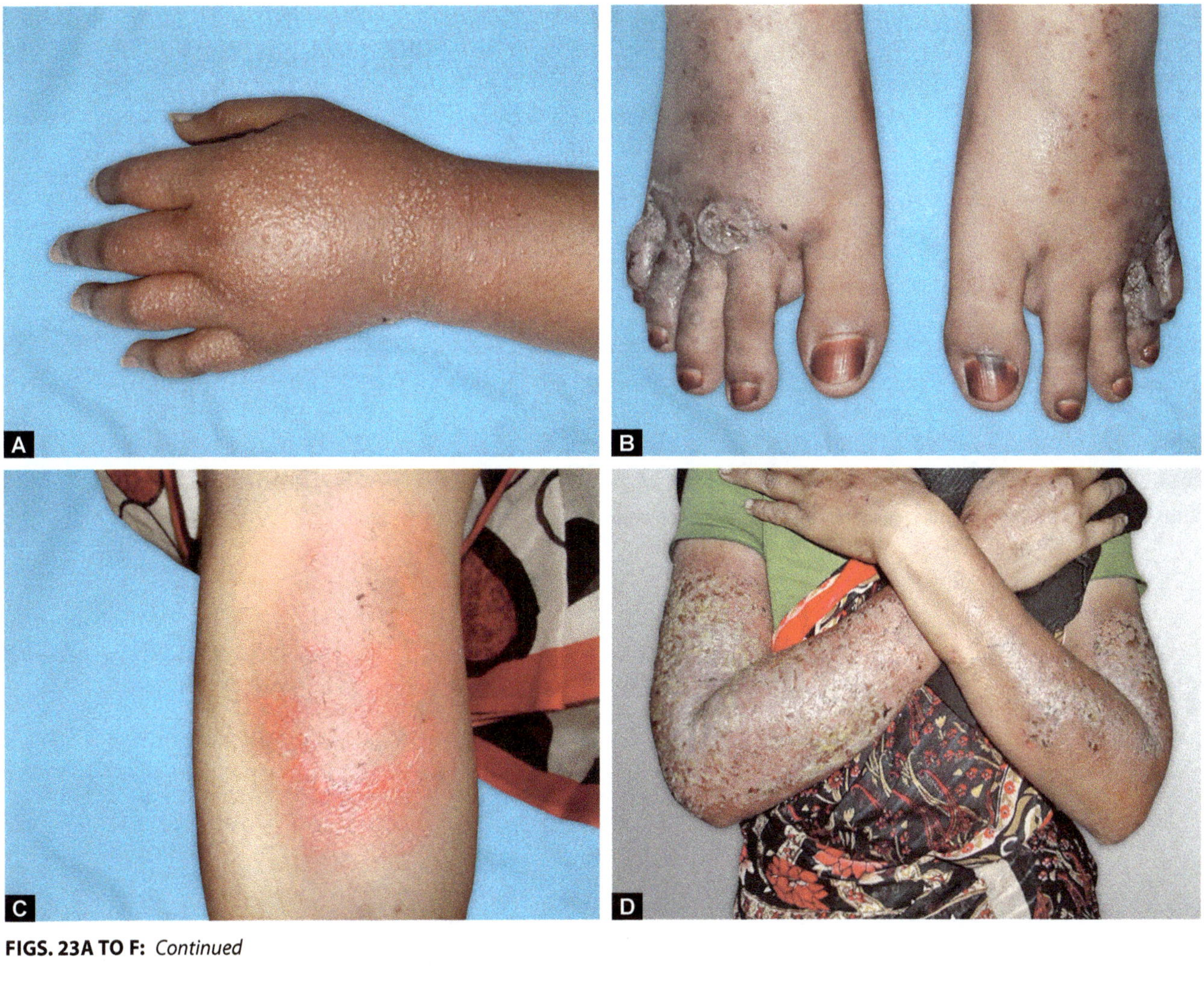

FIGS. 23A TO F: *Continued*

Continued

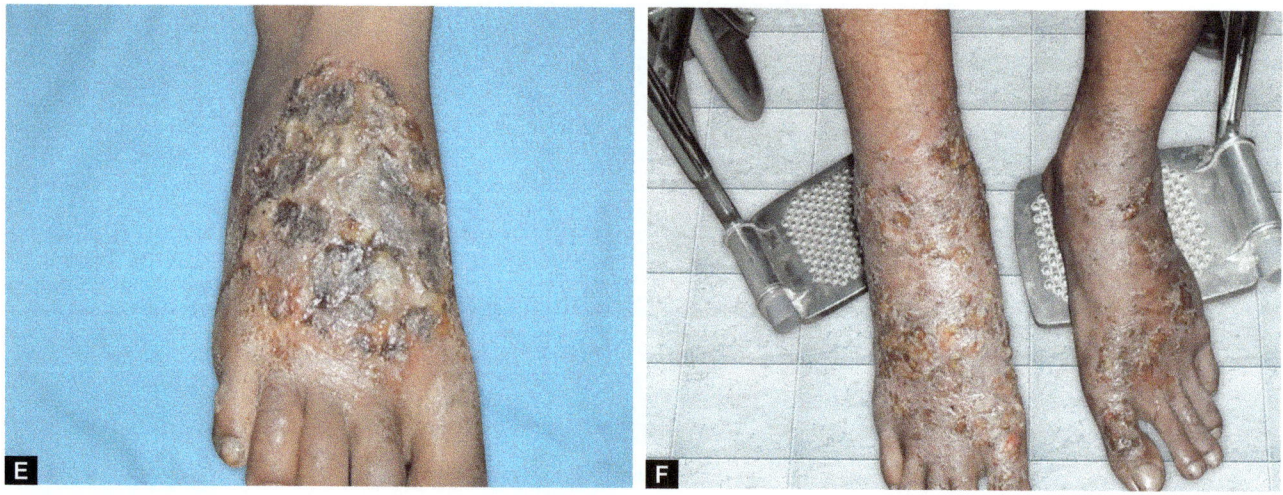

FIGS. 23A TO F: Erythema, edema, vesicles, bulla, and crust formation.

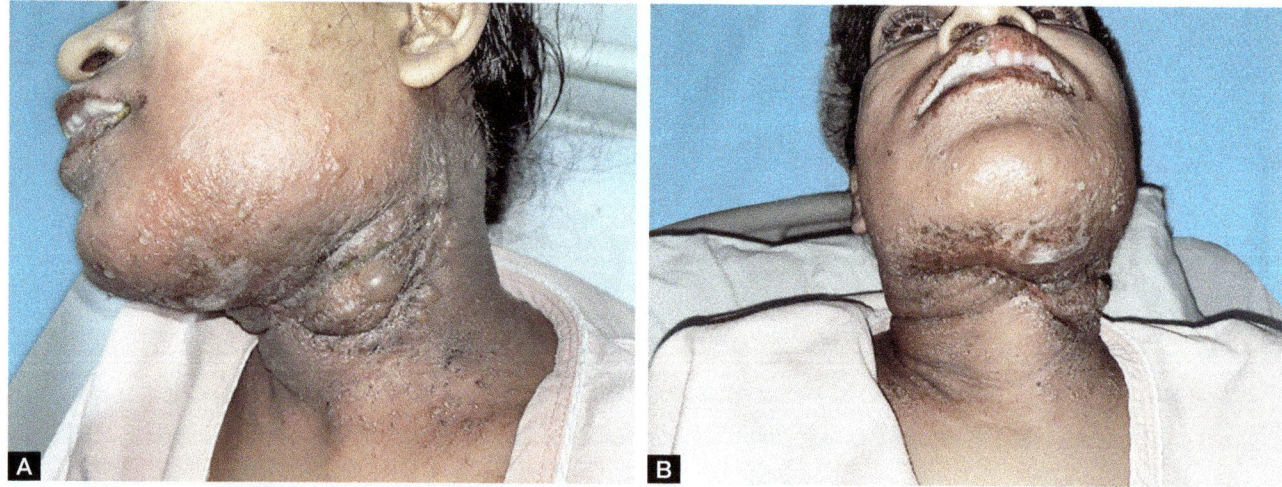

FIGS. 24A AND B: Vesicles, bulla, necrosis, and edema develop after 48 hours of radiation therapy.

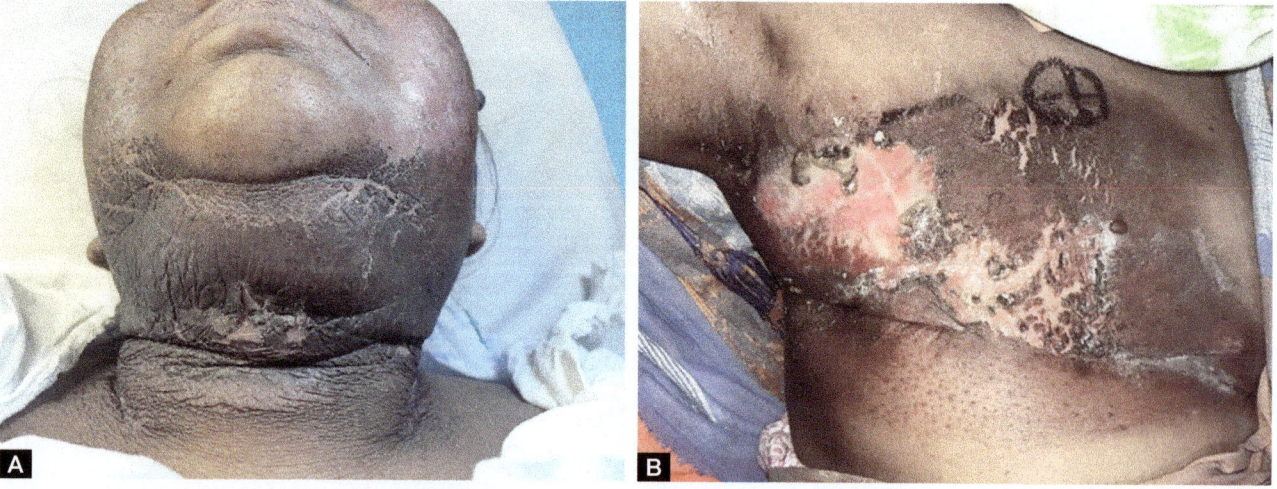

FIGS. 25A AND B: Hyperpigmented and crusted lesion on radiation exposed area.

CHAPTER 5

Psychoneurodermatitis

INTRODUCTION

Some cutaneous disorders are psychiatric in origin. Related to psychopathological cause rather dermatological or organic causes.
- Delusions of parasitosis
- Psychogenic excoriations
- Factitial dermatitis
- Trichotillomania

SKIN SIGNS OF PSYCHIATRIC ILLNESS

- Self-biting (onychophagia) or recurrent manipulation of the nail unit (onychotilomania) **(Figs. 1A and B)**.
- Compulsive repetitive handwashing may produce an irritant dermatitis or pompholyx of the hands **(Figs. 2A and B)**.
- Lip licking produces increased salivation and lip dermatitis **(Fig. 3)**.

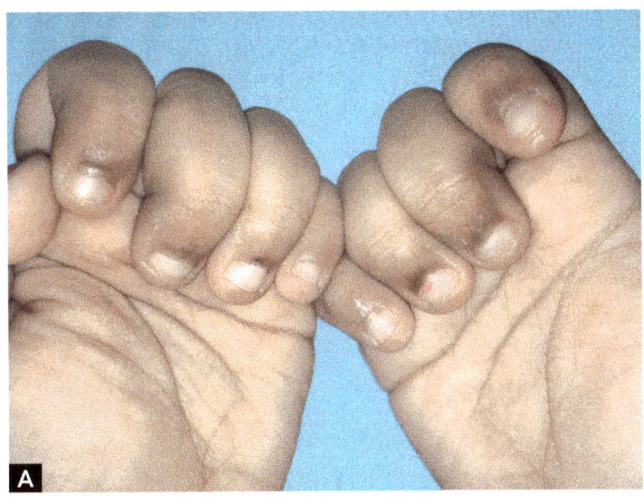

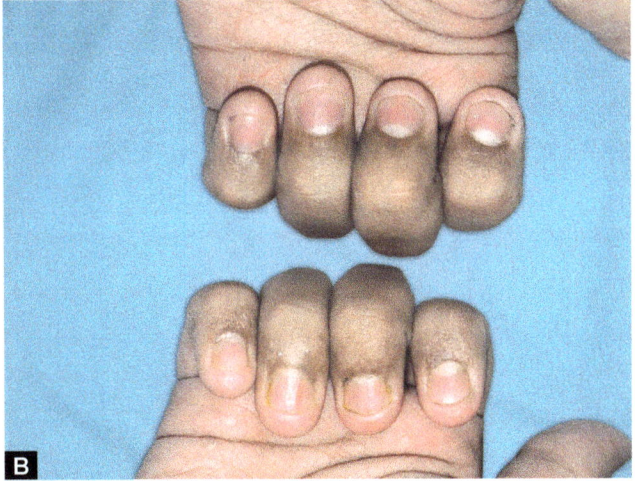

FIGS. 1A AND B: Onychophagia.

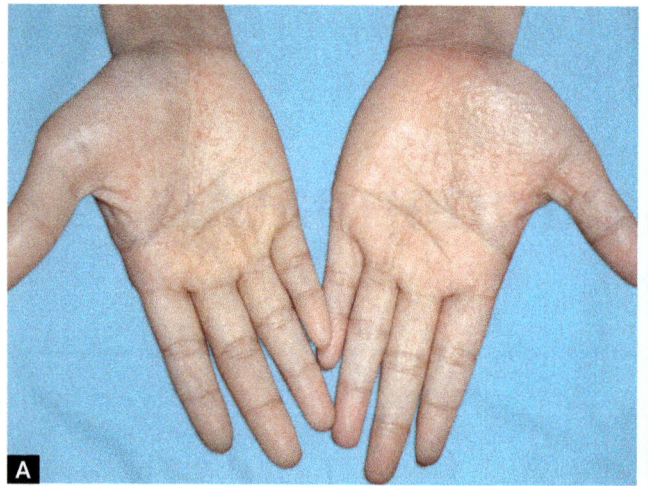
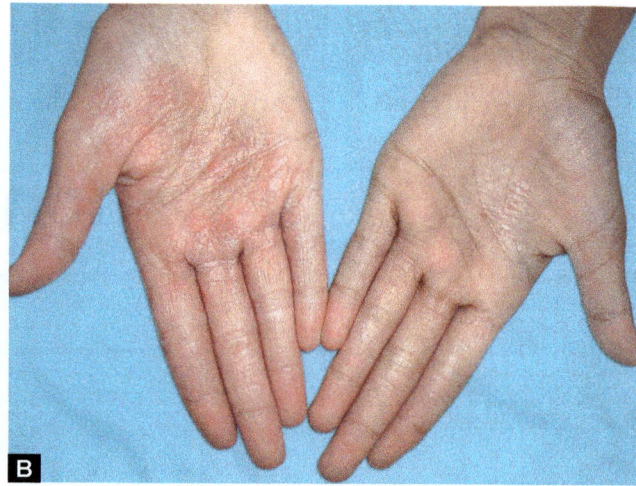

FIGS. 2A AND B: Hand eczema.

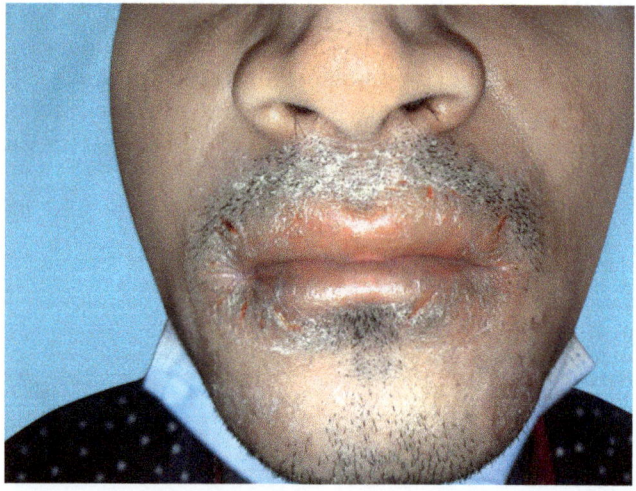

FIG. 3: Lip licking dermatitis.

Pruritus Ani

Pruritus ani is characterized by paroxysms of violent itching, which results in tearing of the affected area **(Figs. 4A and B)**.

Chronic pruritus and rubbing produces lichenification.

Etiology

- Unknown
- *Allergic contact dermatitis*: Drug, fragrance in toilet paper, preservative in moist toilet tissue.
- *Irritant contact dermatitis*: Food (hot spices), failure to clean adequately after bowel.
- *Physical factors*: Hemorrhoids, anal tags, fissure, and fistula.
- Mycotic
- Pinworm

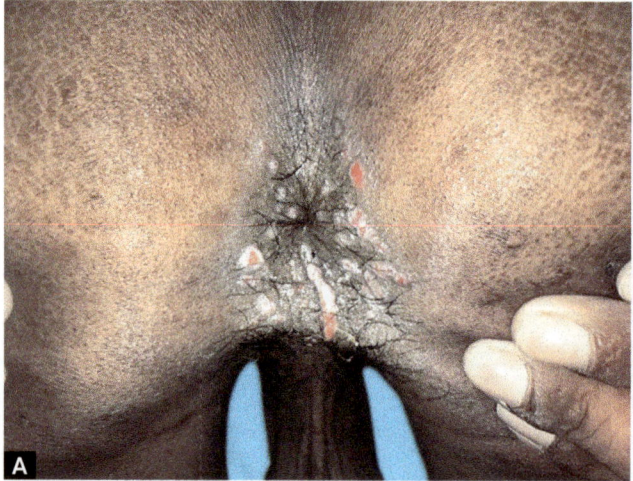
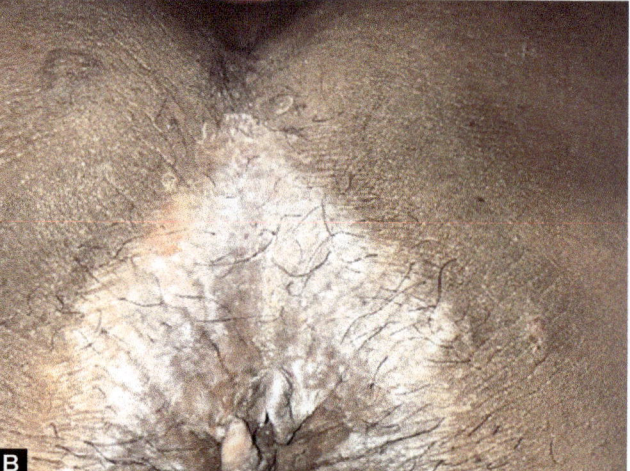

FIGS. 4A AND B: Lichenification, erosion, and ulceration present.

Pruritus Scroti

The scrotum of an adult is a susceptible site for circumscribed neurodermatitis (lichen simplex chronicus) **(Figs. 5A and B)**.

Etiology
- Unknown
- *Allergic contact dermatitis*: Drug, fragrance, soap, and sweat.
- Fungal infection except *Candida*.

Pruritus Vulvae

Pruritus vulvae **(Fig. 6)** is the counterpart of pruritus of pruritus scroti. Causes of chronic vulvar symptoms are:
- *Unspecified dermatitis (54%)*: May include contact dermatitis due to pads, contraceptives, douche solution, fragrance, preservatives in moist towelettes.
- Lichen sclerosus (13%)
- Chronic vulvovaginal candidiasis (10%)
- Dysesthetic vulvodynia (9%)
- Psoriasis (5%)

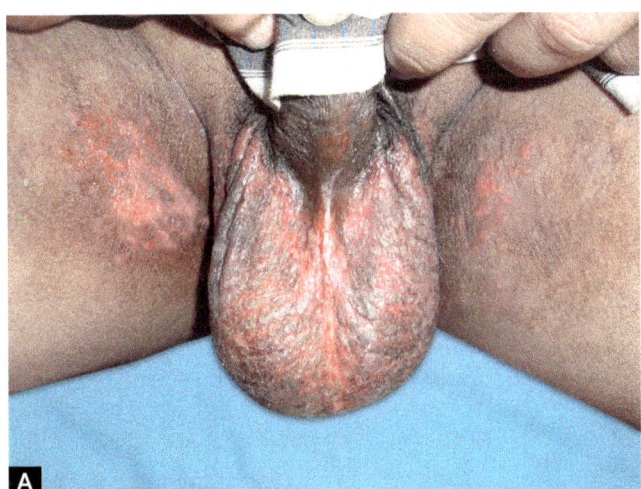
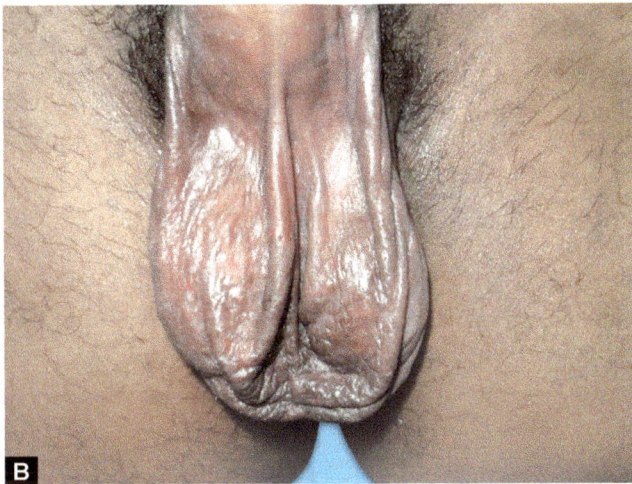

FIGS. 5A AND B: Lichenification, erythema, and hyperpigmentation present.

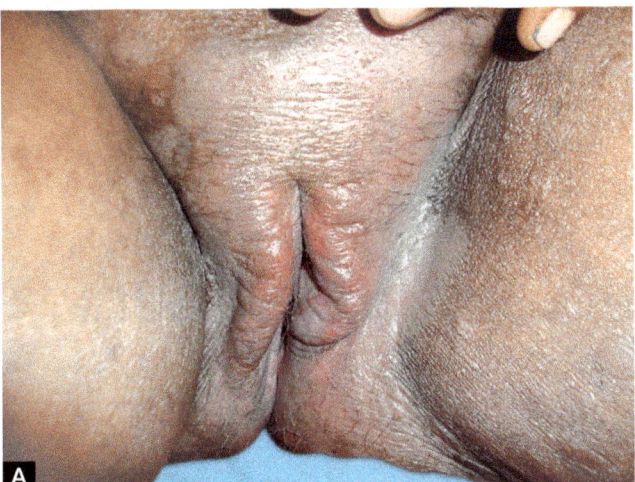
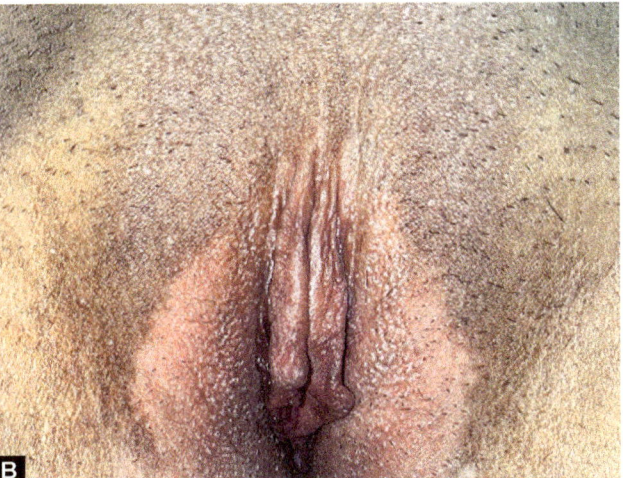

FIGS. 6A AND B: (A) Lichenification, scaly, and hypopigmented plaque; (B) Lichenification, dry, and hypopigmented plaque.

FACTITIOUS DERMATITIS

Factitious dermatitis is the term applied to selfinflicted skin lesions with the intent to elicit sympathy, escape responsibility or correct disability insurance **(Figs. 7 and 8)**.

Psychogenic (Neurotic) Excoriation

- A continuous, repetitive, uncontrollable desire to pick, rub, or scratch skin.
- Favors scalp, face, extensor forearms, shins, and buttocks **(Figs. 9A to D)**.

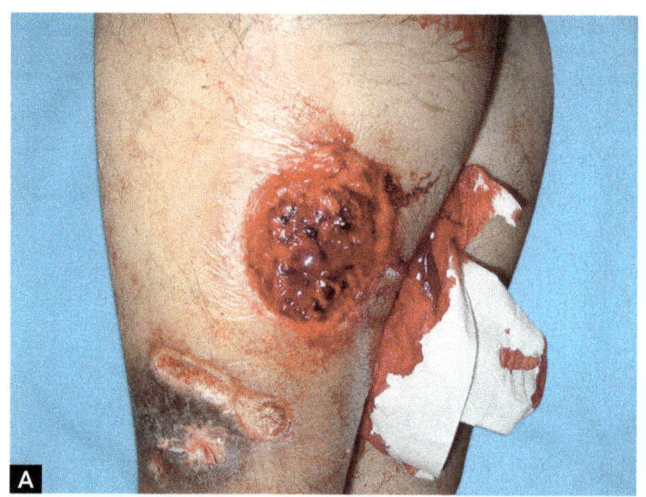
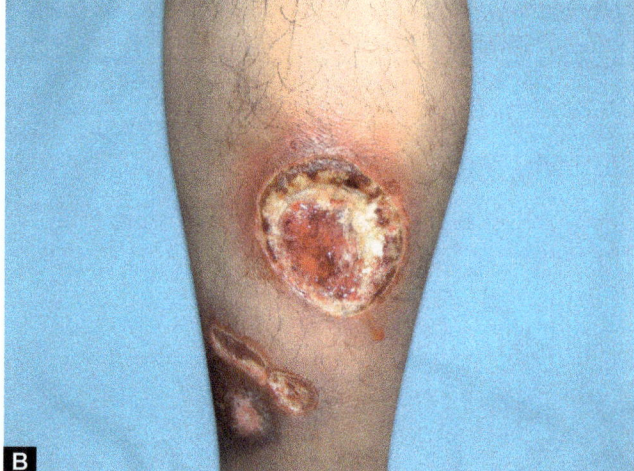

FIGS. 7A AND B: Self-induced ulcer formation by scalpel.

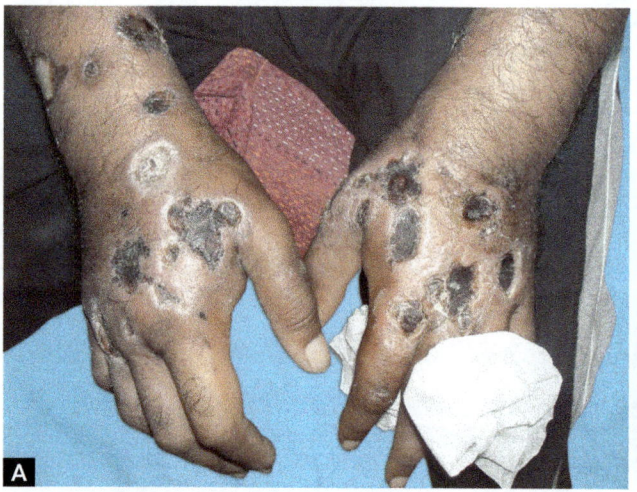
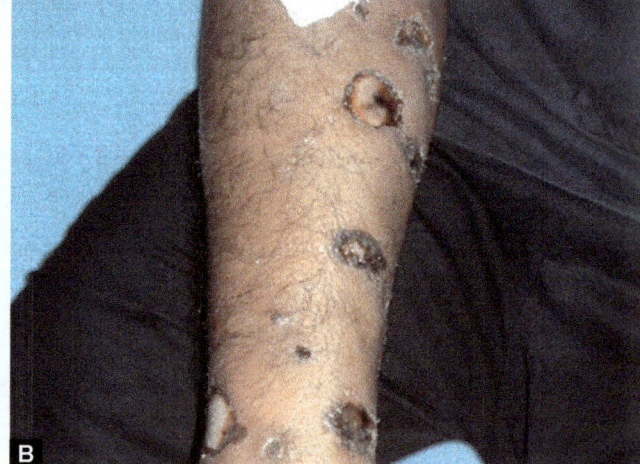

FIGS. 8A AND B: Injecting cocktail (cocaine and pethidine) in skin.

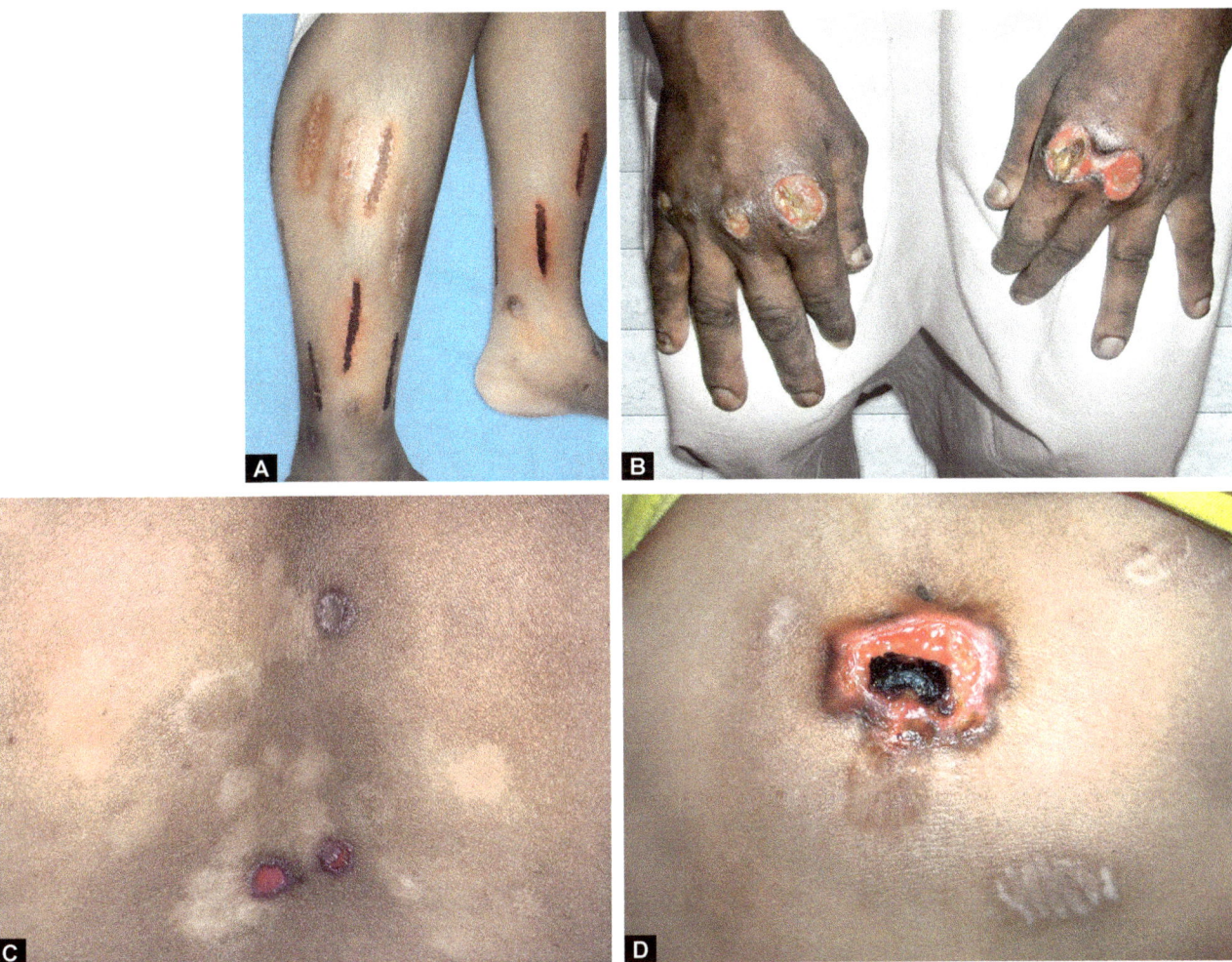

FIGS. 9A TO D: Neurotic excoriations.

■ Lichen Simplex Chronicus

It is also known as circumscribed neurodermatitis. Lichen simplex chronicus (LSC) results from long-term chronic rubbing and scratching, more vigorously than a normal pain threshold wound permits, with the skin becoming thickened and leathery. The normal skin marking becomes prominent and this condition is known as lichenification **(Figs. 10A to D)**.

■ Prurigo Nodularis

- Multiple, discrete, itchy, chronic, firm papulonodules with central scale-crust due to repetitive scratching and picking.
- Lesions usually favor the extensor surfaces of the extremities, upper back, buttocks, but they can be widespread in easily reachable areas **(Figs. 11A and B)**.
- Disruption of the itch-scratch cycle requires symptomatic relief.

Treatment
- Superpotent topical steroid
- Intralesional steroid
- Ultraviolet B (UVB), psoralen and ultraviolet A (PUVA)
- Thalidomide

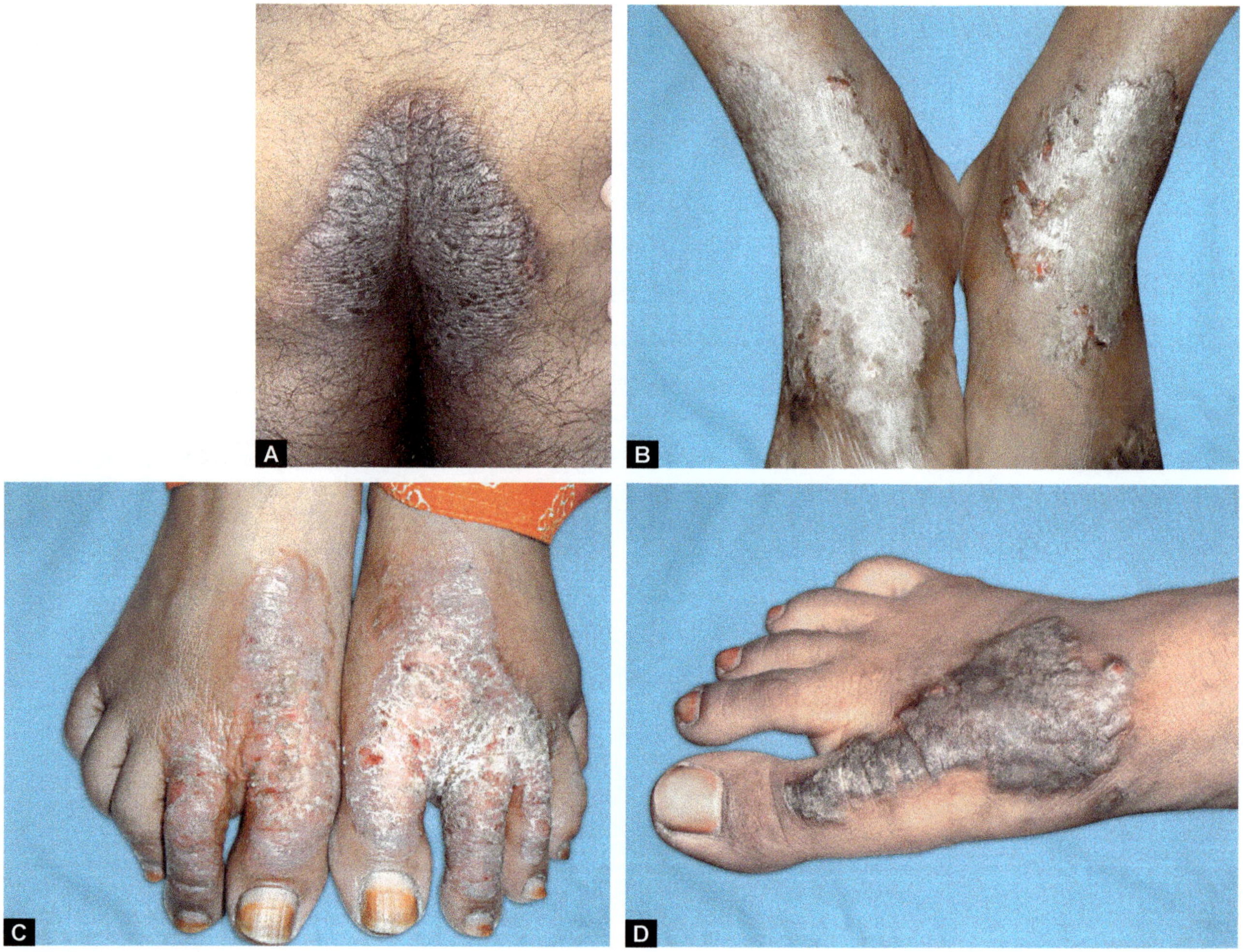

FIGS. 10A TO D: Lichenification, scaly, and hyperpigmentation.

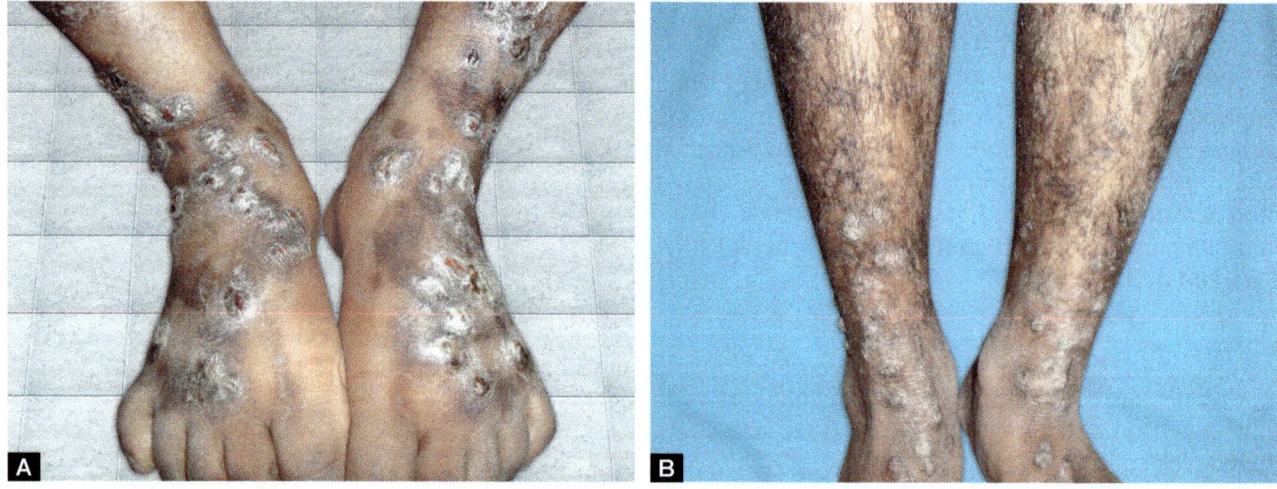

FIGS. 11A AND B: Multiple papulonodular lesions on lower extremity.

Delusions of Parasitosis

Delusional infestation (Ekbom syndrome) is a firm fixation of a person that he or she suffers from a parasitic infestation of the skin. The belief is so fixed that the patient often picks small pieces of epithelial debris from the skin and show these to close contacts and sometimes bring to doctor as proof **(Figs. 12A and B)**.

Trichotillomania

Trichotillomania **(Figs. 13A and B)** or hair pulling disorder is characterized by an abnormal urge to pull out the hair and person do that usually from frontal region of scalp, eyebrows, eyelashes, and the beard.

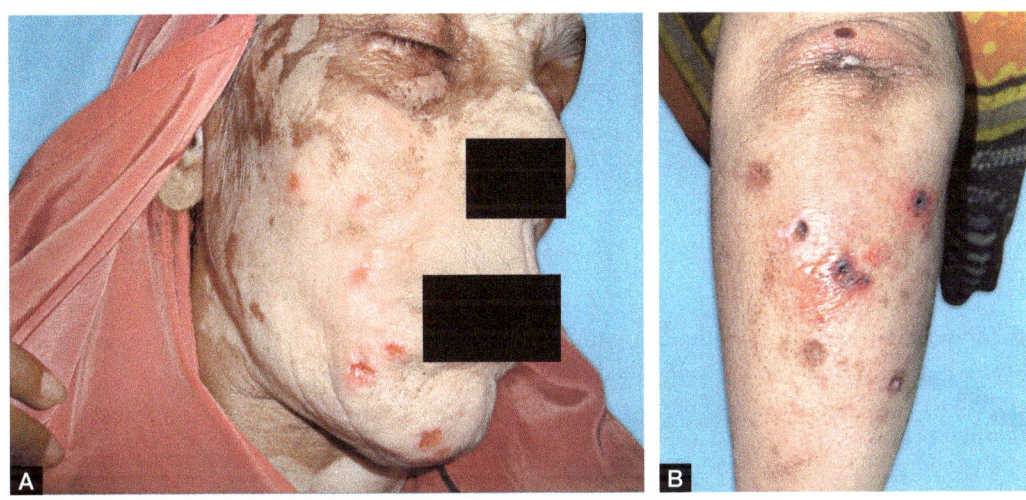

FIGS. 12A AND B: Self-induced ulcers in patients suffering from delusions of parasitosis.

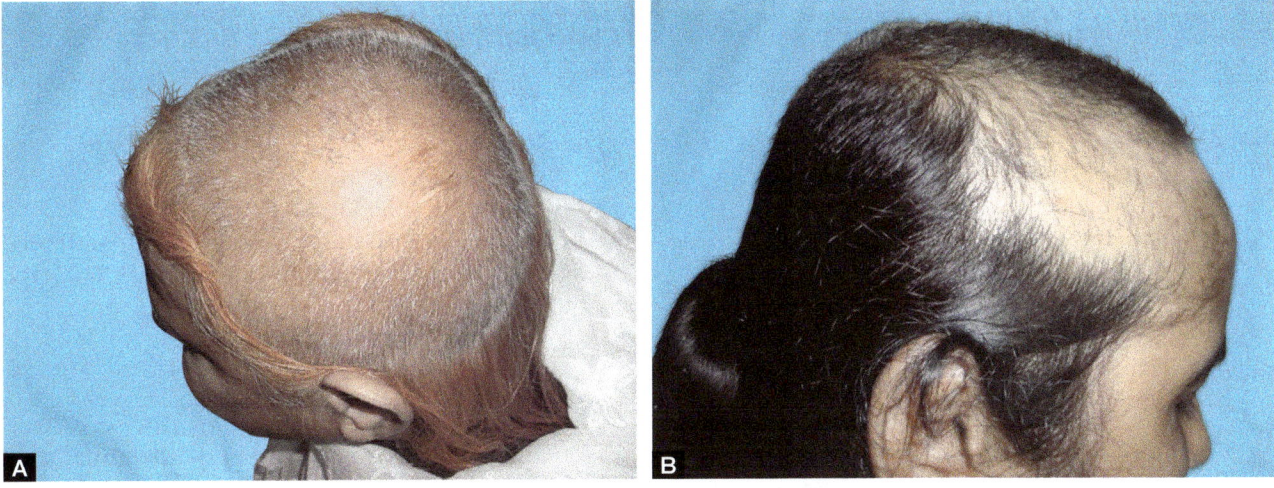

FIGS. 13A AND B: Trichotillomania.

CHAPTER 6

Urticaria and Angioedema

INTRODUCTION

- Urticaria is composed of transient edematous papules and plaques (wheals), usually pruritic. This is due to edema of papillary dermis, the wheals are superficial and well-defined **(Fig. 1)**.
- Angioedema is a larger edematous area that involves the dermis and subcutaneous tissue and is deep and ill-defined **(Figs. 2A to C)**.
- Urticaria and/or angioedema may be acute recurrent or chronic recurrent.

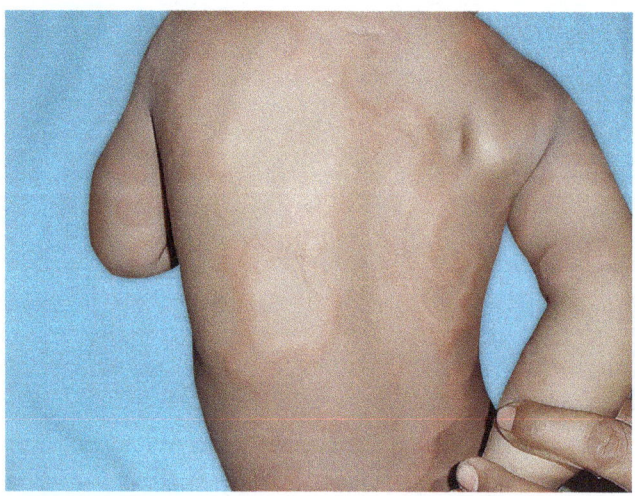

FIG. 1: Wheals.

ACUTE URTICARIA

- Acute onset and occurring over <6 weeks.

Causes

- Infection, e.g., urinary tract infection (UTI), upper respiratory tract infections (up to 40%)
- Drug (up to 10%)
- Food (<1%)
- Idiopathic (up to 50%)

CHRONIC URTICARIA

- Occurring at least twice weekly by ≥6 weeks.

Causes

- Idiopathic (up to 50%)
- Autoimmune (histamine releasing autoantibodies against Fc portion of immunoglobulin E (IgE) (40–50%)
- Chronic infections (e.g., parasite ≤5%)

Investigations

- Complete blood count (CBC) and differential count (DC)
- Urine routine microscopic examination (R/M/E) and culture for *Candida* and bacteria
- Stool R/M/E for parasite

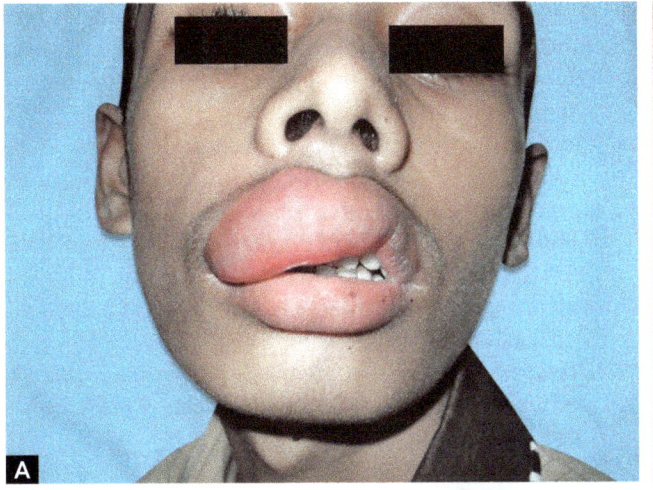
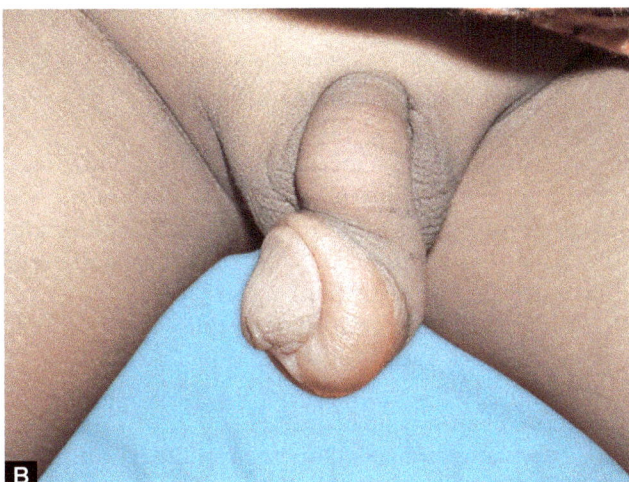
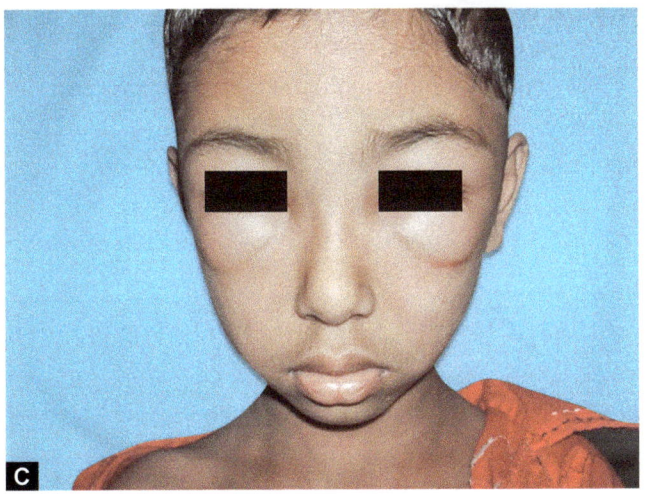

FIGS. 2A TO C: Angioedema.

- *X-ray of teeth*: Root abscess, check for sinusitis.
- Swab scrapping and culture for dermatophytes and *Candida*
- Vaginal swab for diagnosis of trichomoniasis
- Venereal disease research laboratory (VDRL) test
- Biopsy for histopathological examination for excluding vasculitis
- Kidney functions test
- Liver functions test
- Antinuclear antibody (ANA)
- C3 and CH50 levels
- Cryoglobulin, cryofibrinogen and cold hemolysins, if cold urticaria is suspected.
- X-ray, USG of gastrointestinal tract (GIT), and chest for cancer screening
- Photo test for ultraviolet B (UVB), ultraviolet A (UVA), and visible light to exclude solar elastosis.
- Serum thyroid stimulating hormone (TSH)

■ **Treatment**

- *Eliminate any identifiable causes*:
  ○ Avoid physical triggers and drugs that stimulate mast cell degranulation [e.g., aspirin, nonsteroidal anti-inflammatory drugs (NSAIDs), codeine, and morphine].
- *Long-acting nonsedative antihistamine (cetirizine/ levocetirizine)*:
  ○ Increase dose if needed (two- to fourfolds).
  ○ Use of more than one drug (loratadine) can maximize benefit.

If no response:
Plus—Sedating H1 antihistamine (Doxepin 10–50 mg).

If response not adequate:
Plus—Sedating H2 antihistamine (Famotidine).

Special Cases

- *Due to mechanical stimuli*: Pressure urticaria, systemic corticosteroids (prednisolone 30 mg/day).
- Due to temperature change
- *Cold*: Mizolastine 10 mg/day, cyproheptadine 4 mg, doxantrazole, and doxepin.
- *Due to sweating/physical exertions*: Cholinergic > adrenergic urticaria, and exercise-induced anaphylaxis. Hydroxyzine 10 mg tid.
- *For idiopathic urticaria*: Hydroxyzine 10 mg tid and mizolastine 10 mg/day effective.
- Chlorpheniramine maleate 4 mg tid is cheap and effective in most types of urticaria.
- For dermatographism, combination of H1- and H2- receptor antagonists is effective.
- *Cetirizine 10 mg*: Only antihistamine with antieosinophilic property.
- *Tricyclic antidepressants are potent blockers of H1 and H2 receptors*: Doxepin 10–25 mg tid, amitriptyline 10–25 mg tid.
- Ketotifen is effective in cold urticaria, dermatographism, cholinergic urticaria, and idiopathic urticaria.
- *Hereditary angioedema*: Danazol 400 mg/day and stanozolol 2 mg/day.
- *Solar urticaria and porphyria*: Chloroquine.
- *Aquagenic pruritus*: Antihistamines, propranolol, atenolol, selective serotonin reuptake inhibitors (SSRIs), aspirin, pregabalin, montelukast, and UVB/PUVA (psoralen plus ultraviolet A) therapy.
- *Acute severe urticaria/urticarial vasculitis*: Systemic corticosteroids (prednisolone 30 mg/day).
- *Delayed pressure urticaria/urticarial vasculitis*: Indomethacin 50 mg tid, or colchicine 0.6 mg bid, or dapsone 100 mg/day.

Refractory Cases

- Dapsone or colchicine
- Mycophenolate mofetil, methotrexate, cyclosporine, and omalizumab may be given.

CHAPTER 7

Erythema Multiforme, Stevens–Johnson Syndrome, Toxic Epidermal Necrolysis, and Fixed Drug Eruption

ERYTHEMA MULTIFORME

A common reaction pattern of blood vessels in the dermis with secondary epidermal changes characterized by erythematous iris-shaped popular and vesiculobullous lesions. Self-limited, but potentially recurrent disease.

Two forms:
1. Erythema multiforme (EM) minor
2. EM major

Two types of target lesion:
1. *Typical target (**Fig. 1**), three different zones*:
    i. Central dusky purpura

FIG. 1: Typical target in right index finger with vesicles.

 ii. An elevated and edematous pale ring
 iii. Surrounding macular erythema. Best observed on palms and soles.
2. *Atypical target—two zones*:
    i. *EM*: Papular.
    ii. *Stevens–Johnson syndrome (SJS)/toxic epidermal necrolysis (TEN)*: Macular.

■ Precipitating Factors

- *Infectious causes*: Viral; herpes simplex virus (HSV-1 and HSV-2), varicella, adenovirus, human immunodeficiency virus (HIV), hepatitis virus, Cytomegalovirus (CMV), parvovirus B19, and adenovirus.
- *Bacterial*: *Mycoplasma* pneumonia, *Chlamydophila* (chlamydia), *Salmonella, Mycobacterium tuberculosis*.
- *Fungal*: *Histoplasma capsulatum*, dermatophytes.
- *Drugs causing EM major (most frequently)*:
    o Sulfonamide, phenytoin, barbiturate, phenylbutazone, penicillin, and allopurinol.

■ Erythema Multiforme Minor

Typical target lesion ± Papular atypical targets (**Figs. 2 to 5**).
- Acrofacial involvement
- Little or no mucous membrane involvement
- Vesicles, no bulla
- No systemic symptoms
- No progression to TEN
- *Precipitating factors*: HSV and other infectious agents.

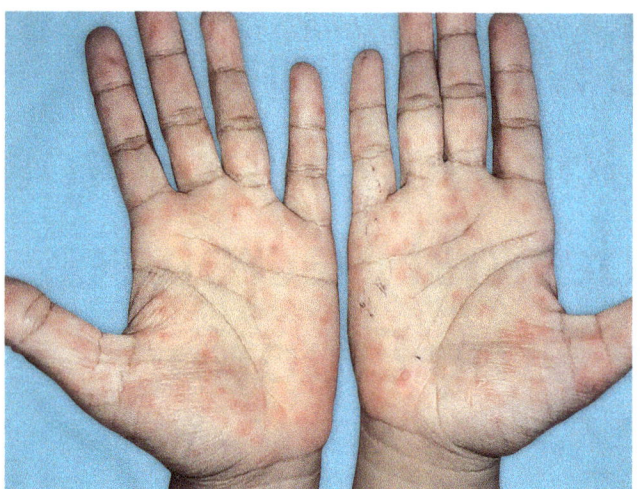

FIG. 2: Papular atypical target on both palms.

Erythema Multiforme Major

Typical target lesion ± Papular atypical targets
- Acrofacial involvement
- Moderate-to-severe mucous membrane involvement
- Vesicles and bulla
- *Systemic symptoms*: Fever, asthenia, and arthralgias.
- No progression to TEN
- *Precipitating factors*: HSV, mycoplasma pneumoniae, other infectious agents, and rarely drugs.

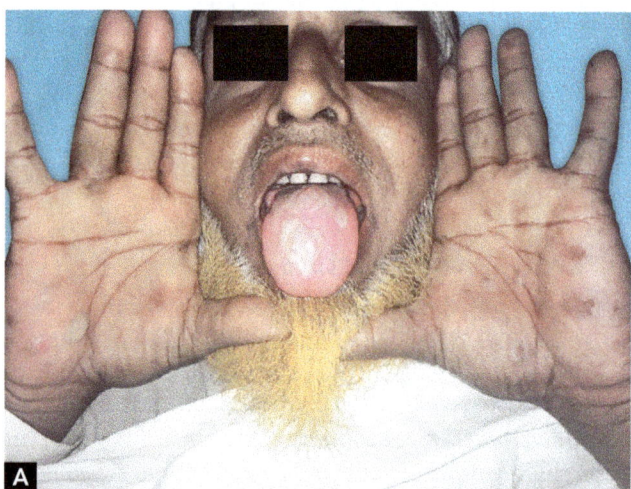
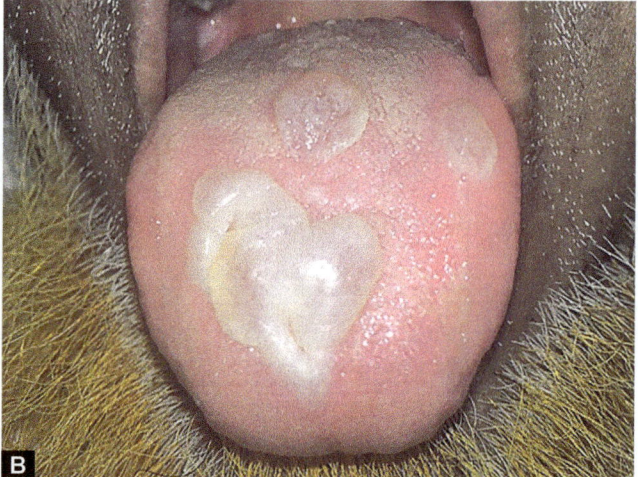

FIGS. 3A AND B: Atypical target on both palm and vesicle–bulla on tongue.

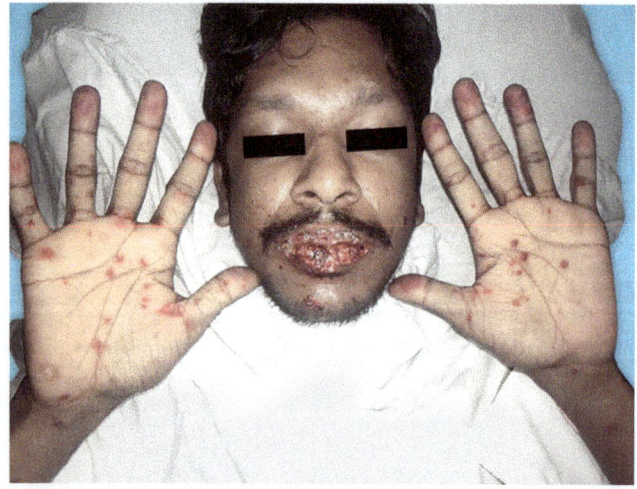

FIG. 4: Mucosal erosion due to rupture vesicle and bulla with atypical target in palms.

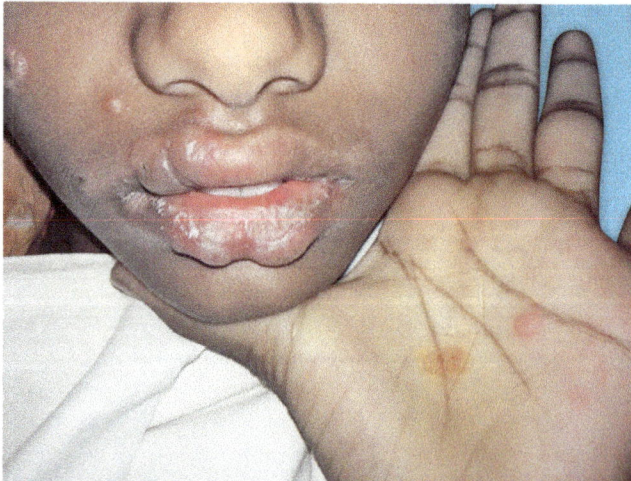

FIG. 5: Atypical target on left palm with vesicles on lips.

STEVENS–JOHNSON SYNDROME

- Dusky macules with or without epidermal detachment
- Macular atypical lesions
- Bullous lesions
- Less than 10% body surface area (BSA) detachment
- Trunk, face, and neck involvement
- Severe mucous membrane involvement
- *Systemic symptoms*: Fever, lymphadenopathy, hepatitis, cytopenia.
- *Progression to TEN*: Possible.
- *Precipitating factors*: Drugs, occasionally *Mycoplasma pneumoniae*, rarely immunizations.

STEVENS–JOHNSON SYNDROME/TOXIC EPIDERMAL NECROLYSIS (FIGS. 6 TO 9)

- Dusky macules with or without epidermal detachment
- Macular atypical lesions
- Bullous lesions
- 10–30% BSA detachment
- Confluence (++) trunk, face, and neck involvement
- Severe mucous membrane involvement
- *Systemic symptoms*: Fever, lymphadenopathy, hepatitis, cytopenia, conjunctivitis can lead to keratitis and ulceration.
- *Progression to TEN*: More likely.
- *Precipitating factors*: Drugs. Onset usually 7–21 days after starting culprit medication.

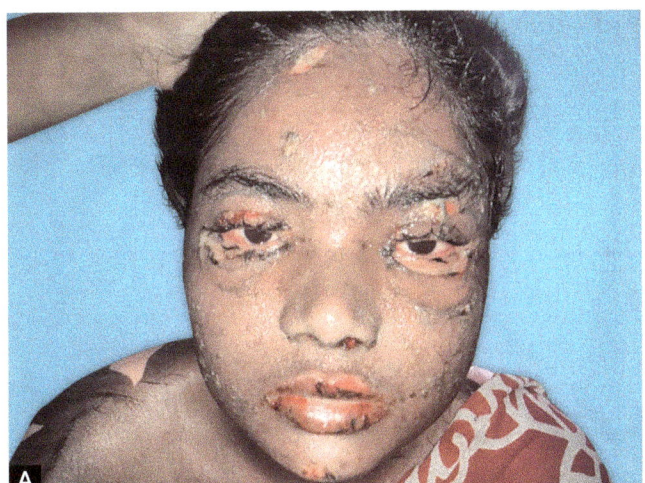
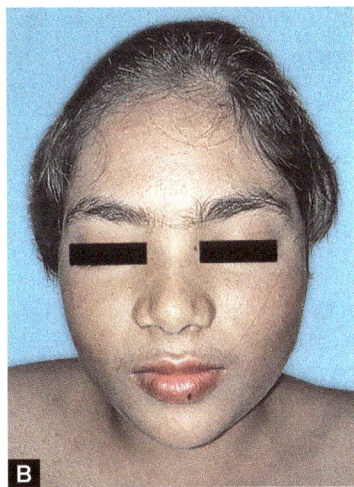

FIGS. 6A AND B: Before and after recovery.

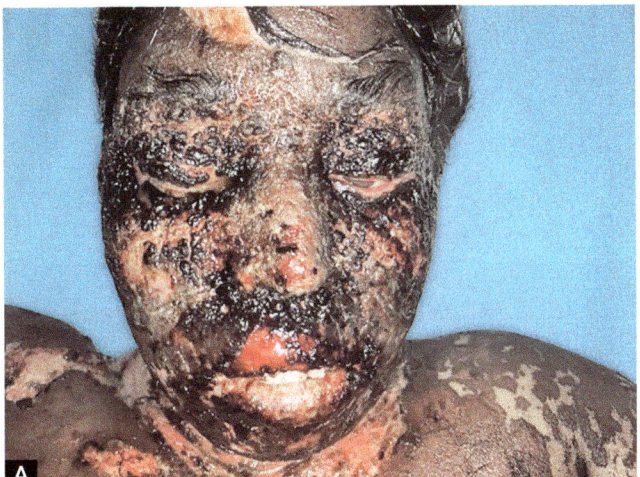
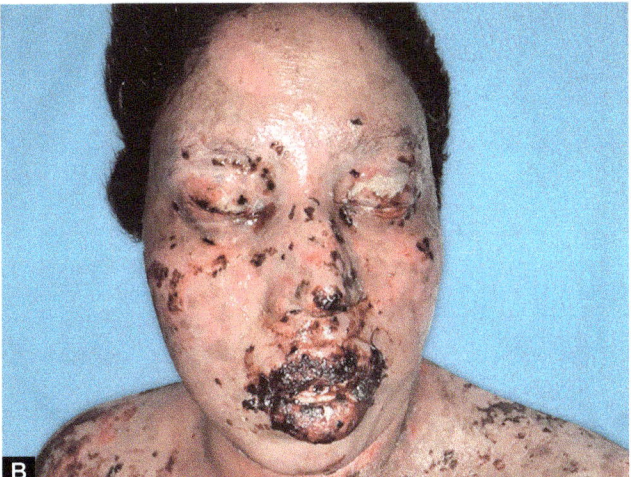

FIGS. 7A TO K: *Continued*

Continued

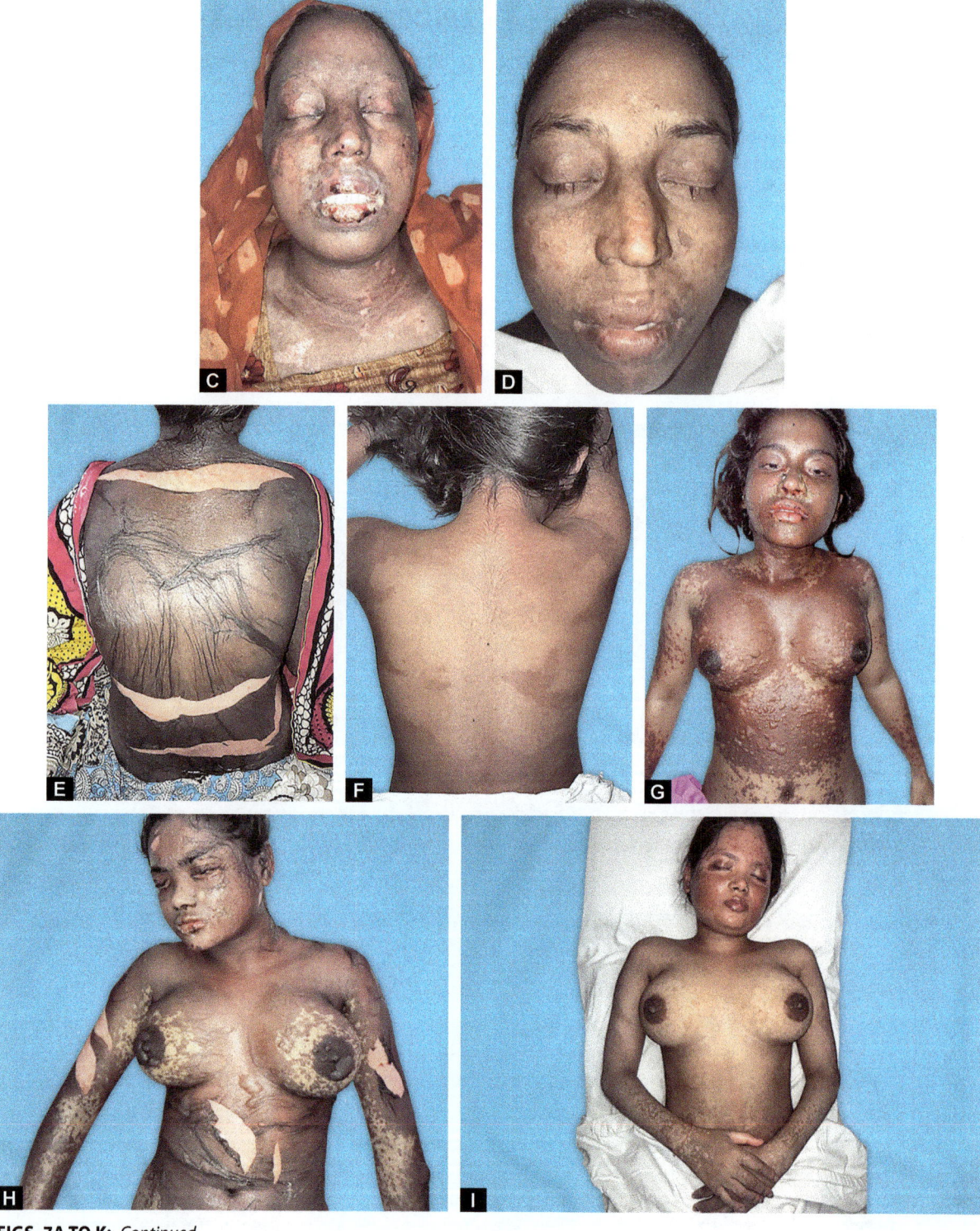

FIGS. 7A TO K: *Continued*

Continued

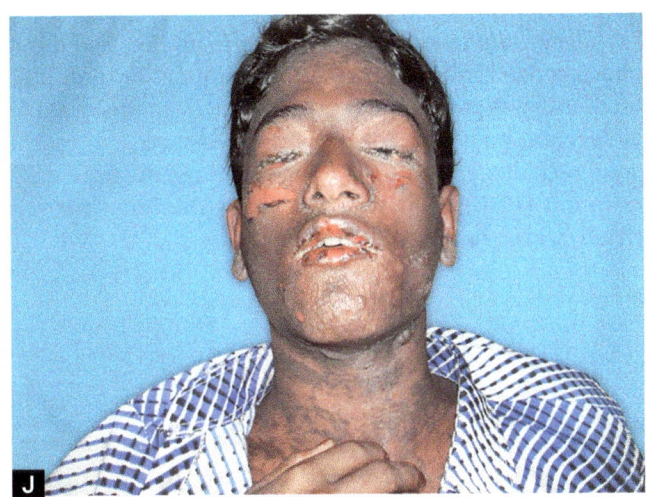
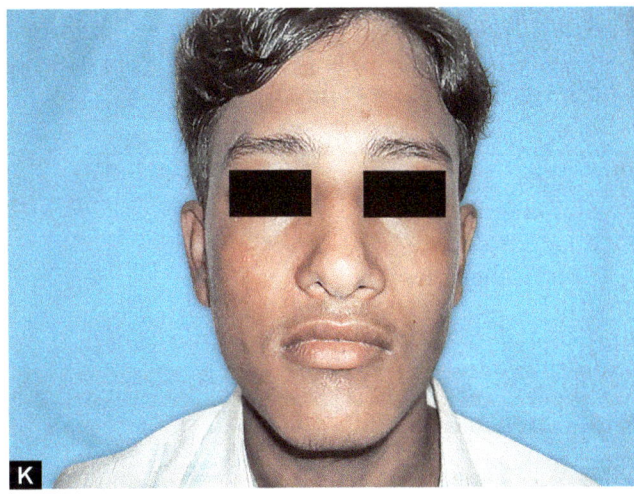

FIGS. 7A TO K: Before and after recovery from toxic epidermal necrolysis (TEN).

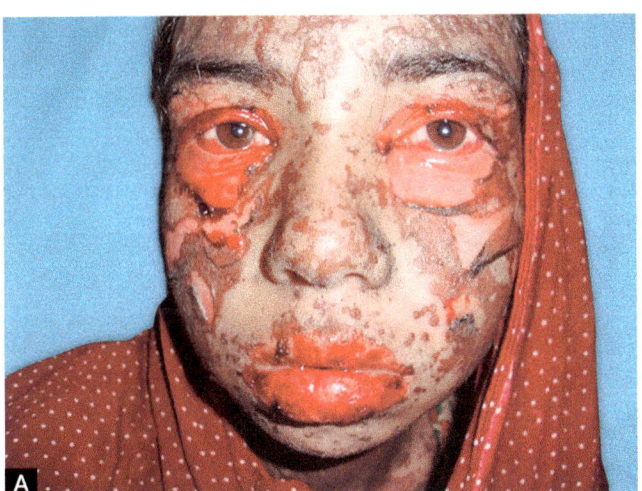
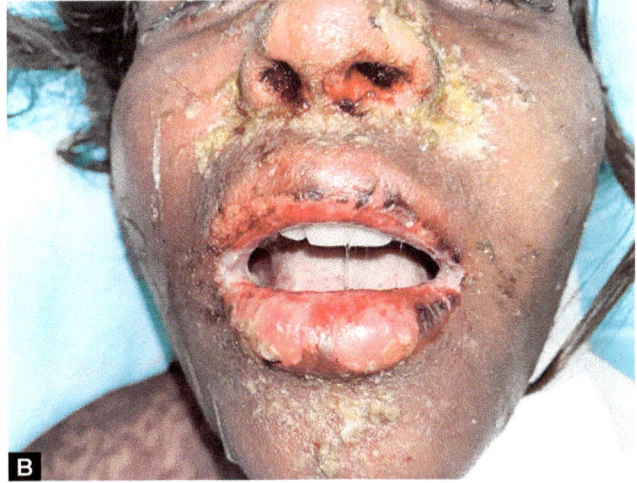

FIGS. 8A AND B: Mucosal and skin erosion.

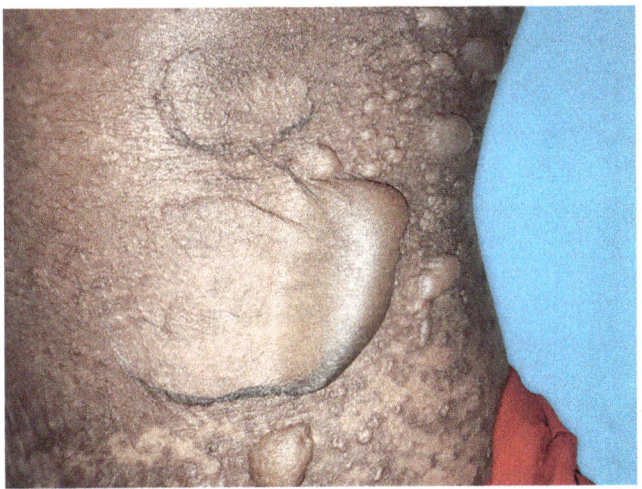

FIG. 9: Vesicle and flaccid bulla.

TOXIC EPIDERMAL NECROLYSIS

- Dusky macules and macular atypical lesions rarely
- Poorly delineated erythematous plaques
- Bullous lesions
- More than 30% BSA detachment
- Confluence (++) trunk, face, neck, and whole body
- Severe mucous membrane involvement may also involve respiratory and gastrointestinal epithelial linings.
- *Systemic symptoms*: Fever, lymphadenopathy, hepatitis, cytopenia, and conjunctivitis can lead to keratitis and ulceration.
- *Precipitating factors*: Drugs. Onset usually 7–21 days after starting culprit medication.

SCORTEN Scale

The SCORTEN scale (SCORe of Toxic Epidermal Necrolysis) is widely used to predict mortality in patients with SJS or TEN **(Tables 1 and 2)**.

Treatment

- Stop culprit drug
- Supportive care
- Specific therapies

FIXED DRUG ERUPTION (FIGS. 10 TO 14)

An adverse cutaneous drug reaction to an ingested drug, characterized by the formation of a solitary or multiples erythematous patch or plaque, then turn into dusky red to violaceous; bulla or eroded lesions often seen.

If rechallenged with the offending drug, the fixed drug eruption (FDE) occurs repeatedly at the identical site (fixed) within hours of ingestion.

TABLE 1: SCORTEN scale (prognostic factors and points).

Prognostic factors	Points
Age >40 years	1
Heart rate >120 beats/minute	1
Cancer or hematological malignancy	1
Body surface area on day 1 >10%	1
Serum urea level >10 mmol/L	1
Serum bicarbonate level <20 mmol/L	1
Serum glucose level >14 mmol/L	1
(SCORTEN: SCORE of Toxic Epidermal Necrolysis)	

TABLE 2: SCORTEN scale (score and mortality rate).

Score	Mortality rate (%)
0–1	3.2
2	12.1
3	35.8
4	58.3
≥5	90
(SCORTEN: SCORE of Toxic Epidermal Necrolysis)	

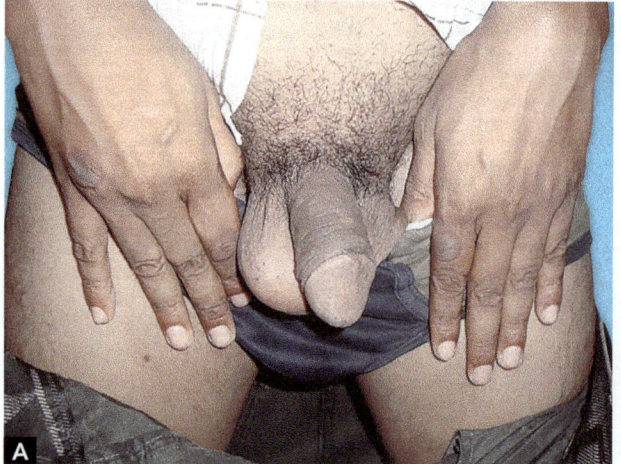
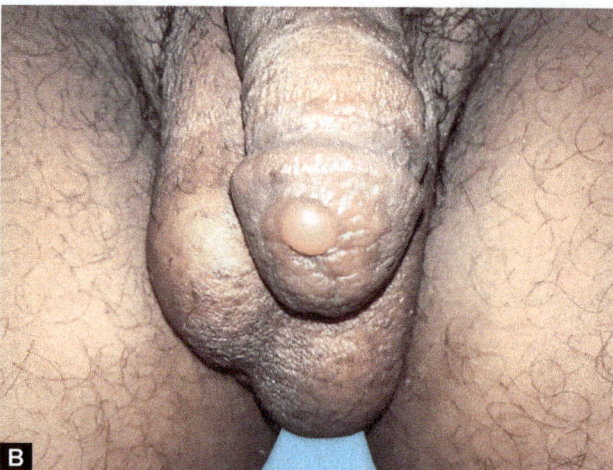

FIGS. 10A AND B: History of same type of vesicle bulla after taking fluconazole.

CHAPTER 7 Erythema Multiforme, Stevens–Johnson Syndrome, Toxic Epidermal Necrolysis, and Fixed Drug Eruption

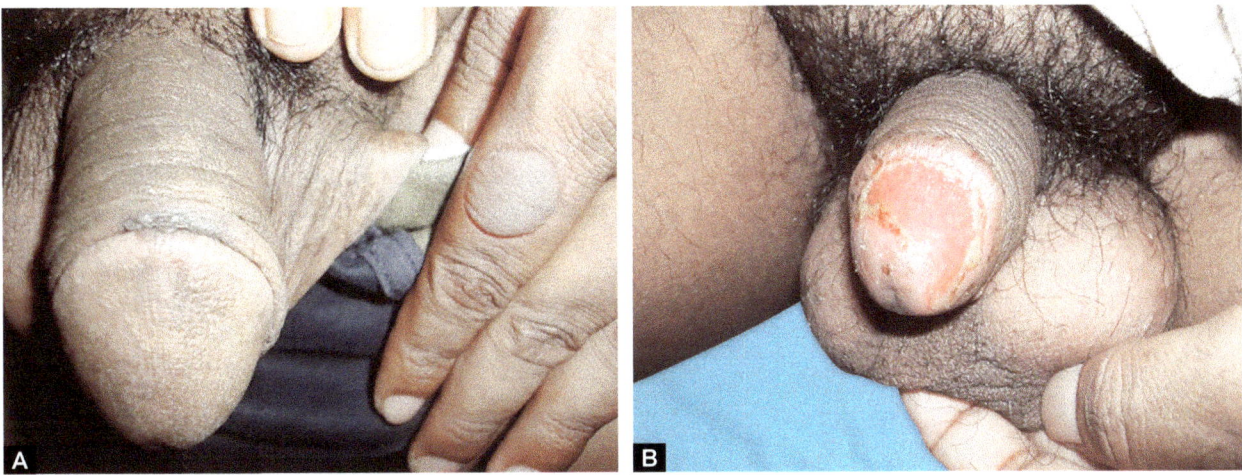

FIGS. 11A AND B: Vesicle, bulla, and erosion due to ingestion of naproxen.

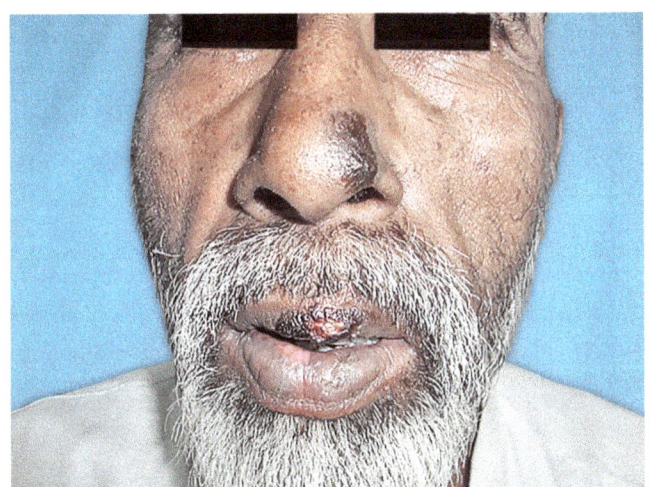

FIG. 12: Mucosal and skin erosion and rust due to ciprofloxacin.

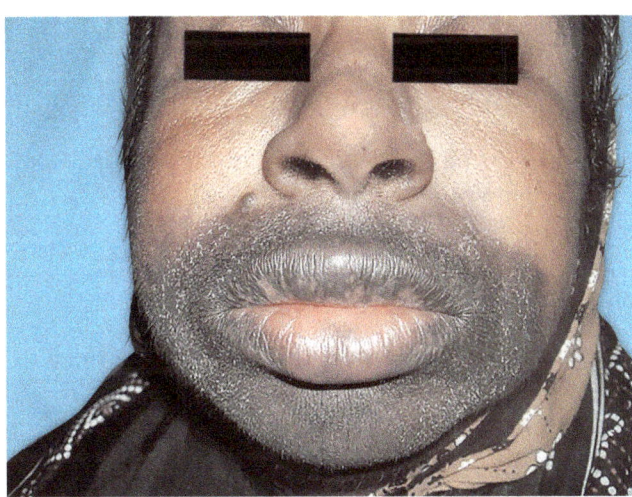

FIG. 13: Perioral darkening gradually worsens due to tetracycline.

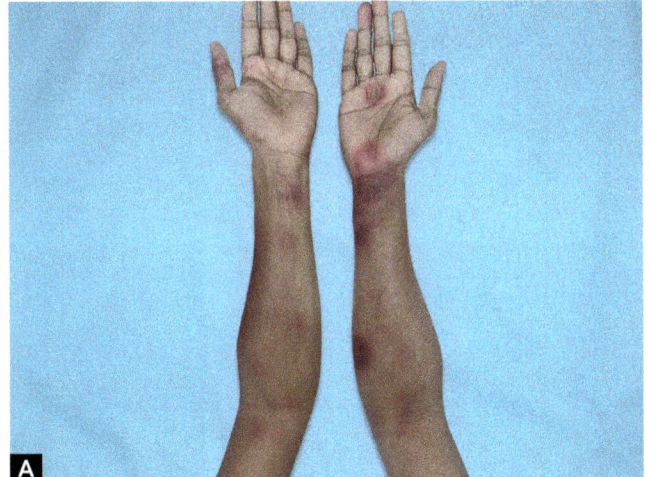

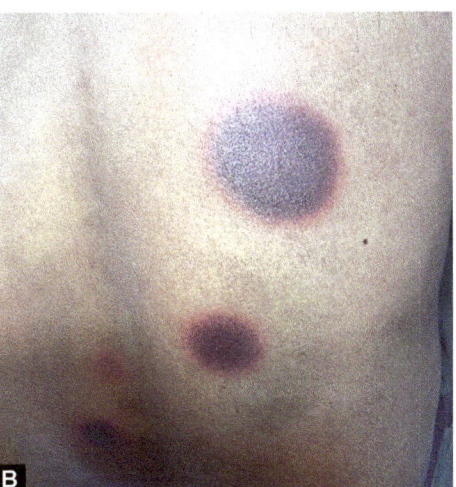

FIGS. 14A AND B: Fixed drug eruption.

Common Drugs

- Tetracyclines
- Minocycline
- Doxycycline
- Fluconazole
- Ciprofloxacin
- Sulfonamides
- *Other sulfa drugs*: Naproxen, barbiturates, oral contraceptive pills, quinine, quinidine, phenolphthalein, and food color-yellow.

Chemotherapy Induced Dyspigmentation (Figs. 15 and 16)

Many chemotherapeutic agents such as bleomycin, doxorubicin, daunorubicin, and alkylating agents such as cyclophosphamide and busulfan causes various patterns of cutaneous hyperpigmentation.

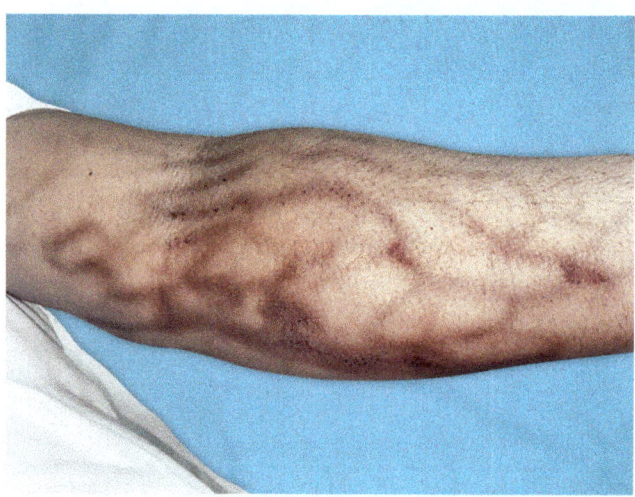

FIG. 15: Methotrexate induced vascular hyperpigmentation.

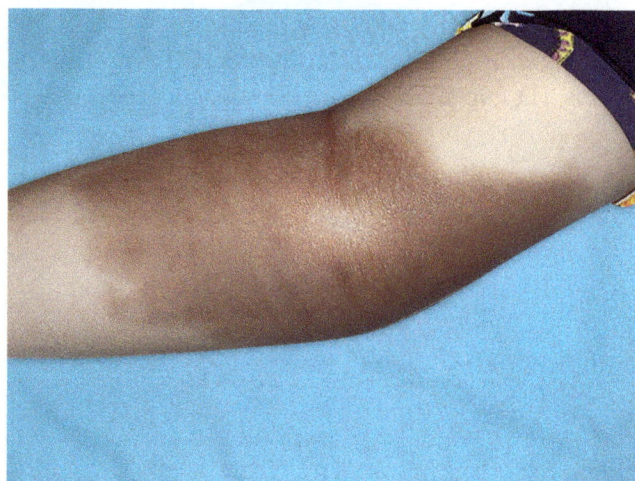

FIG. 16: Hyperpigmentation due to extravasation of methotrexate during infusion.

CHAPTER 8

Environmental and Occupational-related Dermatoses

CHRONIC ARSENICOSIS

Millions of tubewells were dug beginning in the 1960s and 1970s financed by the United Nations International Children's Emergency Fund (UNICEF) and the World Bank in Bangladesh and West Bengal (India) in an effort to combat poor quality surface drinking water that was causing fatal diarrhea and to provide enough water for agriculture. The wells, however, were dug without testing for metal impurities in the environment as the tests were not mandatory until years later and wells became contaminated with arsenic.

The problems began appearing in the 1980s and included arsenicosis, which is the collective name for the symptoms of chronic consumption of arsenic.

The estimated dose of arsenic that can cause keratosis and skin cancer is about 0.5–1 g regardless of whether it is from arsenal medicine (acute poisoning) or accumulated through drinking water with small amounts of arsenic of about 0.4–0.6 mg/L or 400 μg daily over many months or years.

The World Health Organization (WHO) maximal recommendation or allowable level of arsenic in drinking water is 50 μg or 0.05 mg/L.

Mechanism of Action

- Arsenate binds with protein/enzyme that have sulfhydryl group and hamper their physiological work.
- Arsenate inhibits adenosine triphosphate (ATP) production by competing phosphate group in oxidative phosphorylation.
- It interferes in Krebs cycle.
- *Interferes in hemoglobin (Hb) synthesis*: Develops anemia.
- *It has mutagenic/carcinogenic action*: Cancer develops in skin, urinary bladder, liver, kidney, and urinary bladder, etc.

The latent period for papules to become noticeable was as early as 6 months when it is acquired from drinking water highly contaminated with arsenic. But, patients do not usually seek medical advice until after about 10-24 years when an extensive full-blown keratosis or malignancy develop.

Clinical Manifestation of Chronic Arsenic Poisoning

Nonspecific Lesions

- Contact dermatitis such as lesions, folliculitis, ulceration, and pyoderma in skin.
- Conjunctivitis, rhinitis, and nasal septum perforation are due to airborne arsenic dust and fumes.

Specific Lesions

Small hypopigmented macules intermingled with diffuse brown pigmentation of the skin, specially on trunk and extremities presenting as characteristic "rain drops in a dusty road" pattern. Some cases have only small white macules on the trunk and extremities resembling idiopathic guttate hypomelanosis.

Staging of Chronic Arsenic Poisoning (Figs. 1 to 4)

- Stage 0—No skin lesions.
    - Arsenic level in hair is high, may be up to 20 μg/g.
- Stage I—≥6 months.
    - *Melanosis or darkening of skin*: Generalized, localized, spotted, diffuse, or raindrop pigmentation.
- Stage II—Up to 2.5 years after exposure of contaminated water.
    - Numerous pinhead to 0.5 cm flesh-colored keratotic papules.
- Stage III—2.5-6 years after exposure.
    - Keratotic papules become larger up to 1-1.5 cm covered with yellowish keratotic plaques on the center and slight swelling.
- Stage IV—Tumor stage
    - 10 years after exposure
    - Bowen's disease **(Fig. 4)**
    - 24 years of exposure

Basal cell epithelioma and squamous cell carcinoma, depending on the concentration of arsenic level in well water and duration of drinking water.

Investigations

- Direct evidence of arsenic hair >1 mg/kg
- Nail >1 mg/kg
- Urine >0.1 mg/kg
- Blood >0.0025 mg/L

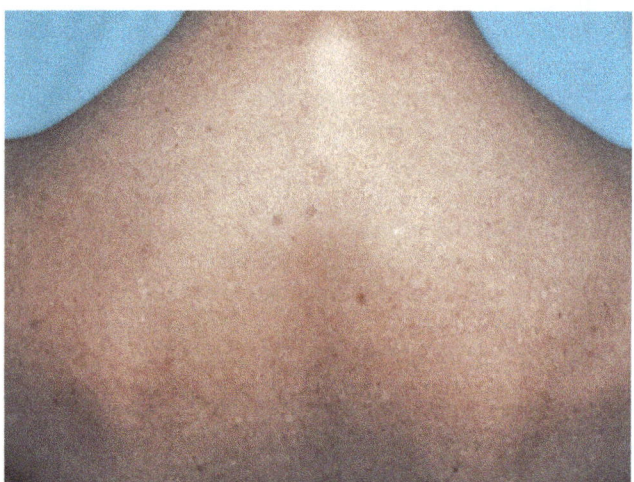

FIG. 1: Raindrop melanosis.

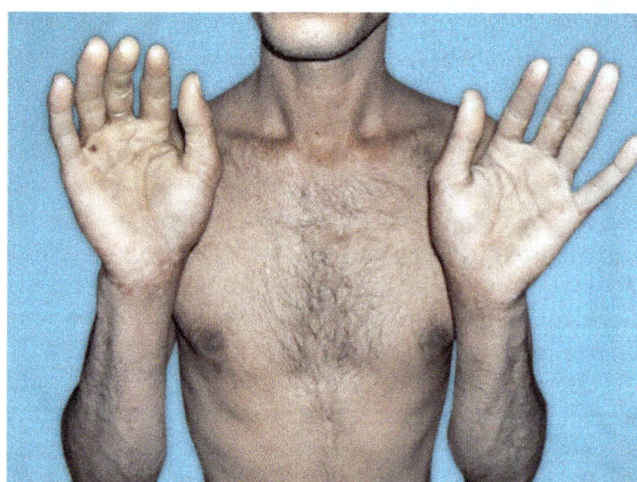

FIG. 2: Raindrop melanosis and hyperkeratosis on both palms.

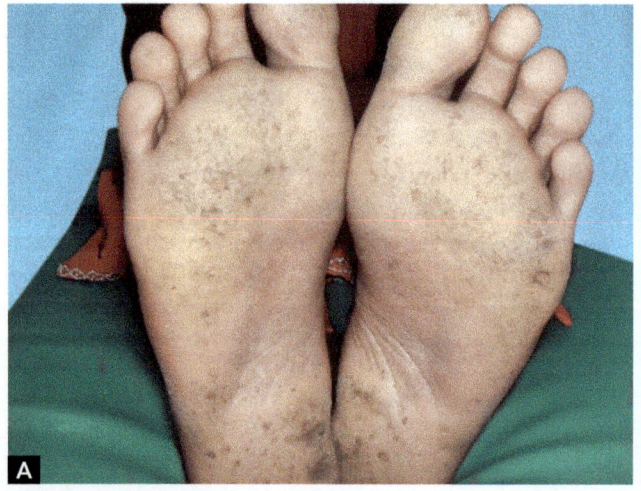

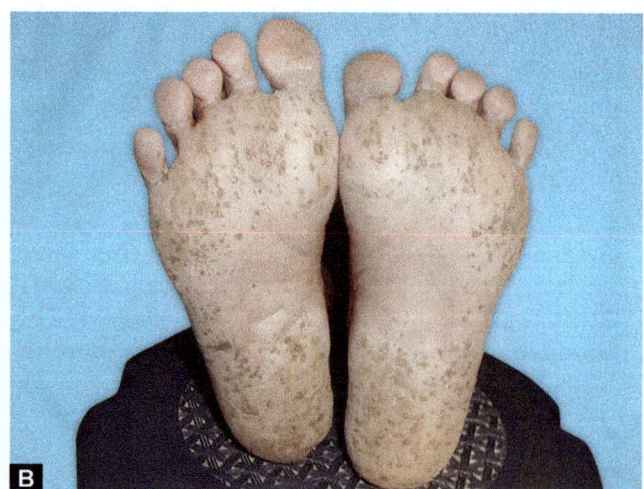

FIGS. 3A AND B: Hyperkeratosis on sole.

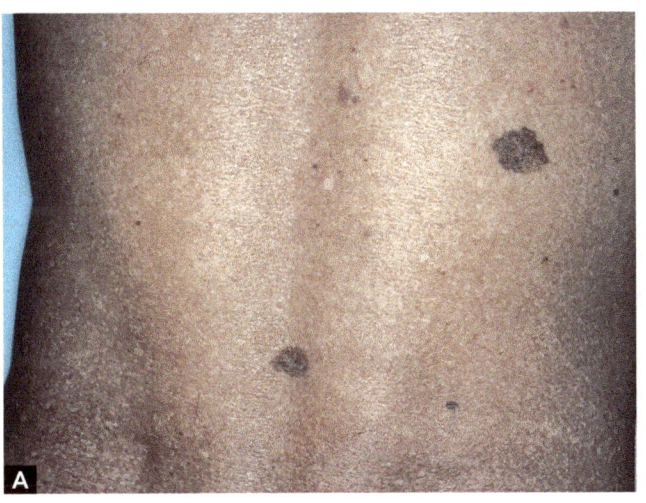
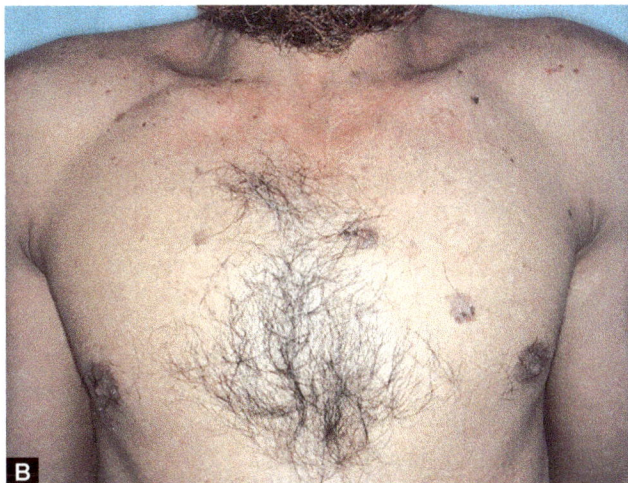

FIGS. 4A AND B: Bowen's disease and raindrop melanosis.

Treatment

Preventive Measures
- Social awareness and motivation about disease and drinking water
- Provision of safe drinking water
- Counseling of patient and family
- Political commitment

Medical Measures
- Stage 0, I—No treatment.
  If high level of arsenic in hair and nail (may be up to 20 µg/g):
  ○ Dimercaprol (BAL) 100 mg/day intramuscular for 10 days, or
  ○ D-penicillamine 100 mg/day for 2–4 months.
  New drugs: Dimercaptosuccinic acid and N-acetylcysteine.
- Stage II—Observe.
- Stage III—Etretinate 25 mg bid for 6 months
  ○ Liquid nitrogen
  ○ Desiccation and curettage or debulking by electrocautery, CO_2 laser.
  ○ Excision of suspicious lesion.
- Stage IV—Follow stage III, plus.
  ○ Excision of Bowen's disease, squamous cell carcinoma (SCC), basal cell carcinoma (BCC), or malignant melanoma **(Figs. 5 to 8)**.
  ○ Aminolevulinic acid plus photodynamic therapy or 5-fluorouracil for:
    – Bowen's disease
    – Mohs micrographic surgery in invasive cancers
  ○ Role of antioxidants or vitamins controversial
  ○ Management of complications.

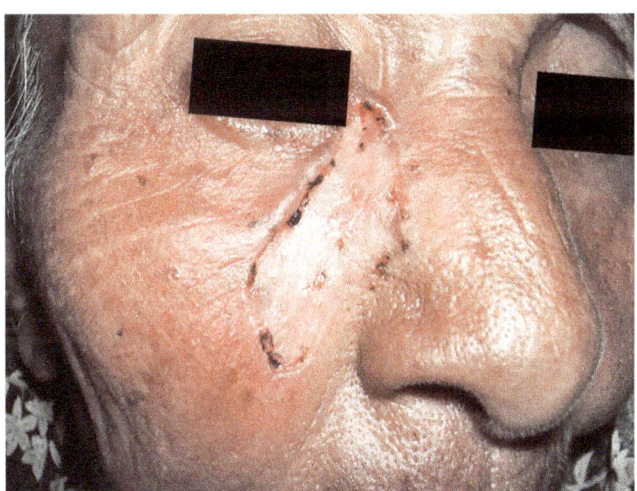

FIG. 5: Basal cell carcinoma.

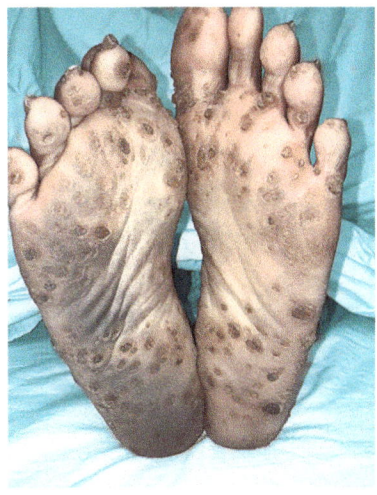

FIG. 6: Punctate hyperkeratosis.

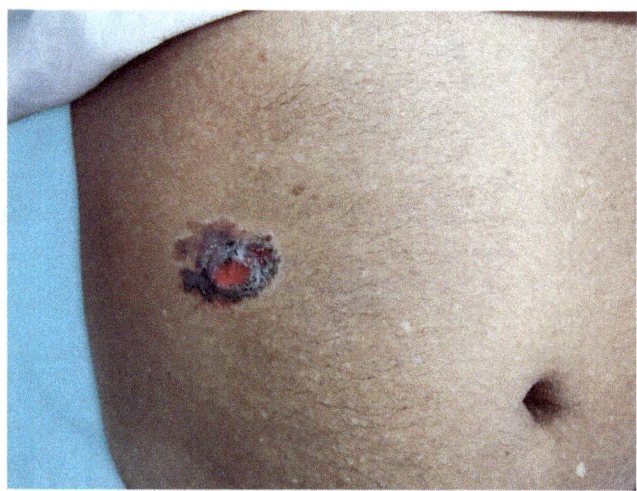

FIG. 7: Squamous cell carcinoma (SCC) with raindrop melanosis.

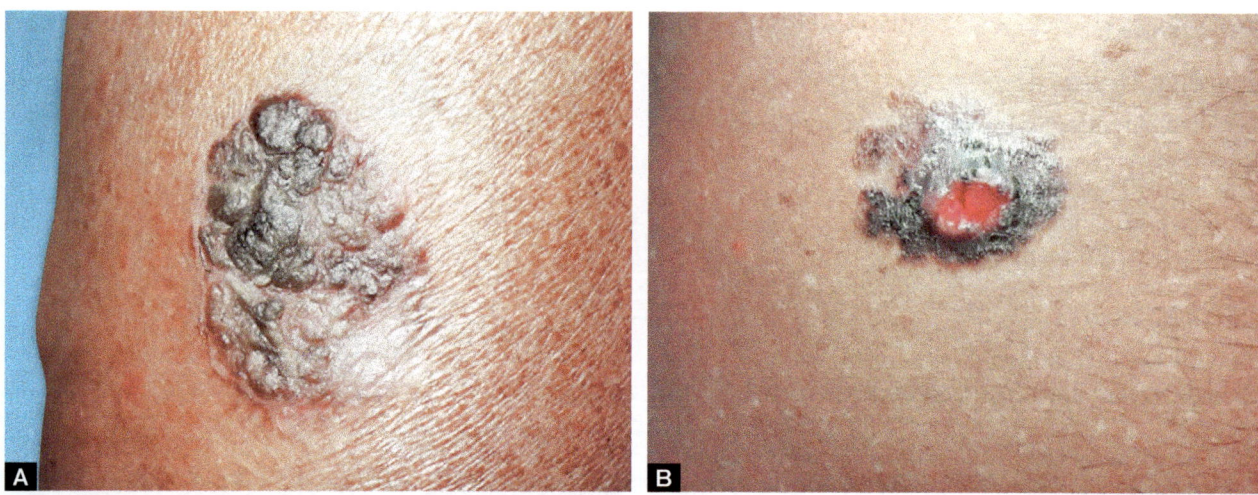

FIGS. 8A AND B: Squamous cell carcinoma (SCC).

CHAPTER 9
Endocrine, Metabolic, and Nutritional Diseases

PREGNANCY-INDUCED DERMATOSES

Polymorphic Eruption of Pregnancy: Pruritic Urticarial Papules and Plaques of Pregnancy

- Usually begins in third trimester, most often in primigravidae (76%) (usually 1-2 weeks before delivery).
- No increased risk of fetal morbidity or mortality
- *Estimated occurrence*: 1:120-240 pregnancies.
- Unknown etiology
- *Lesions*:
  o Erythematous papules (1-3 mm) **(Figs. 1A to C)**
  o Quickly coalescing into urticarial plaques
  o Tiny vesicles (2 mm) may occur in the plaque but no bullae.
  o Target lesion is present in 19% of cases.
  o Pruritus is the main symptom.
- Differential diagnosis—pemphigoid gestationis, drug reaction, allergic contact dermatitis, viral exanthem, erythema multiforme (EM) minor, and scabies.
- Site—over striae distensae **(Fig. 2)**, abdomen, buttocks, thighs, upper inner arms, and lower back
- Management consists of topical steroids and antihistamine (cetirizine).
- Oral prednisolone in doses of 10-40 mg/day has been used for severe cases.

Pustular Psoriasis of Pregnancy (Figs. 3A and B)

- Previously called impetigo herpetiformis.
- Clinically and histopathologically indistinguishable from pustular psoriasis of von Zumbusch
- Burning, snorting, and not itching
- May have hypocalcemia and decreased vitamin D levels.
- Systemic corticosteroid is treatment of choice.

Pemphigoid Gestationis

- A rare pruritic and polymorphic inflammatory bullous dermatosis of pregnancy **(Fig. 4)**
- Externally pruritic vesicular eruption
- Site—abdomen, also on mucous membrane
- Onset—4th to 7th month of pregnancy, but can also occur in the first trimester.
- May recur in subsequent pregnancies.
- Can be exacerbated by use of estrogen and progesterone therapy.
- Prednisolone 20-40 mg/day is given, but sometimes higher doses are required. Prednisolone is tapered gradually during the postpartum period.
- Some patients can be managed with antihistamine and topical glucocorticoids.

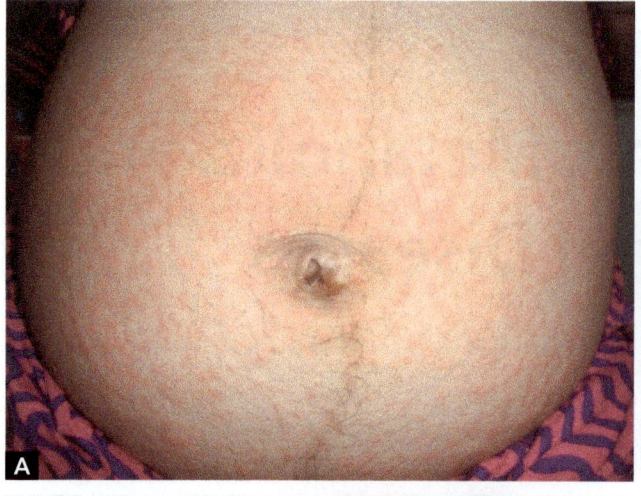
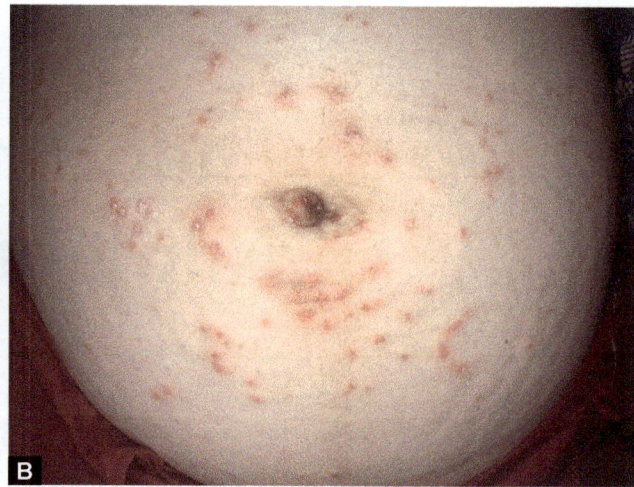
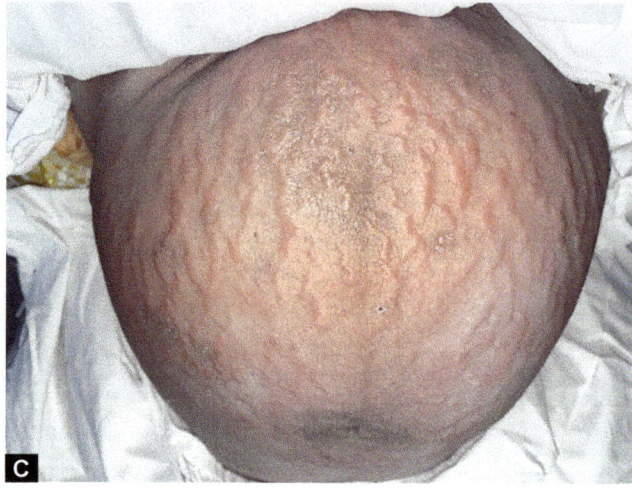

FIGS. 1A TO C: Erythematous papules and tiny vesicles on abdomen.

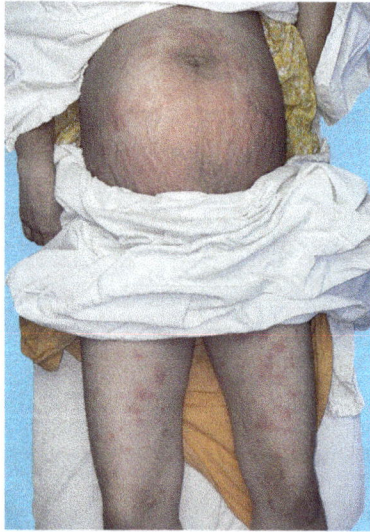

FIG. 2: Erythematous papules and plaques on striae distensae of abdomen and thigh.

Prurigo of Pregnancy

- Now classified as part of the atopic eruption of pregnancy (AEP) spectrum.
- It is very common.
- It consists of flares of atopic dermatitis. It presents either with eczematous or prurigo lesions.

Cholestasis of Pregnancy

- Due to increased level of serum bile acids.
- Occurs in third trimester.
- *Leading symptom*: Pruritus.
- Most severe during night.
- Cutaneous lesions are invariably absent, but excoriations in severe cases (**Figs. 5 and 6**).
- *Treatment*: Ursodeoxycholic acid and plasmapheresis.
- Fetal risks include prematurity, intrapartum distress, and fetal death.

CHAPTER 9 Endocrine, Metabolic, and Nutritional Diseases

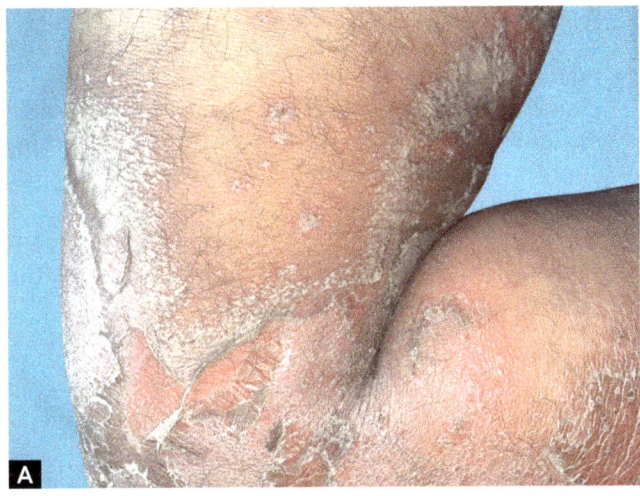
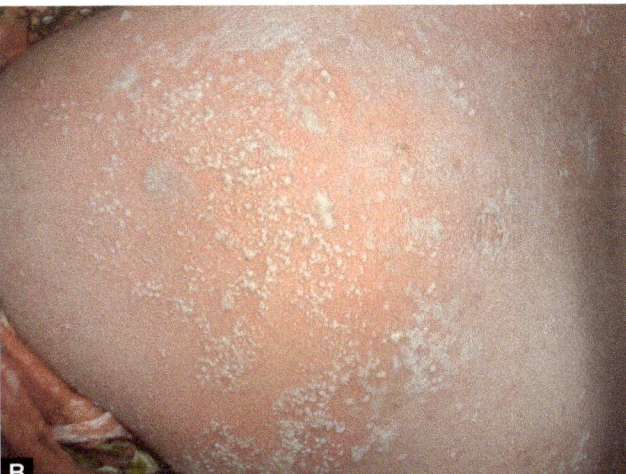

FIGS. 3A AND B: Multiple sterile pustules with erythematous base.

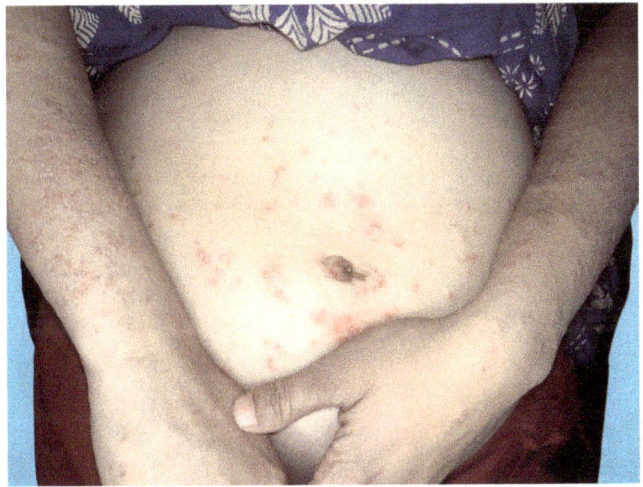

FIG. 4: Papules, vesicles, and bullae on abdomen.

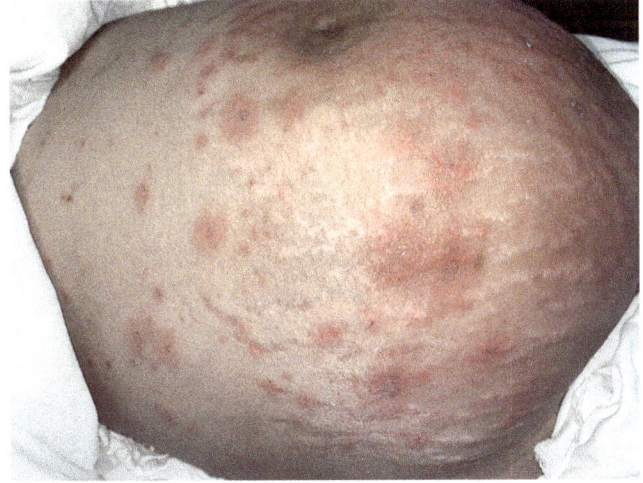

FIG. 5: Dry, erythematous papules, plaques, and eroded lesions on abdomen.

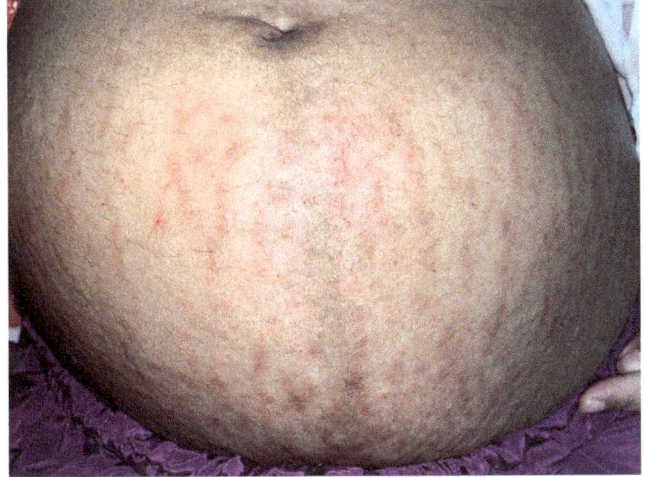

FIG. 6: Erosions and excoriations are the late features of cholestasis of pregnancy.

PREGNANCY-INDUCED STRIAE

- Also known as striae gravidarum **(Fig. 7)**, these are a specific form of atrophic linear scar that represents connective tissue changes during pregnancy of skin of abdomen due to rapid expansion of uterus as well as sudden weight gain during pregnancy.
- About 90% of women are affected.
- Topical tretinoin ≥0.05% has demonstrated up to 47% improvement and fractional erbium (2,940 nm) lasers have consistently demonstrated 50–75% improvement in pregnancy-induced striae.

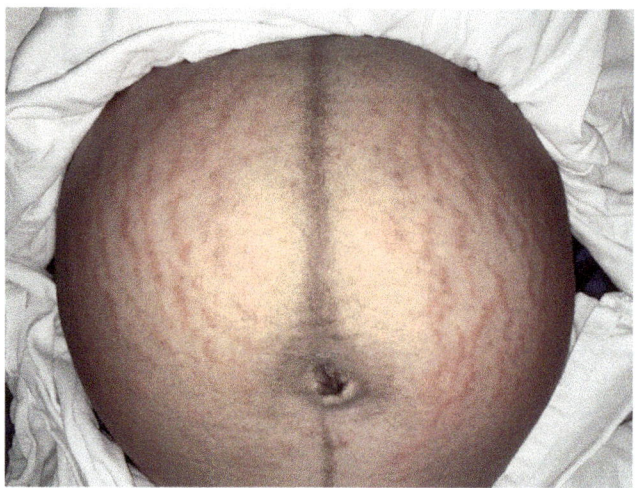

FIG. 7: Striae gravidarum.

OBESITY

- Defined as body mass index (BMI) >30 kg/m².
- Predisposing genetic syndromes that result in an earlier childhood onset include Prader-Willi syndrome, Bardet-Biedl syndrome, Alström syndrome, and Wilson-Turner syndrome.
- Predisposing endocrine conditions include Cushing disease, Cushing syndrome, polycystic ovarian syndrome, and insulin resistance.
- Acquired obesity is at epidemic level, especially in highincome populations.

■ Cutaneous Lesions

The cutaneous lesions are described in **Figures 8 to 16**.

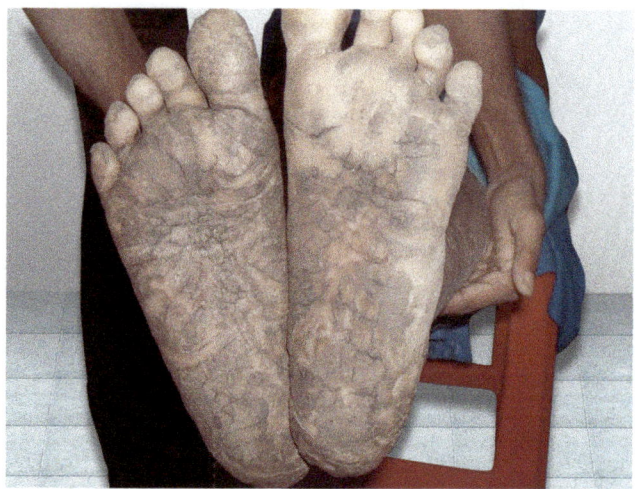

FIG. 8: Plantar hyperkeratosis.

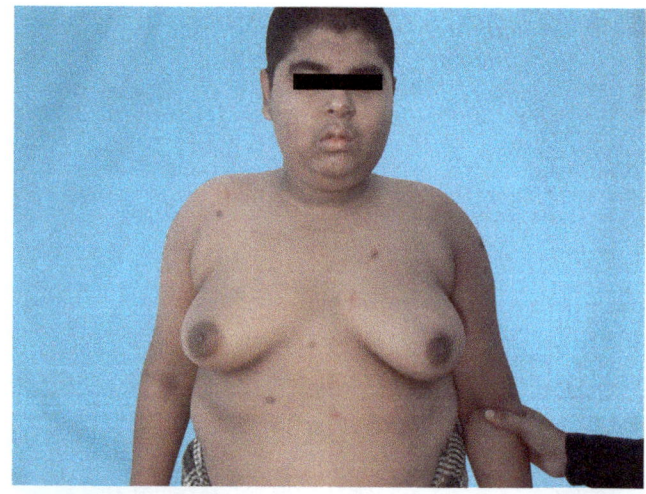

FIG. 9: Gynecomastia.

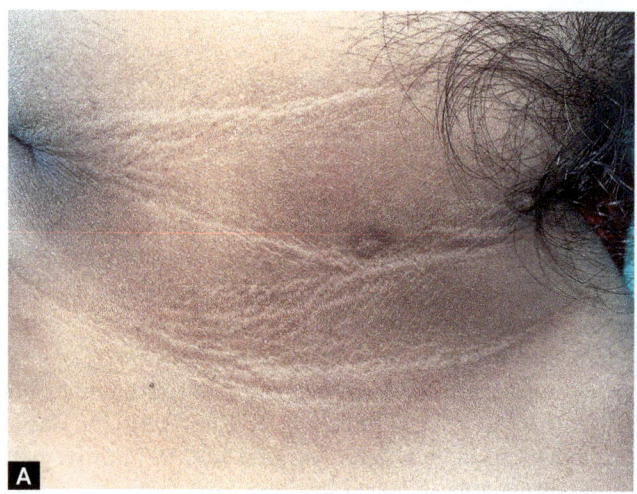

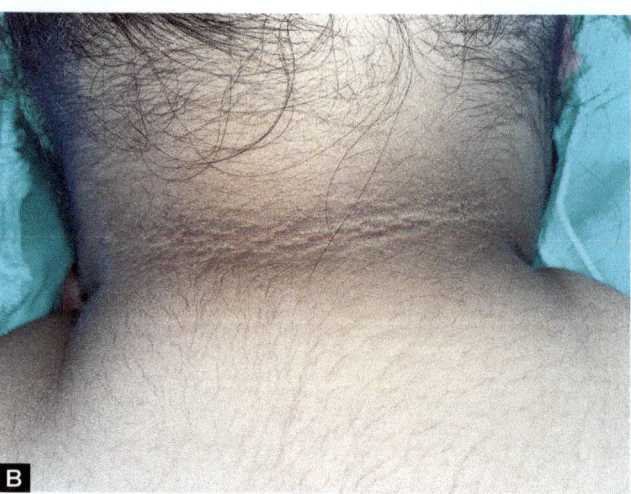

FIGS. 10A AND B: Cutaneous lesions.

CHAPTER 9 Endocrine, Metabolic, and Nutritional Diseases

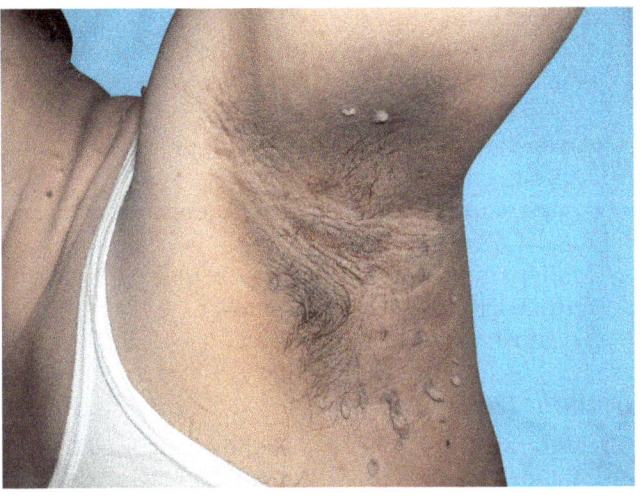

FIG. 11: Acrochordons.

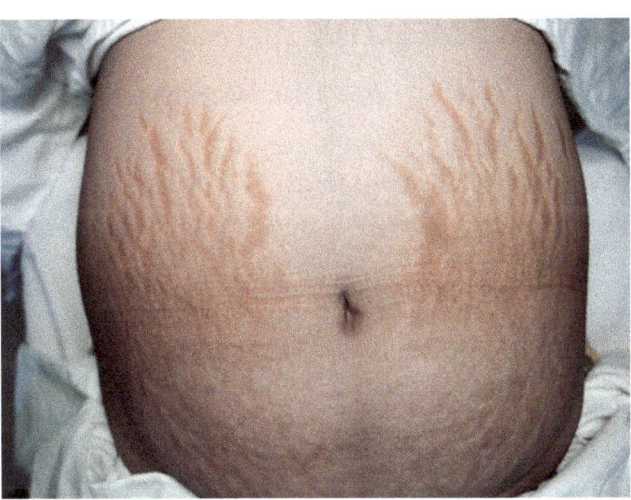

FIG. 12: Striae distensae.

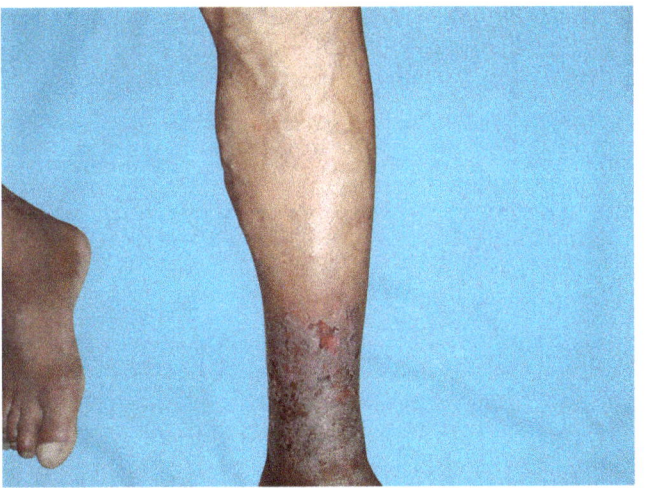

FIG. 13: Stasis dermatitis.

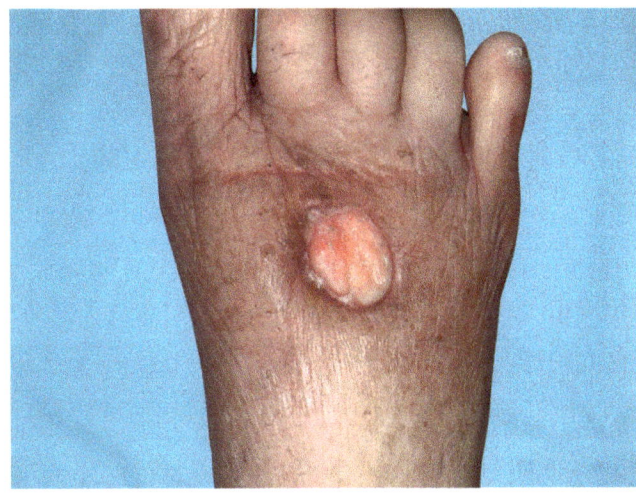

FIG. 14: Leg ulcer.

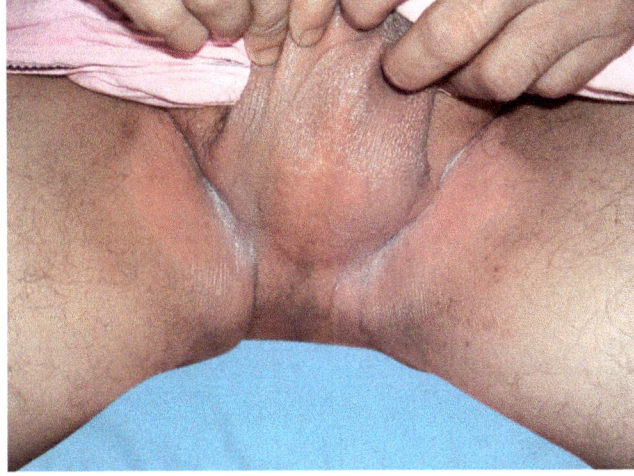

FIG. 15: Intertrigo.

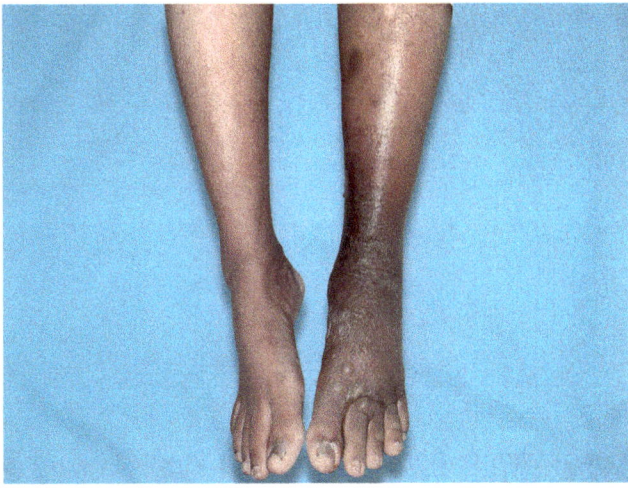

FIG. 16: Lipodermatosclerosis.

DIABETES MELLITUS

■ Skin Findings Associated with Diabetes Mellitus

Acanthosis Nigricans (Figs. 17A and B)
- Asymmetrical revelry thickening and hyperpigmentation of skin.
- Sites—neck, axilla, groin, and other body folds.
- *Related to*:
  - *Endocrine disorders*:
    - Insulinresistant type 2 diabetes mellitus (T2DM)
    - Hyperandrogenic states
    - Acromegaly or gigantism
    - Cushing disease
    - Hypogonadal syndrome with insulin resistance
    - Addison disease
    - Hypothyroidism
- Associated with obesity. Obesity produces insulin resistance.
- Drugs—nicotinic acid, stilbestrol, glucose OCPL, and diethylstilbestrol.
- Malignancy—paraneoplastic, usually of gastrointestinal tract (GIT) or lymphoma.
- Treatmentassociated disorder

Diabetic Dermopathy
Circumscribed, atrophic, and slightly depressed lesions on anterior lower legs **(Figs. 18A and B)**.

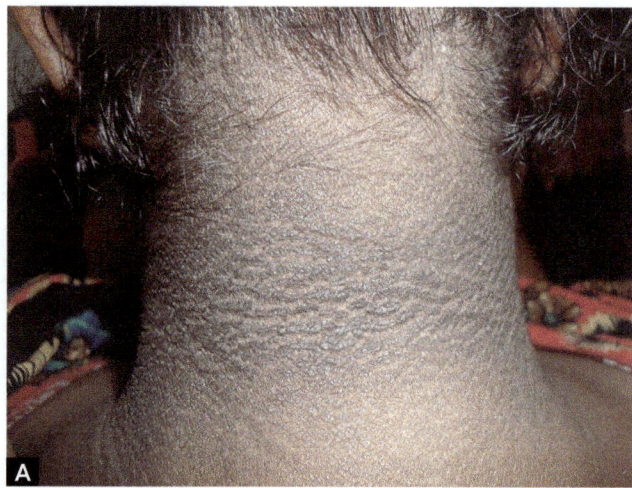
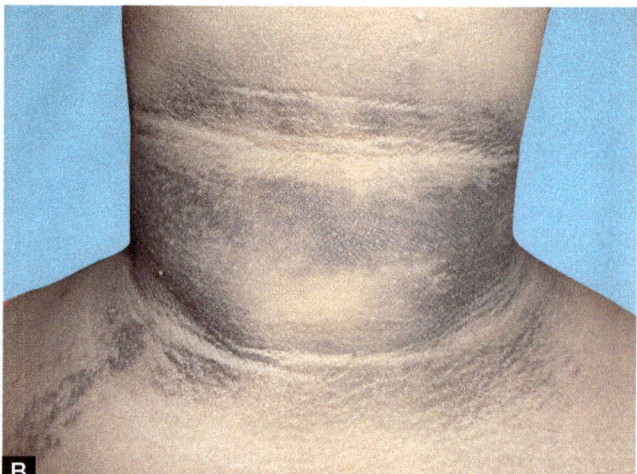

FIGS. 17A AND B: Acanthosis nigricans.

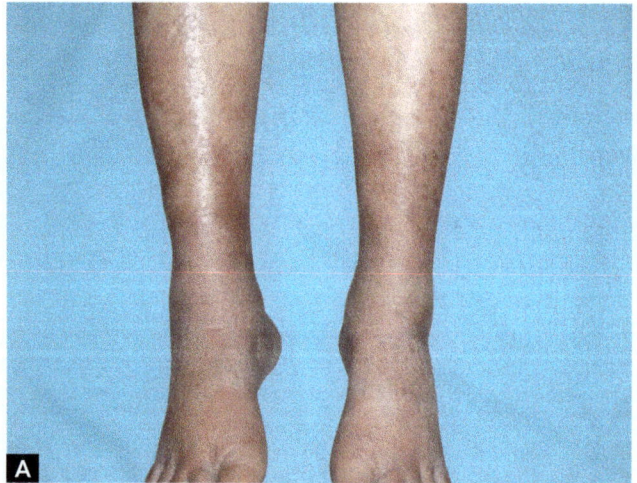
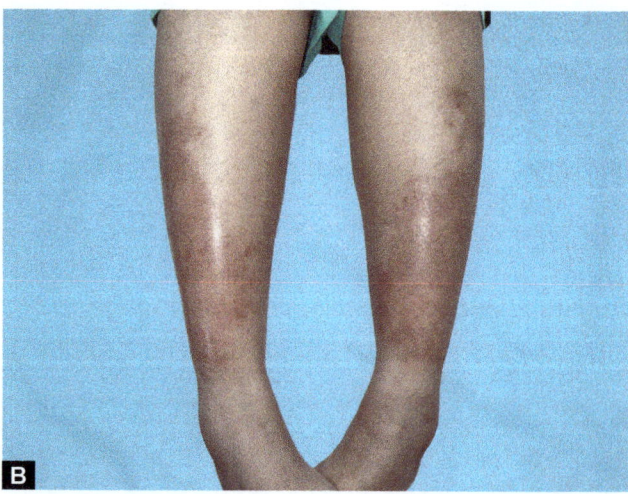

FIGS. 18A AND B: Dry, atrophic, and slightly depressed lesions on anterior lower legs.

Adverse Cutaneous Drug Eruption

- *Insulin*:
  - Local reaction—lipodystrophy.
  - Arthus-like reaction with urticarial lesion.
  - Systemic reactions—urticaria and serum sickness-like lesion.
- *Oral hypoglycemic agents*:
  - Exanthematous eruption
  - Urticaria
  - Erythema multiforme
  - Photosensitivity

Calciphylaxis (Fig. 19)

Progressive cutaneous necrosis associated with small and medium-sized vessel calcifications.

Necrobiosis Lipoidica (Fig. 20)

Sharply circumscribed, multicolored plaques occurring on the anterior and lateral surfaces of the lower legs.

Infections

The various infections are given in **Figures 21 to 30**.

Scleredema Diabeticorum

Poorly demarcated scleroderma indurations of skin and subcutaneous tissue of the upper back, neck, and proximal extremities.

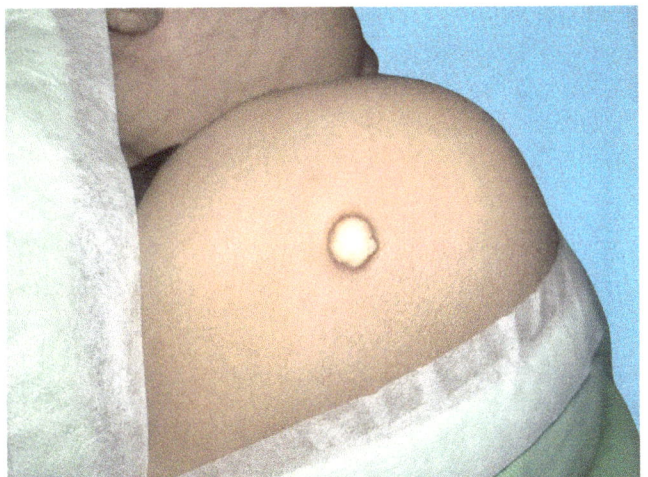

FIG. 19: Calciphylaxis.

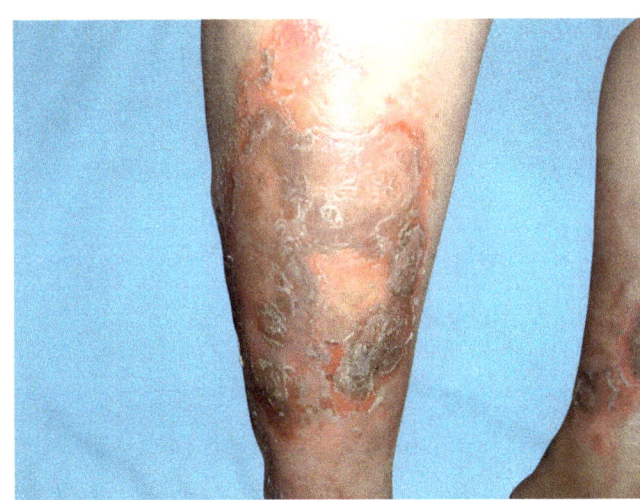

FIG. 20: Necrobiosis lipoidica.

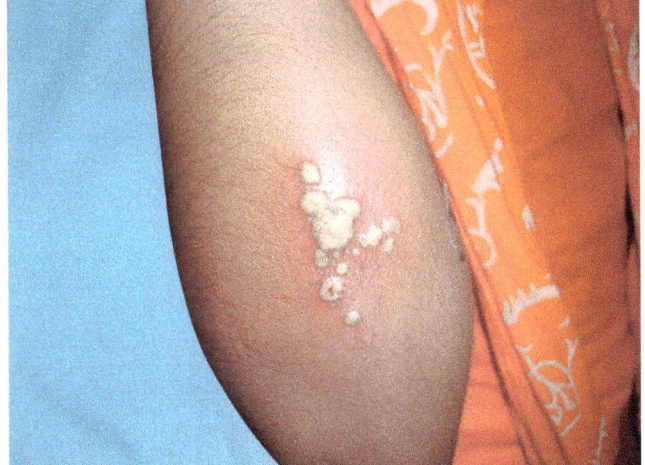

FIG. 21: Furuncles.

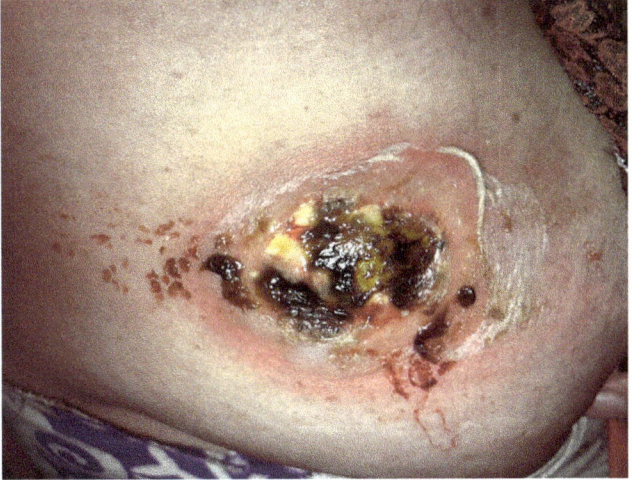

FIG. 22: Carbuncles.

74 CHAPTER 9 Endocrine, Metabolic, and Nutritional Diseases

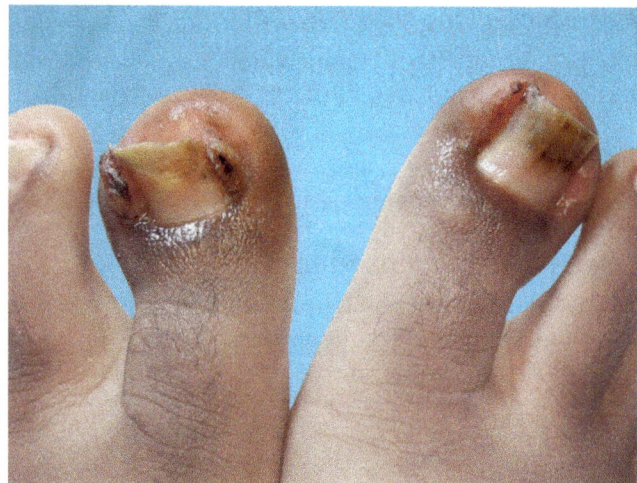

FIG. 23: Paronychia.

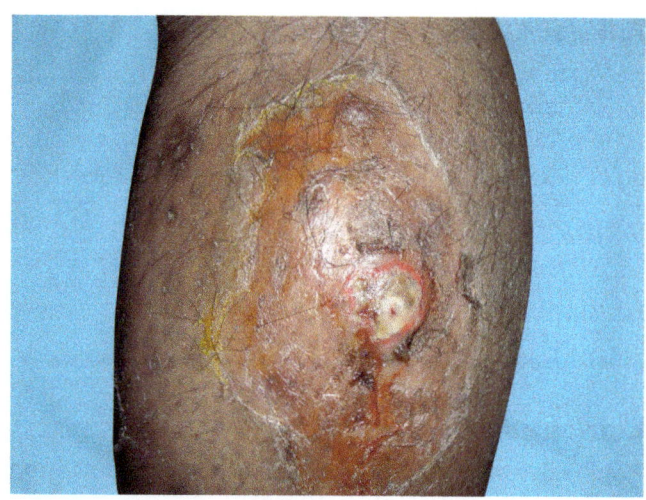

FIG. 24: Wound/ulcer infections.

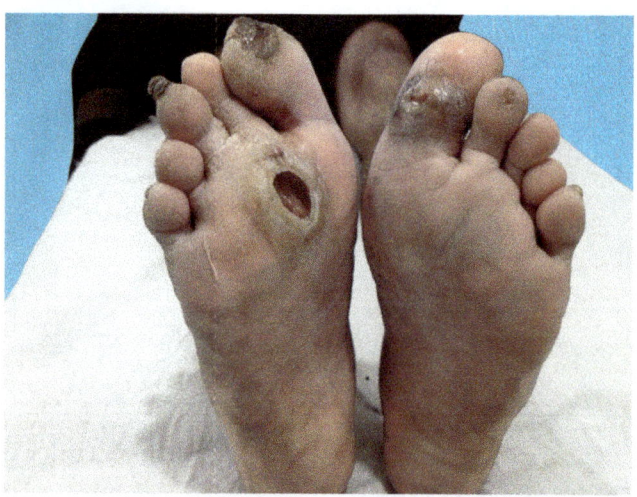

FIG. 25: Anesthetic ulcers.

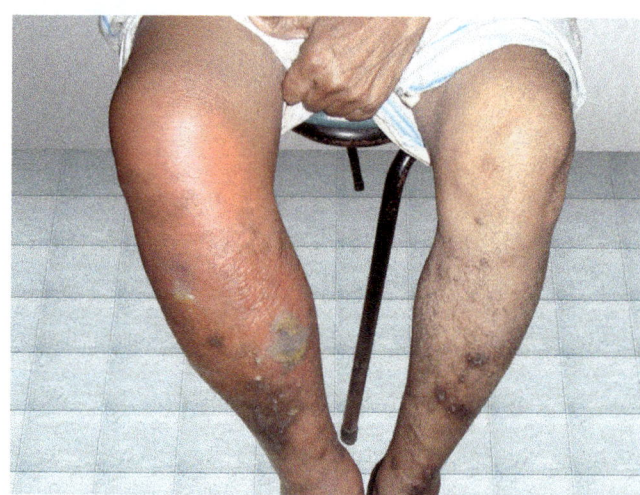

FIG. 26: Cellulitis.

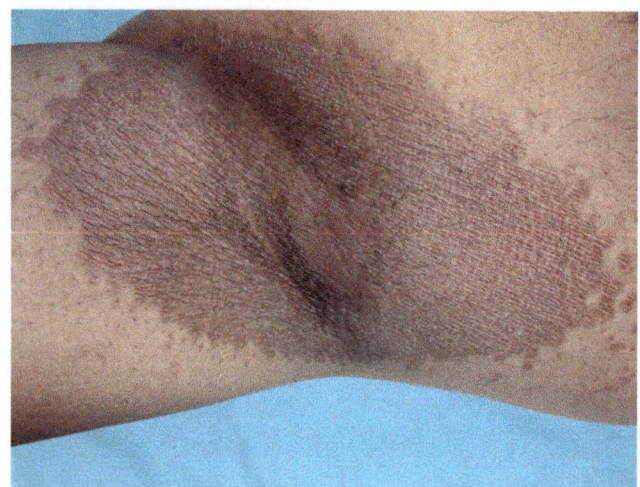

FIG. 27: Erythrasma.

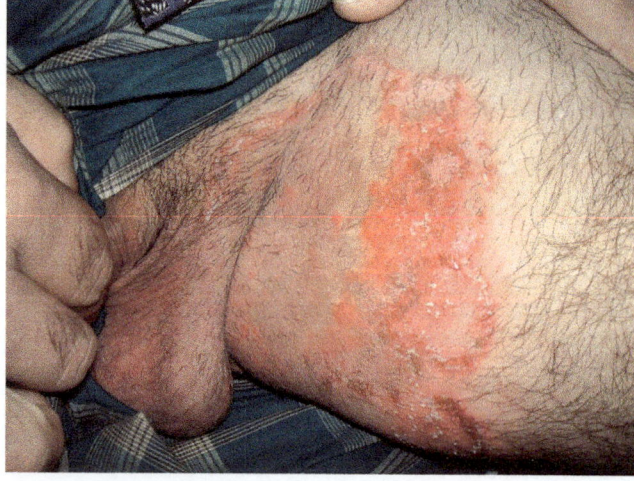

FIG. 28: Dermatophytes.

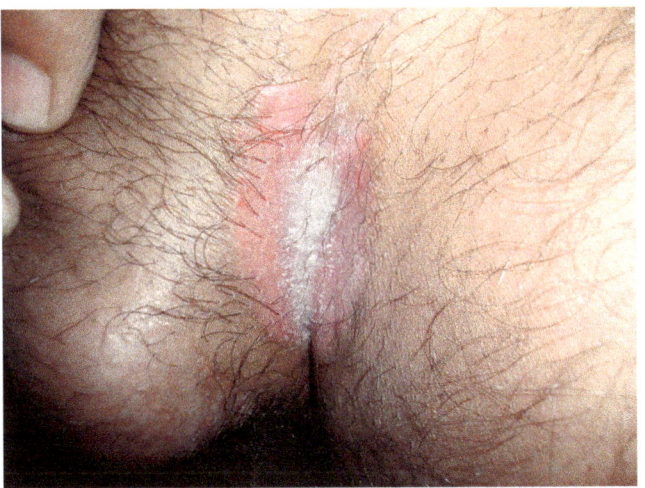

FIG. 29: Candidiasis.

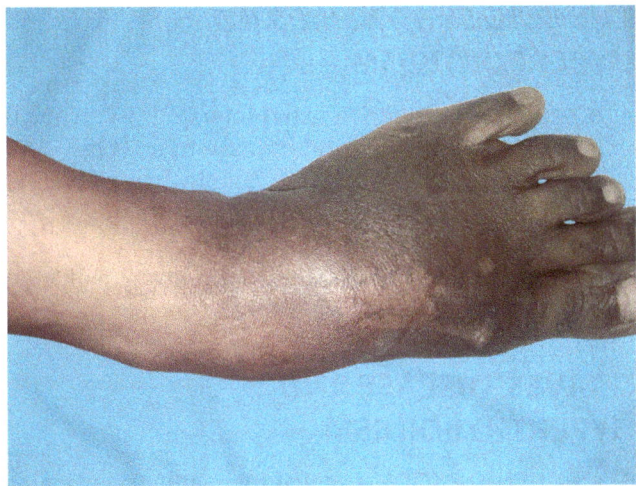

FIG. 30: Peripheral vascular disease.

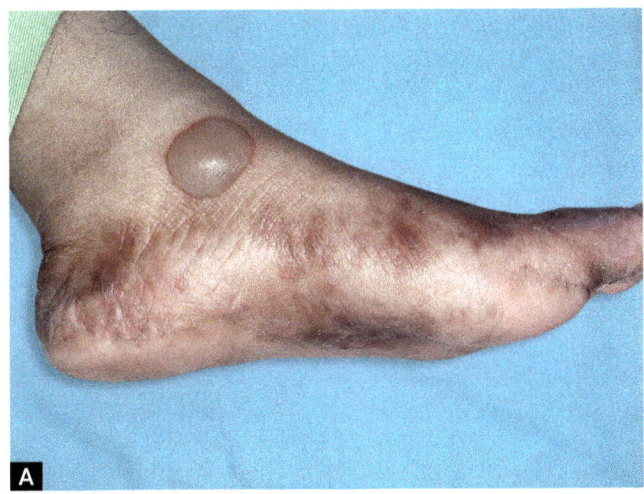

FIGS. 31A AND B: Diabetic bullae.

Diabetic Bullae (Figs. 31A and B)

Large and intact bullae arise spontaneously on the lower legs, feet, dorsa of hands, and fingers on noninflamed base.

Perforating Disorders

The perforating disorders are given in **Figure 32**.

Diabetic Foot and Diabetic Neuropathy

Diabetic neuropathy is the most common complication of diabetes mellitus (DM), affecting as many as 50% of patients with type 1 diabetes mellitus (T1DM) and type 2 diabetes mellitus (T2DM). Diabetic peripheral neuropathy involves the presence of symptoms or signs of peripheral nerve dysfunction resultant anesthetic ulcers **(Fig. 25)**.

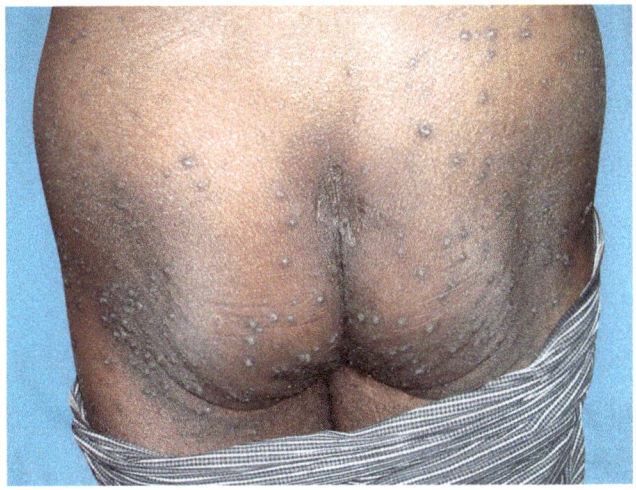

FIG. 32: Perforating disorders.

CUSHING SYNDROME AND HYPERCORTICISM

- Cushing syndrome is characterized by truncal obesity, moon face, abdominal striae **(Figs. 33A to D)**, hypertension, decrease carbohydrate tolerance, protein catabolism, psychiatric disturbances, and amenorrhea and hirsutism in females.
- It is associated with excess adrenocorticoids of endogenous or exogenous source.

GRAVES' DISEASE AND HYPERTHYROIDISM

Graves' disease (GD) is a disorder with three major manifestations: (1) Hypothyroidism with diffuse goiter, (2) Ophthalmology, and (3) Dermopathy.

■ Dermopathy (Pretibial Myxedema)

- Early lesions—bilateral, asymmetric, firm, nonpitting nodules and plaques that are pink, colored, or purple.
- Late lesions—confluence of early lesions results in grotesque involvement of entire legs and dorsum of feet. Smooth surface with orange peel-like appearance, later becomes verrucous.
- Fingers show acropachy.
- *Ophthalmology*:
  - Stare, lid lag, and lid retraction.
  - Proptosis, ophthalmoplegia, congestive oculopathy, chemosis, conjunctivitis, and periorbital swelling.
  - Potential risk of corneal ulceration, ophthalmoplegia, ocular muscle weakness, convergence, strabismus, and diplopia.
- Thyroid—diffuse toxic goiter, asymmetric, and lobular.

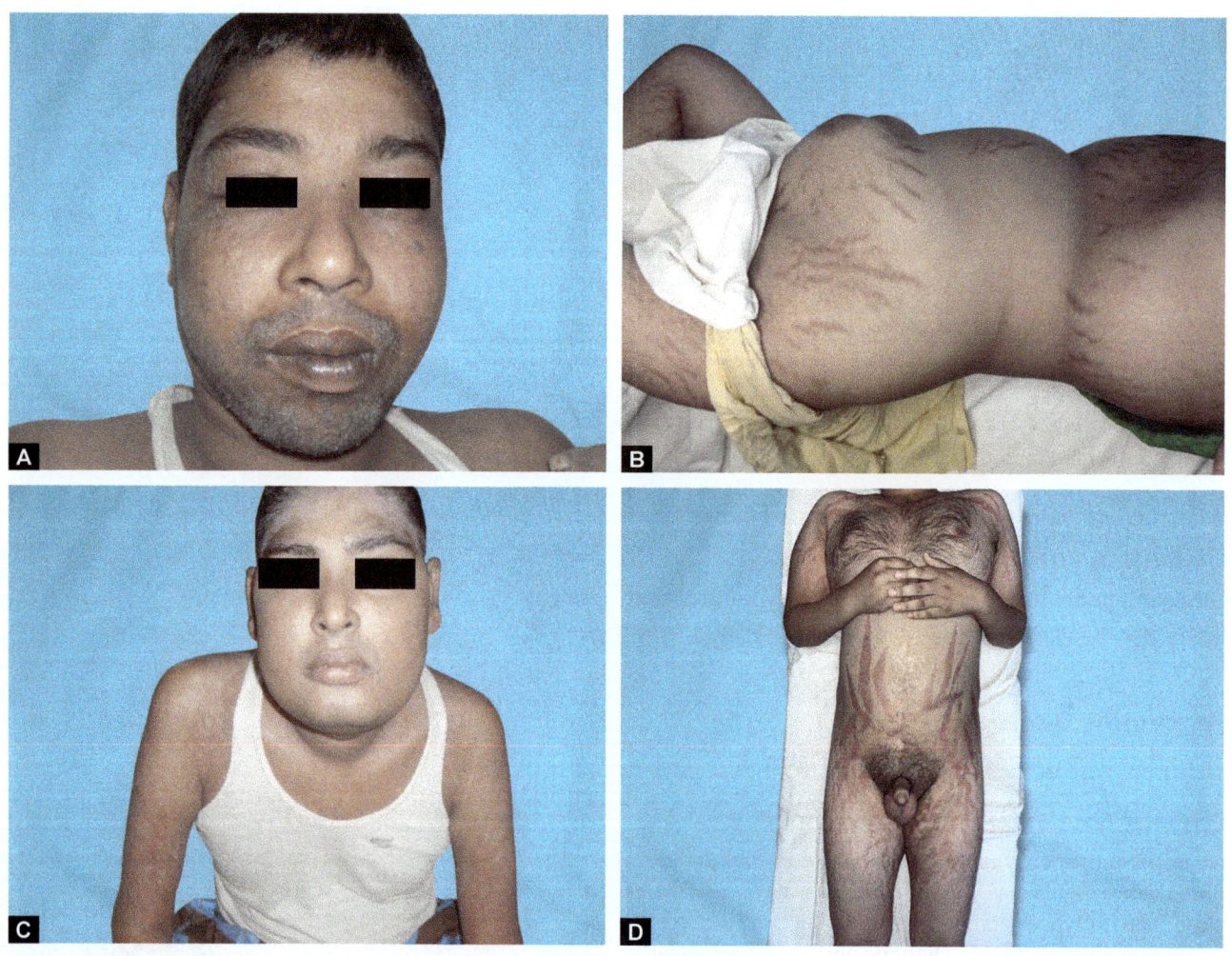

FIGS. 33A TO D: Moon face, striae, and skin atrophy.

CHAPTER 9 Endocrine, Metabolic, and Nutritional Diseases

HYPOTHYROIDISM AND MYXEDEMA

- *Myxedema* results from insufficient production of thyroid hormones.
- *Clinical features*: Fatigue, lethargy, cold intolerance, constipation, stiffness and cramping of muscles, carpal tunnel syndrome, menorrhagia, slowing of intellectual and motor activity, decline in appetite, increase in weight, and deepening of voice.
- Dull, expressionless facies, with puffiness of eyelids. Skin appears swollen, cool, waxy, dry, coarse, and pale with increase in skin creases.
- Palm and soles are orange due to carotenemia.
- Hair is dry, coarse, brittle, thinning of scalp, beard and sexual areas, eyebrow: alopecia of lateral onethird.
- Nail is brittle and slow growing.
- Large, smooth, red, and clumsy tongue
- Management is by replacement therapy.

ADDISON'S DISEASE

- It is a syndrome resulting from adrenocortical insufficiency.
- Characterized by progressive generalized brown, hyperpigmentation, slowly progressive weakness, fatigue, anorexia, and frequently GI symptoms (vomiting and diarrhea).
- *Skin findings*:
    o Generalized brown hyperpigmentation around the eyes, face, dorsa of hands, nipples, in the linea nigra (abdomen), axilla, and anogenital areas **(Figs. 34A to D)**.
    o Brown hyperpigmentation is gingival or buccal mucosa, creases of palm, bony prominences, and scar area.
- *Screen test*: Serum plasma cortisol level 30–60 minutes after administering 250 μg cosyntropin intramuscularly or intravenous.

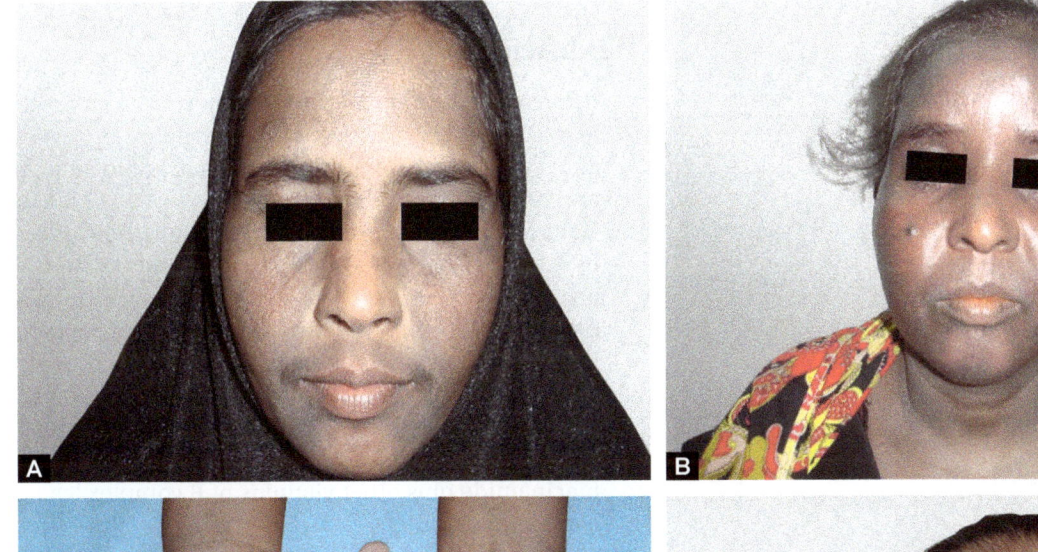
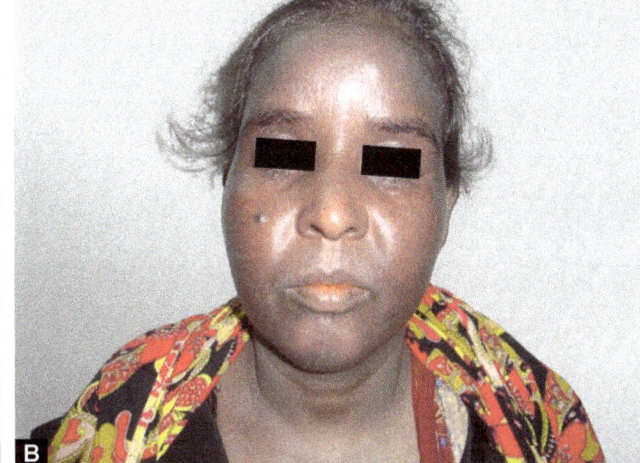
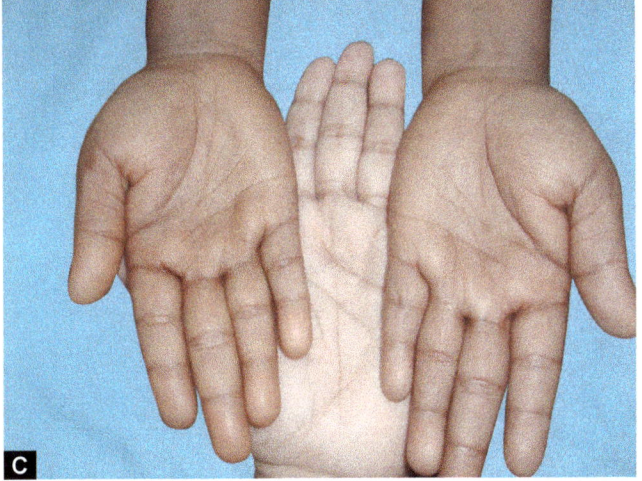
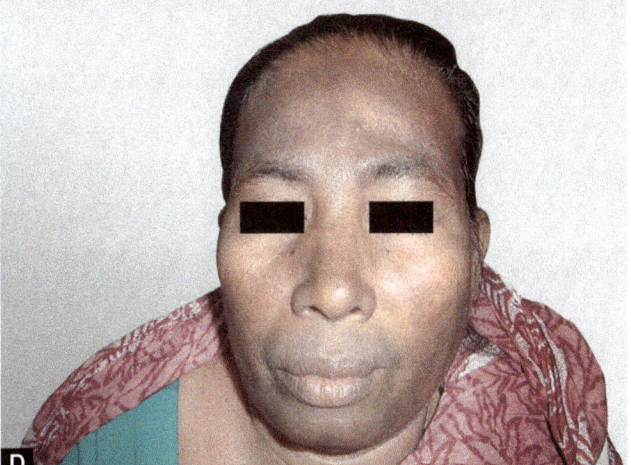

FIGS. 34A TO D: Hyperpigmentation on different areas in Addison's disease.

XANTHOMAS

- Xanthomas are yellow-brown, pinkish, or orange macules, papules, plaques, nodules, or infiltrations in tendons.
- Histologically—accumulations of xanthoma cell—macrophages containing droplets of lipids.
- *Causes*:
  - Primary hyperlipidemia
  - Secondary hyperlipidemia
  - Unknown
- Most common is xanthelasma **(Fig. 35)**. This is in most cases unrelated to hyperlipidemia.
- Skin lesions are a symptomatic, soft, and polygonal yellow-orange papules and plaques located to upper and lower eyelids and around inner canthus.
- Eruptive xanthomas **(Figs. 36A and B)**
- *Treatment*: Laser excision, electrodesiccation, or topical application of trichloroacetic acid. Recurrences are not common.

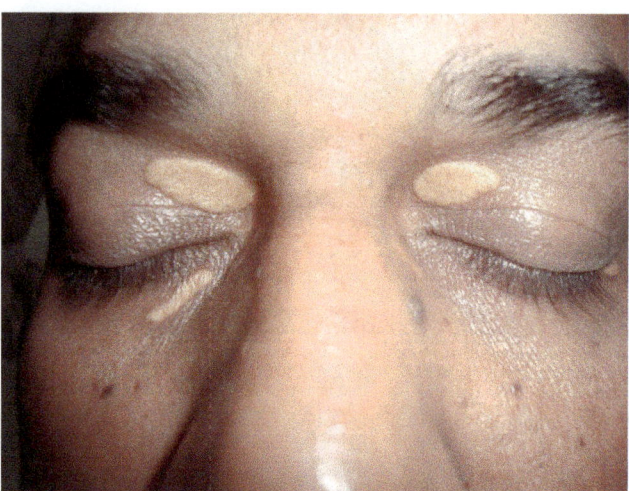

FIG. 35: Xanthelasma.

ZINC DEFICIENCY AND ACRODERMATITIS ENTEROPATHICA

- *Acrodermatitis enteropathica (AE)*: Autosomal recessive genetic disorder of zinc absorption, presenting in infancy, characterized by acral dermatitis (face, hands, feet, and acrogenital areas) **(Figs. 37 and 38)**.
- Acquired zinc deficiency occurs in older people due to dietary deficiency or failure of intestinal absorption.
- Brightly red eczematous lesions evolving into vesicobullous, pustular, erosive, and crusted lesions. Later, scalp, hands, feet, flexural region, and trunk may be involved.
- *Hair and nails*: Diffuse alopecia, graying of hair, paronychia, and loss of nail.
- *Mucous membrane*: Red, glossy tongue, superficial aphthous-like lesions, and secondary oral candidiasis.
- Treatment management is by dietary and intravenous zinc salt supplementation.

PELLAGRA

- Pellagra is related to niacin deficiency.
- *3Ds*: Dermatitis, Diarrhea, and Dementia.
- Skin changes are determined by exposure to sunlight and pressure.
- Generalized itching and erythema on the dorsum of the hand, neck, and face. Vesicles and bullae may erupt and break, so that crust occurs and lesions become scaly **(Figs. 39A and B)**. Later, skin becomes indurated, lichenified, rough, covered by dark scales and crusts, cracks, and fissure also present and a sharp demarcation from normal skin.
- *Management*: Oral administration of 100–300 mg niacinamide plus other vitamins of B complex lead to complete resolution.

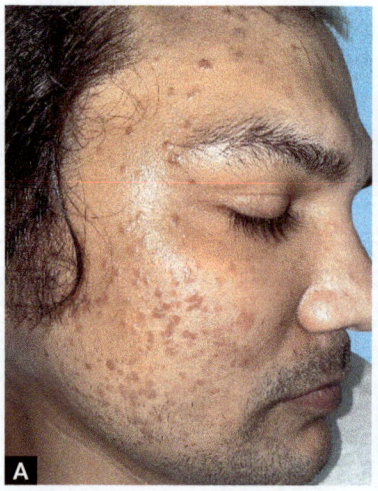 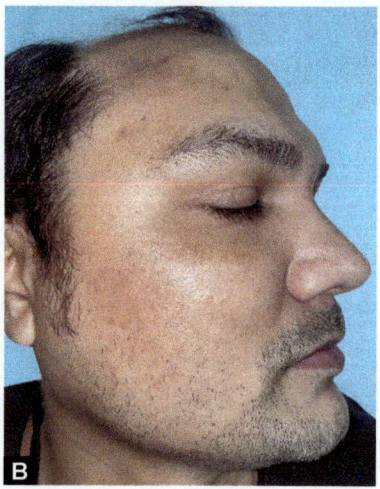

FIGS. 36A AND B: Eruptive xanthomas (before and after systemic lipid lowering agent).

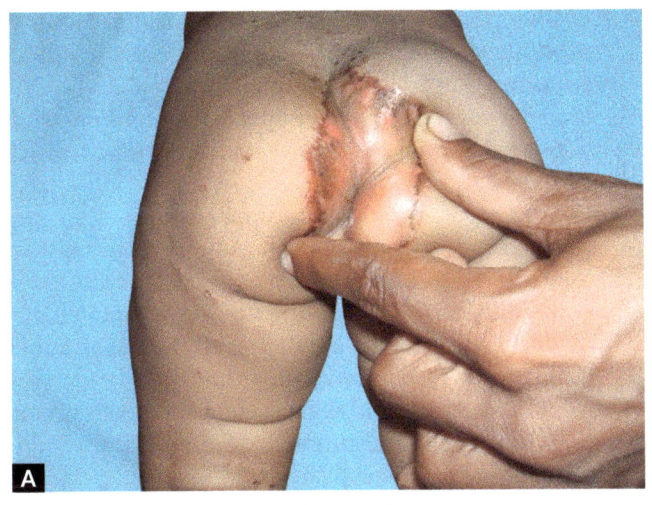
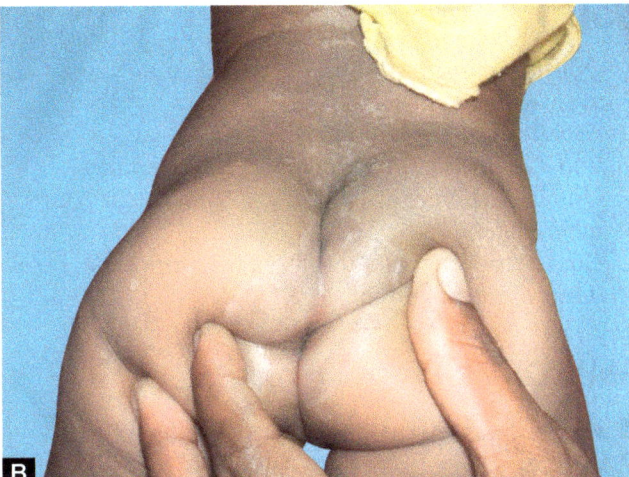

FIGS. 37A AND B: Before and after zinc therapy.

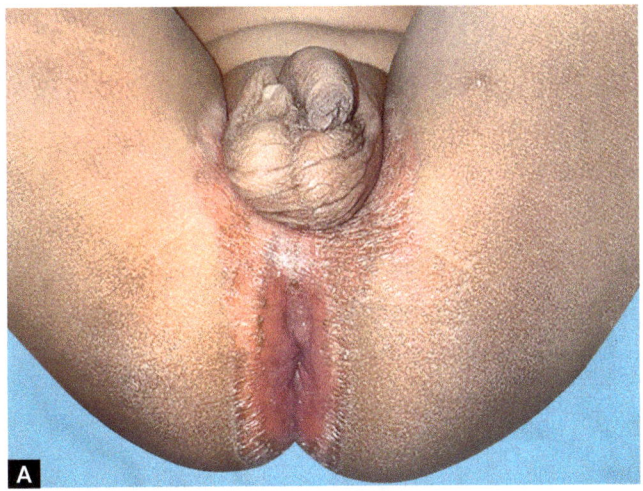
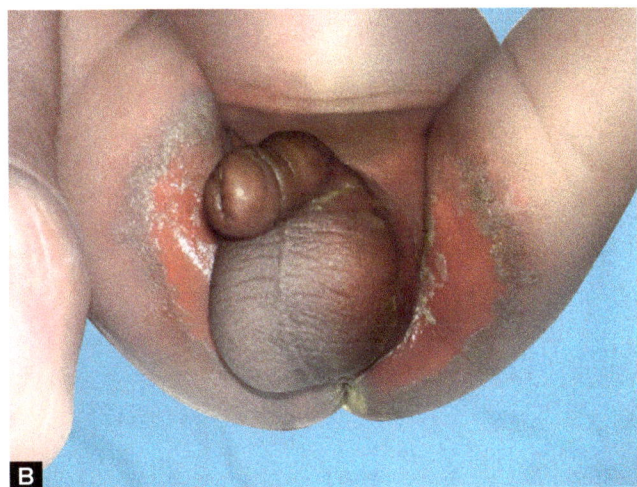

FIGS. 38A AND B: Mucosal erosion on perianal region.

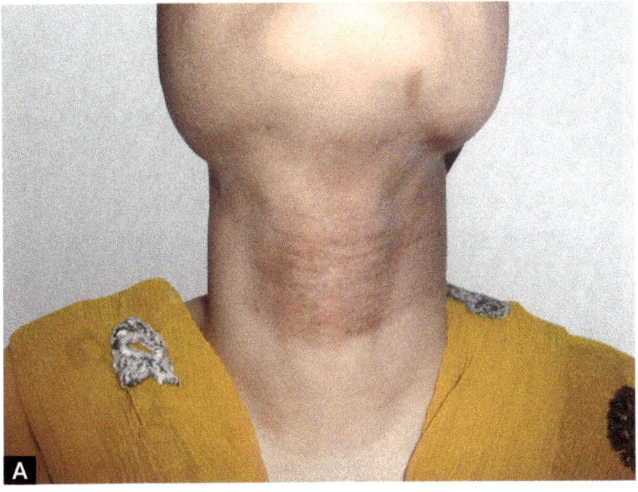
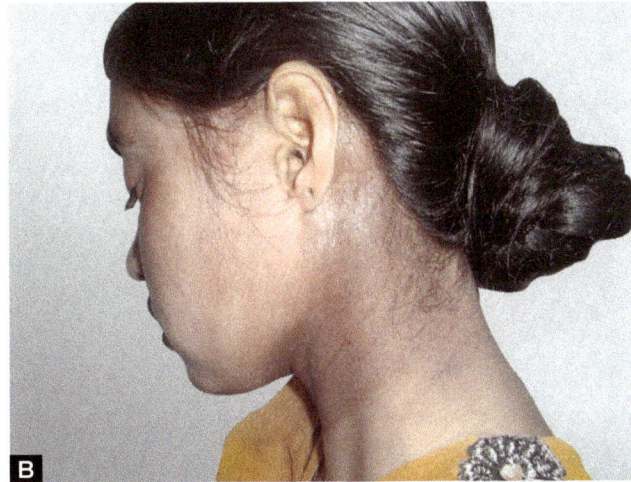

FIGS. 39A AND B: Scaly crusted band-like plaque around the neck.

GOUT

- Due to deposition of monosodium urate crystal in synovial fluid and joints.
- Usually occurs in middle age.
- Usually affects a single joint in lower extremities.
- Usually first metatarsophalangeal joint can also affect other fingers.
- Gout may occur with or without hyperuricemia, renal disease, and nephrolithiasis.

AMYLOIDOSIS

Localized Cutaneous Amyloidosis

- *Three major forms of primary localized cutaneous amyloidosis are*: (1) Macular, (2) Lichenoid, and (3) Nodular amyloidosis **(Figs. 40 to 42)**.
- Both macular and rashes amyloidosis are due to rubbing, scratching, or friction and have a rippled appearance as well as hyperpigmentation.
- Macular form favors the upper back of adults while lichenoid form favors the extensor surface of the extremities.
- Deposition of amyloid in the upper dermis.
- Nodular amyloidosis presents as one or more waxy skin colored to pinkorange plaques or nodules. Most commonly in the trunk or extremities; may chance of develop systemic amyloidosis. So, longitudinal evaluation is recommended.
- Deposition of amyloid eye is seen in cutaneous tumors (e.g., basal cell carcinoma, dermatofibroma, and intradermal melanocytic nevi).

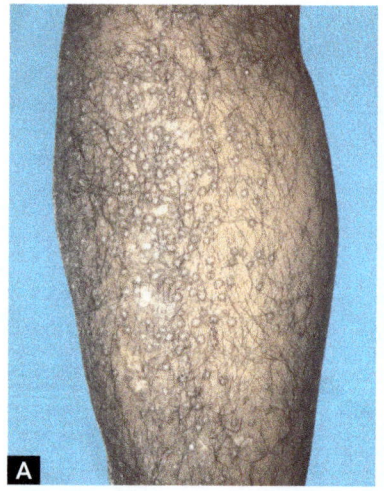
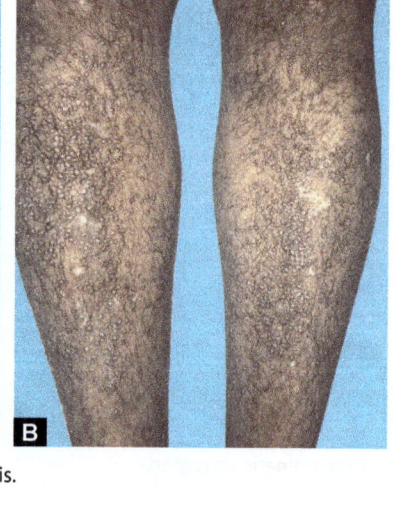

FIGS. 40A AND B: Lichenoid amyloidosis.

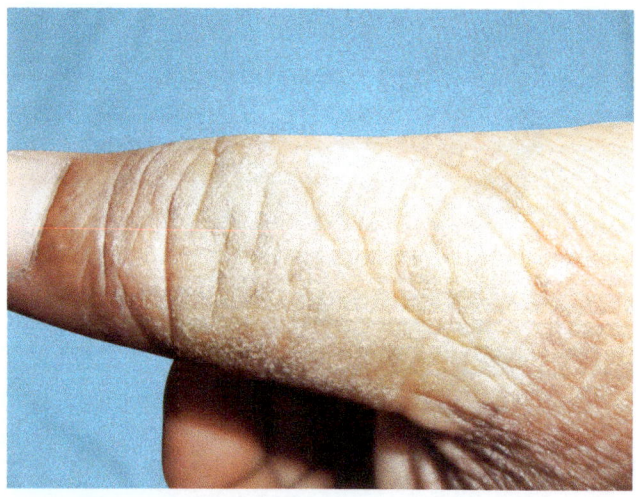

FIG. 41: Plaque amyloidosis.

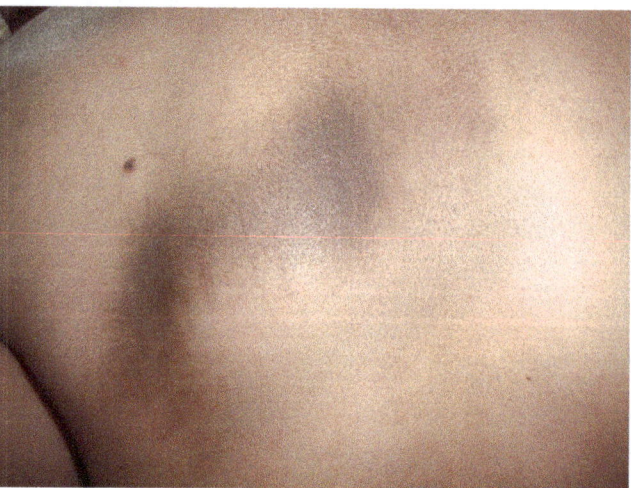

FIG. 42: Macular amyloidosis.

PORPHYRIA

Dysfunction of the enzymes involved in heme synthesis.

Porphyria Cutanea Tarda

- Most common form of cutaneous porphyria. Finding typically appears during third to fourth decades of life.
- Dysfunction of uroporphyrinogen decarboxylase is usually acquired (type 1) but can be inherent in autosomal dominant manner (type 2).
- Photosensitivity, skin fragile, erosion, vesicobullae, milia, and scar in sunexposed areas **(Fig. 43)**, especially on the dorsal aspect of the hand.
- Hyperpigmentation
- Hypertrichosis
- *Doctor's prescription*: Diagnosis is confirmed by the presence of a pinkish-red florescence in urine under a Wood's lamp.
- *Medical prescription*:
  o Photoprotection—cloth and sunscreen (contain titanium dioxide and zinc oxide—block visible light).
  o Phlebotomy—500 mL blood every 2-3 weeks interval.
  o Oral antimalarial

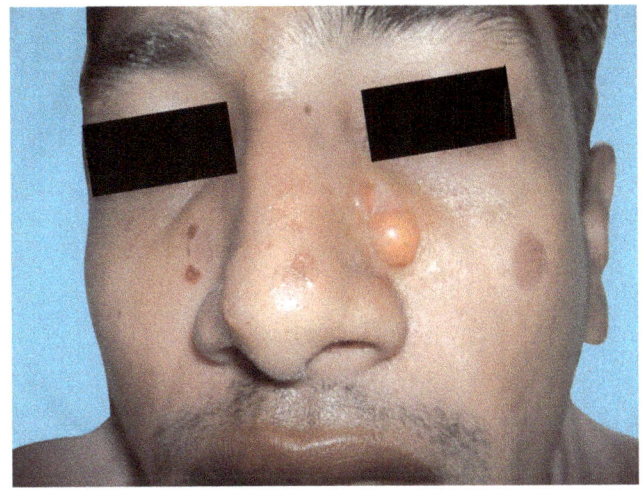

FIG. 43: Skin fragile, erosion, vesicobullae, milia, and scar on face.

CALCINOSIS CUTIS

- Deposition of amorphous, insoluble calcium salts within skin **(Figs. 44 and 45)**.
- Often related to autoimmune connective tissue disease (AICTD), particularly systemic sclerosis and childhood dermatomyositis.

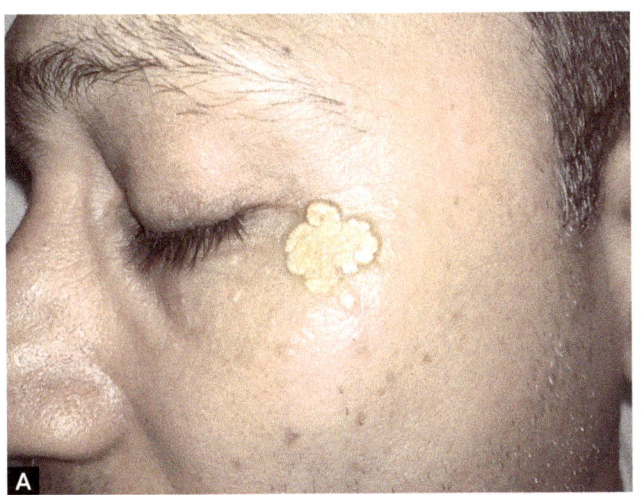
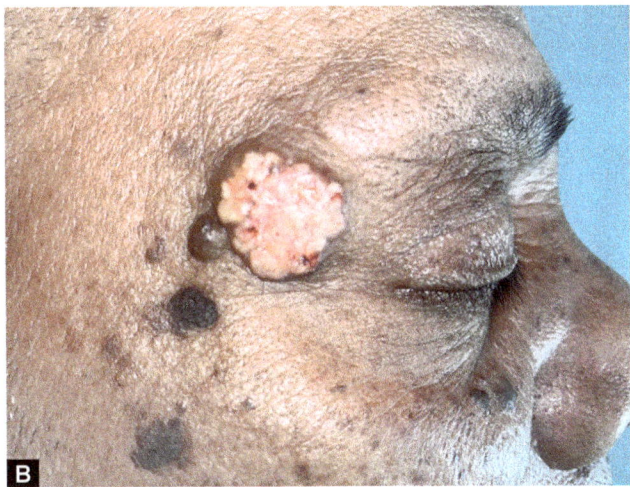

FIGS. 44A AND B: Dystrophic calcification on face.

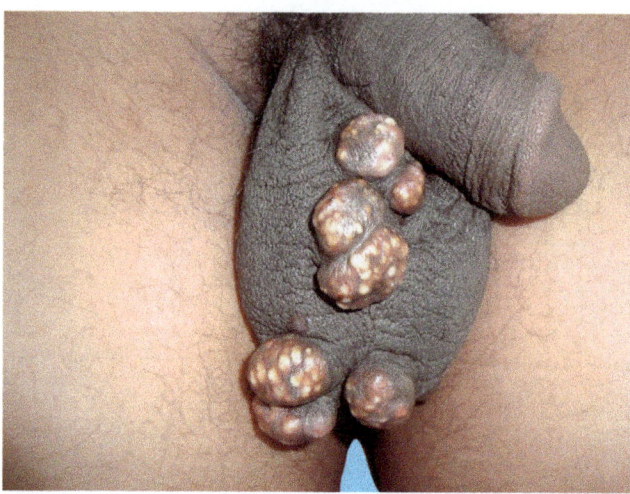

FIG. 45: Calcification in steatocystoma multiplex.

- Cutaneous tremors or cysts, e.g., pilomatricomas, pilar cysts.
- Infections, especially when cysts from around larvae or worms.
- Panniculitis, e.g., pancreatic, lupus profundus, and subcutaneous fat of the newborn.
- Genetic disorders, e.g., pseudoxanthoma elasticum and Ehlers–Danlos syndrome.

CHAPTER 10
Genetic Diseases of Skin (Genodermatosis)

ICHTHYOSES

- Disorders of cornification which are characterized by a defective epidermal barrier due to abnormal differentiation and/or desquamation of keratinocytes.
- Acquired ichthyoses are associated with malnutrition, hypothyroidism, sarcoidosis, lymphoma, leprosy, or human immunodeficiency virus (HIV) infection.
- Congenital one usually has a genetic basis.

Ichthyoses Vulgaris

- Autosomal semidominant inheritance
- Mild ichthyoses with a heterozygous filaggrin (FLG) mutation and severe ichthyoses with mutation in both FLG alleles.
- Filaggrin deficiency results in impaired mutation of cornified keratinocytes, increased transepidermal water loss resulting in mild-to-moderate scaling that favors the extensor extremities ranging from fine white scales to large adherent scales (especially on lower legs, trunk, scalp, and forehead) **(Figs. 1A and B)**.
- It typically becomes apparent during infancy or early childhood and improves by adulthood; worsens in cold dry environment.
- *Differential diagnosis*: Xerosis, acquired ichthyoses, and X-linked ichthyoses.
- *Management*:
  ○ Emollients (especially those containing ceramides plus other lipids)
  ○ Keratolytic agents (urea, lactic acid, and salicylic acid)

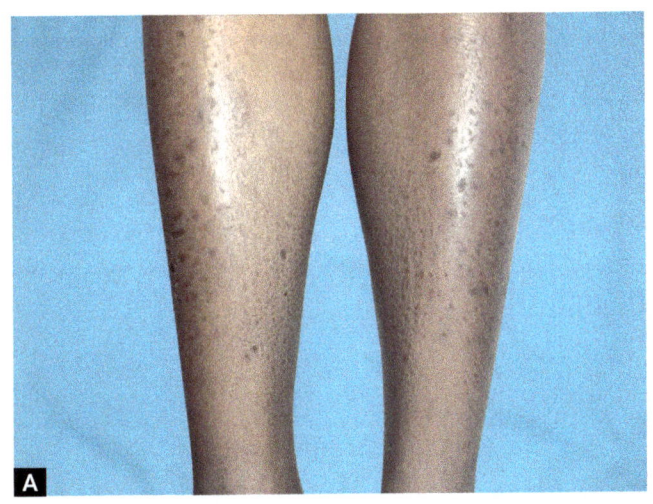
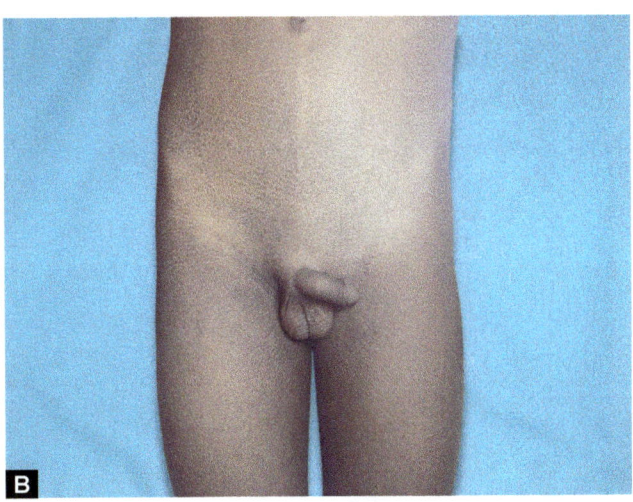

FIGS. 1A AND B: Fine white scales on lower extremities and abdomen.

X-linked Ichthyoses

- It occurs in male.
- *X-linked recessive disorder*: Steroid sulfatase deficiency resulting with failure to shed senescent keratinocytes, clinically present with hyperkeratosis.
- Onset soon after birth
- Large, prominent, and dirty brown scales on the neck, extremities, trunk, and buttocks **(Figs. 2A to D)**
- Involvement of flexural regions
- Absence of palm and sole involvement
- Corneal opacity develops during 2nd to 3rd week in 50% of adult males.
- Cryptorchidism develops in 20% of individuals.
- There is no improvement with age.

Lamellar Ichthyoses

- Often present at birth as collodion baby.
- Autosomal recessive disorder
- Heat intolerance
- Collodion baby—encased in a translucent collodion-like membrane. Clean in a few weeks.
- Ectropion and eclabion
- Generalized erythroderma
- Large parchment-like hyperkeratosis over entire body **(Figs. 3A to C)**. Fracturing of hyperkeratosis plate results in a tessellated (file-like) pattern.
- There is no improvement with age.

Acquired Ichthyoses

- Associated with leprosy **(Fig. 4A)**, Hodgkin's disease, non-Hodgkin's lymphoma **(Fig. 4B)**, acquired immunodeficiency syndrome (AIDS), sarcoidosis, systemic lupus erythematosus (SLE), dermatomyositis, mixed connective tissue disease (MCTD), drugs, eosinophilic fasciitis, and graft-versus-host disease.
- *Drugs responsible*: Nicotinic acid, triparanol, butylphenol, dixyrazine, and nafoxidine.

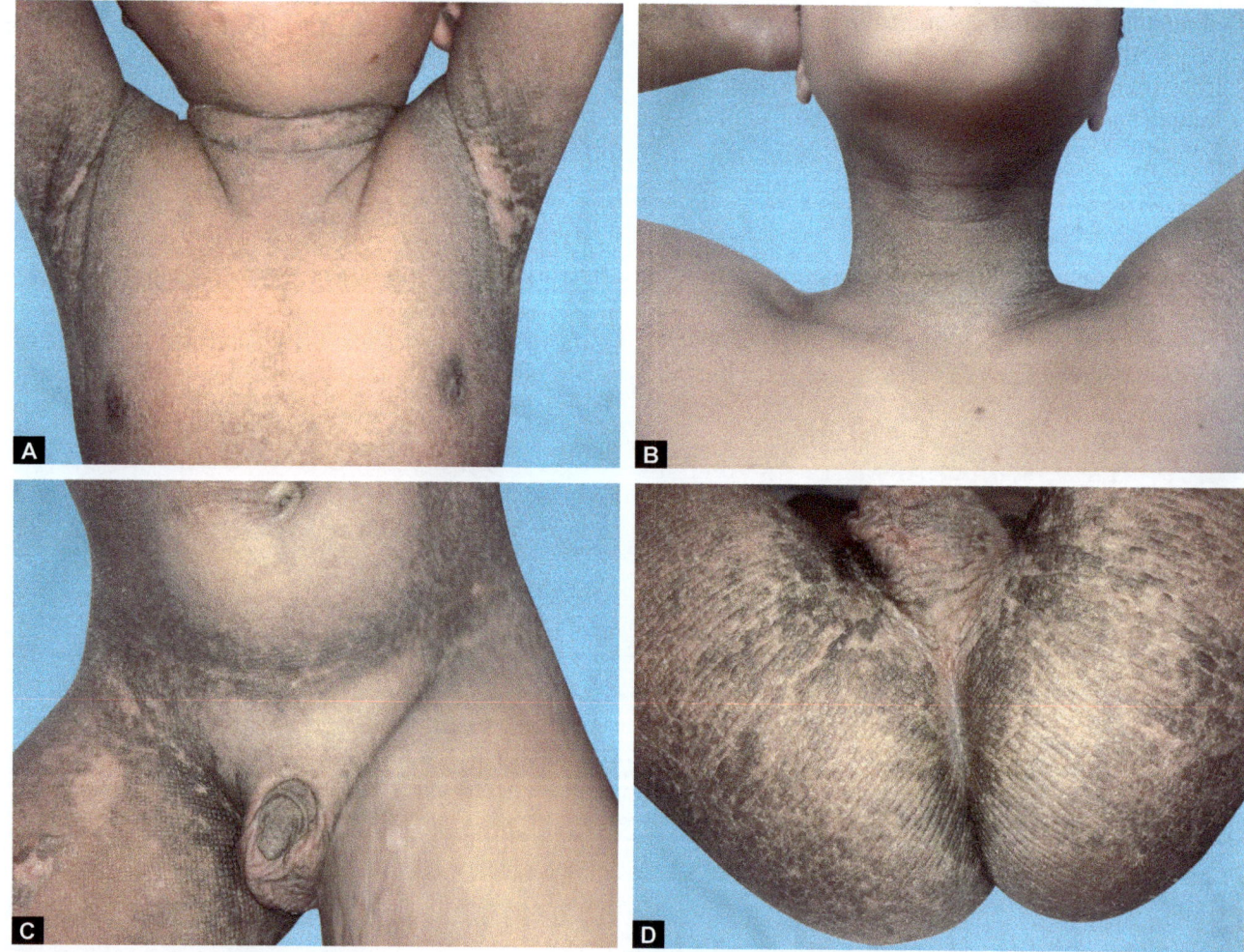

FIGS. 2A TO D: Large, prominent, and dirty brown scales on the neck (dirty neck), axilla, extremities, trunk, and buttocks.

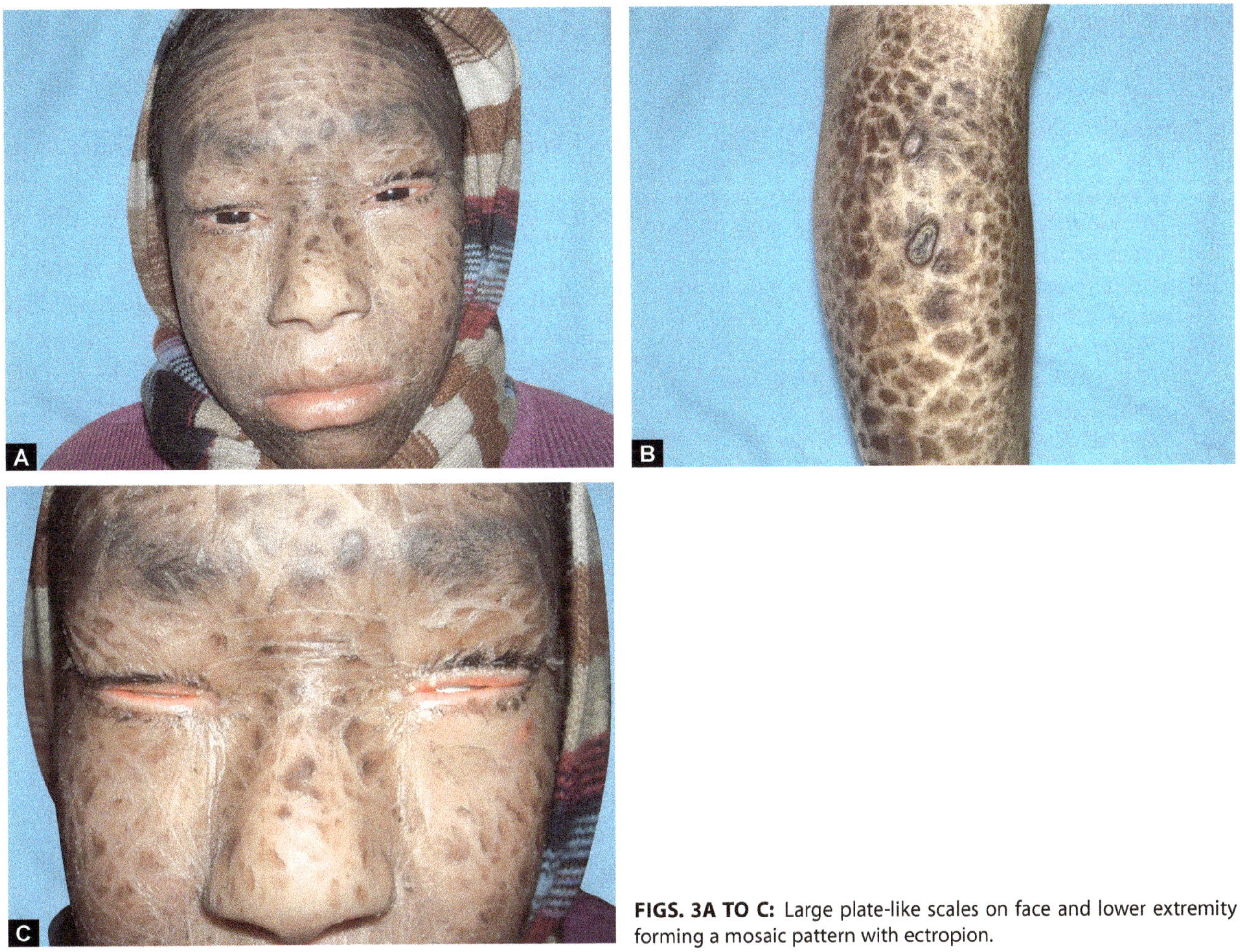

CHAPTER 10 Genetic Diseases of Skin (Genodermatosis)

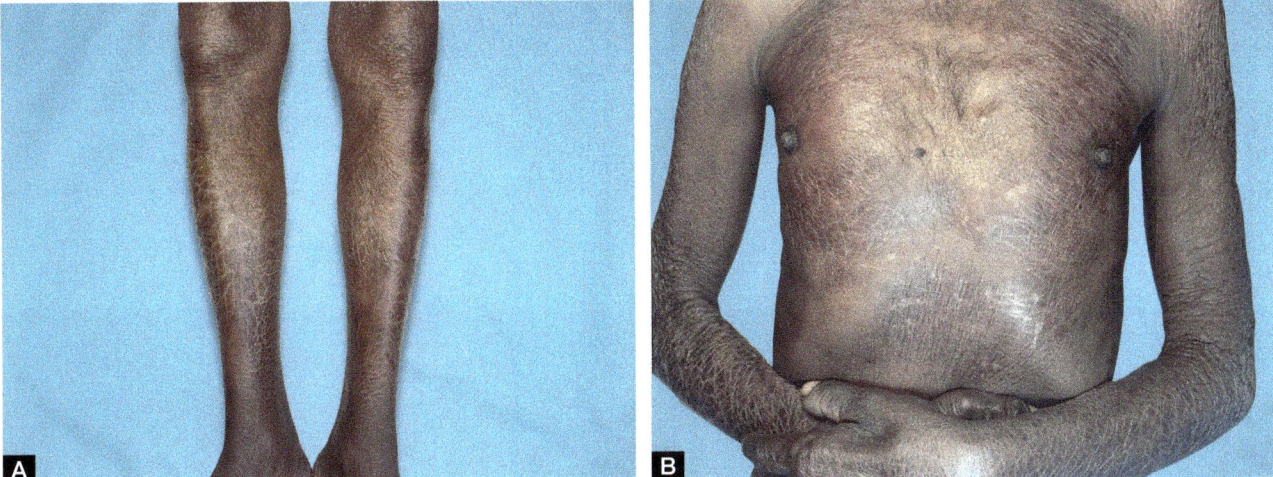

FIGS. 3A TO C: Large plate-like scales on face and lower extremity forming a mosaic pattern with ectropion.

FIGS. 4A AND B: Acquired dark brown scales over lower extremities and trunk due to leprosy and non-Hodgkin's lymphoma, respectively.

KERATODERMA

Palmoplantar Keratodermas

- *Diffuse palmoplantar keratoderma (PPK)*:
  - Confluent over the entire palmoplantar surface. Onset by early childhood in hereditary forms.
  - Thick and yellow hyperkeratosis that may be warty or verrucous **(Figs. 5A and B)**.
- *Focal PPK*: Primarily in areas of friction or pressure.
- *Punctate PPK*:
  - *Treatment*:
    - Keratolytics (salicylic acid 4-6% in petroleum) and urea 40%
    - Mechanical debridement
    - Topical or oral retinoids
    - Treatment of secondary fungal and bacterial infections

DARIER DISEASE

- Rare autosomal dominant inherited disease with late onset.
- Multiple discrete scaling, crushed, and pruritic papules mainly in seborrheic and flexural areas **(Figs. 6A to D)**. Hypopigmented macules may be prominent in texture, especially in darker skin type.
- Itching, malodorous, and disfiguring also involving nails and mucous membrane (whitish papules). Distal notching with longitudinal erythronychia.
- Squamous cell carcinoma (SCC) develops in long-standing untreated or maltreated cases **(Figs. 7A to C)**.
- Chronic course often worse in summer.
- Exacerbating factors include sunlight, heat, occlusion, sweat, and bacterial colonization.

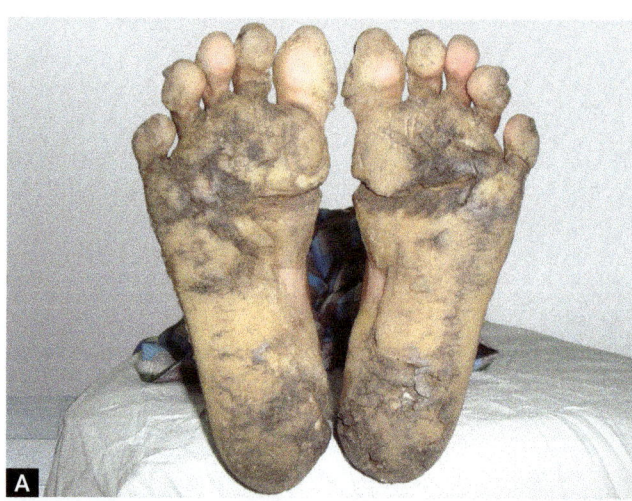
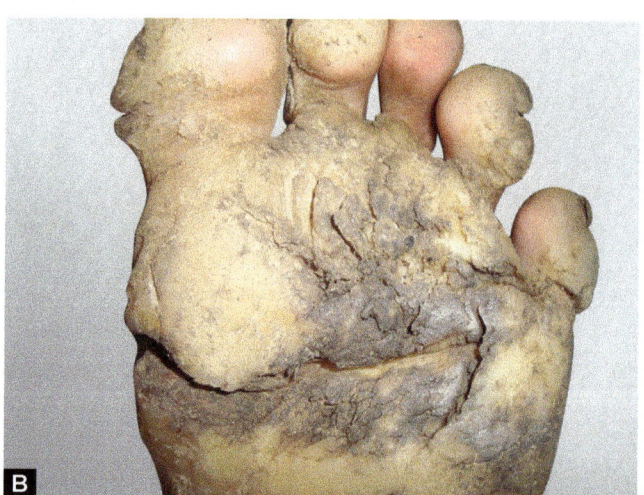

FIGS. 5A AND B: Diffuse hyperkeratosis with fissure.

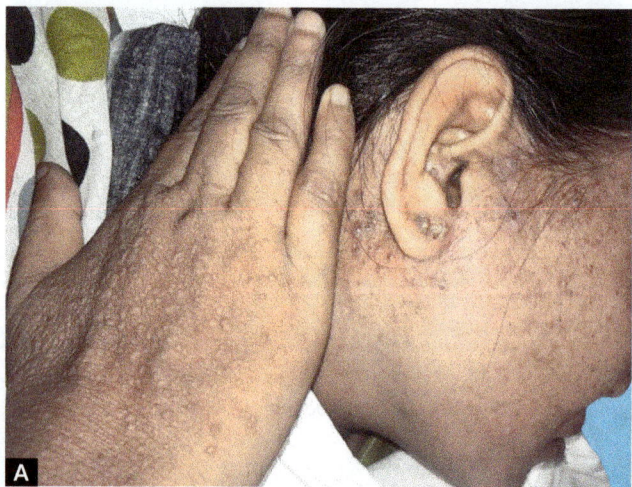
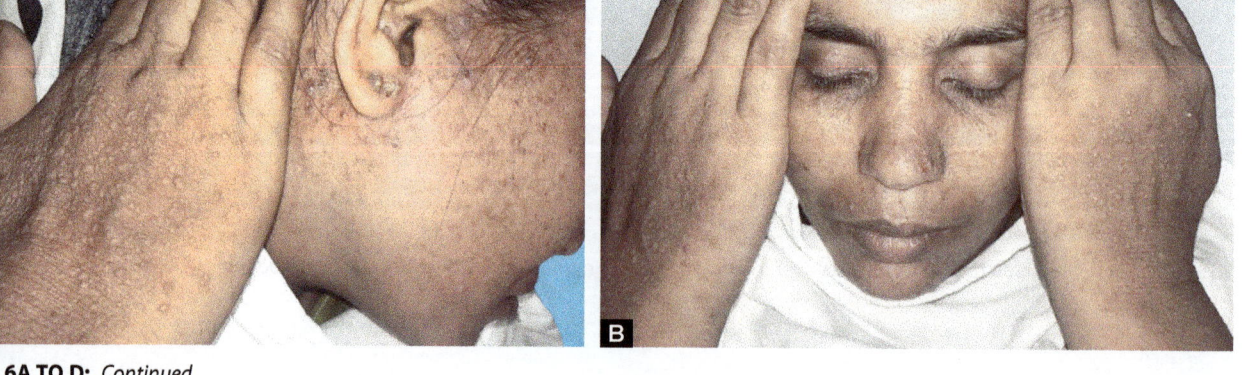

FIGS. 6A TO D: *Continued*

Continued

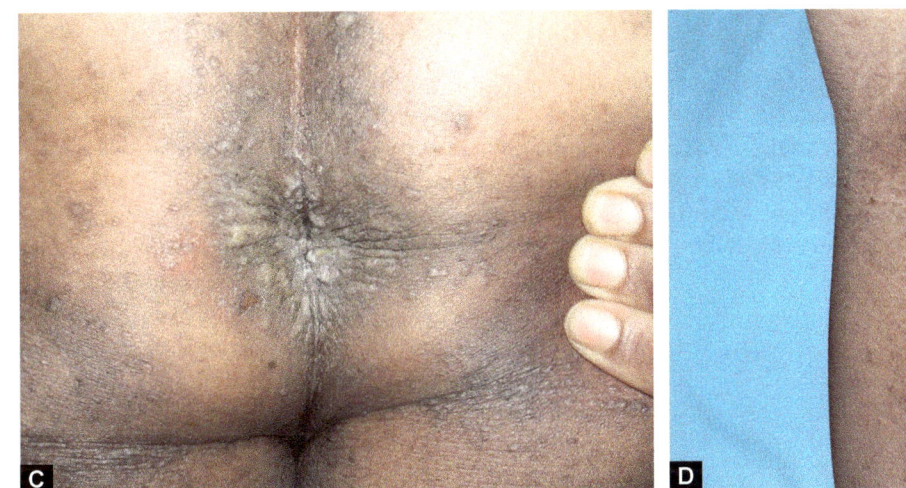
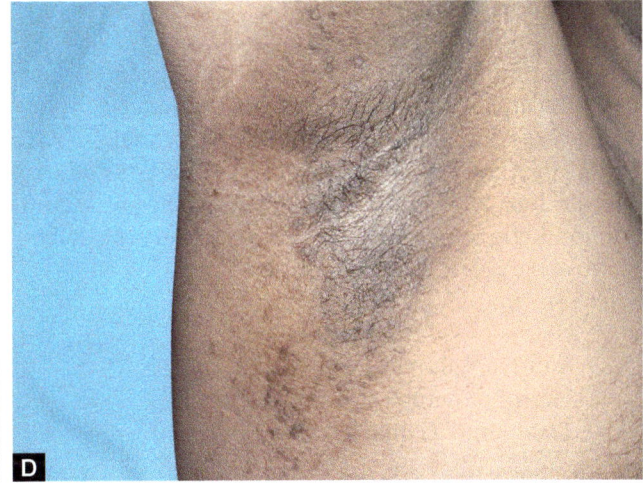

FIGS. 6A TO D: Keratotic papules over face, trunk, perianal, and axillae.

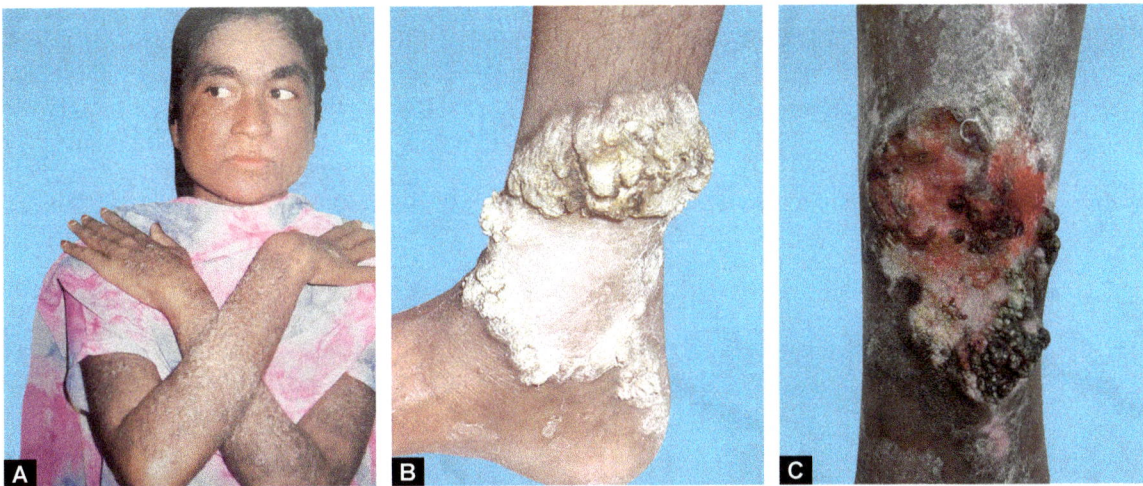

FIGS. 7A TO C: Extensive involvement and squamous cell carcinoma (SCC) develops in long-standing untreated or maltreated cases.

- Whitish papule of the oral mucosa
- *Differential diagnosis*: Seborrheic dermatitis, Grover's disease, benign familial pemphigus, pemphigus foliaceus, and blastomycosis.
- *Treatment*:
    - General—covering of entire body by cloth, sunscreen.
    - Antimicrobial cleansers
    - Keratolytic emollient
    - Topical retinoid + Topical corticosteroids (CS)
    - Oral retinoids
    - Topical and oral antibiotics
    - Systemic antifungal and antiviral

HAILEY–HAILEY DISEASE (FIG. 8)

- Also known as familial benign chronic pemphigus
- Autosomal dominant

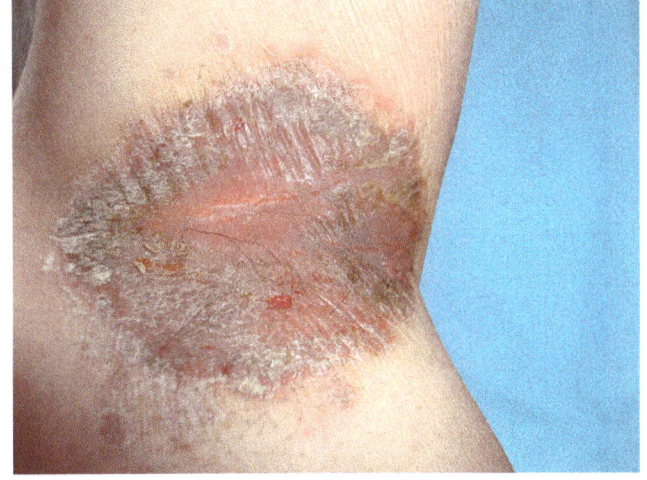

FIG. 8: Hailey–Hailey disease.

- Onset in the second or third decade, but sometimes into fourth and fifth decades.
- Variable course with remission and flare.
- Submammary regions, inguinal folds, axilla, and scrotal area are the major site of involvement.
- Exacerbating factors include friction, heat, sweat, and bacterial colonization. It also includes moist, malodorous plaques with erosions, fissures, and flaccid blisters and circinate plaques with crowded or crusted border.
- *Treatment*:
    - General—lightweight clothing
    - Antimicrobial cleansers
    - Intermittent topical/intralesional CS
    - Treatment of complications

CHRONIC MUCOCUTANEOUS CANDIDIASIS (FIGS. 9A TO C)

- Group of immune deficient characterized by recurrent and severe infection of the skin, nails, and mucous membrane with *Candida albicans* and susceptible to other infections.
- Clinical manifestations include recalcitrant oral thrush, dystrophic nails, and granulomatous plaques with scale crust favoring the scalp, face, and skin folds.
- Onset usually before the age of 6 years.
- Systemic fluconazole, or itraconazole, or ketoconazole is necessary to control chronic mucocutaneous candidiasis (CMCC). Course is typically prolonged, repeated, and gives at higher doses than usual recommended doses.

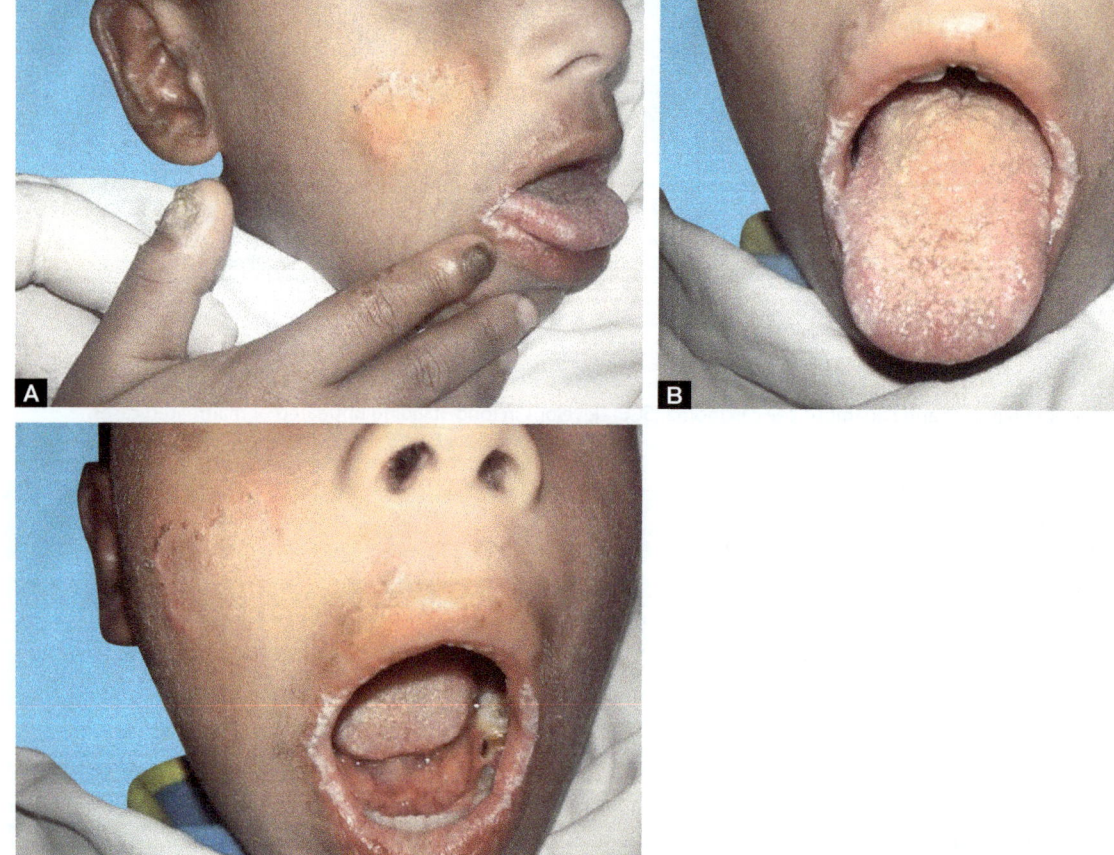

FIGS. 9A TO C: Chronic mucocutaneous candidiasis.

NEUROFIBROMATOSIS TYPE I

- It is also known as von Recklinghausen disease.
- Incidence of approximately 1 in 3,000 births.
- Neurofibromatosis is an autosomal dominant trait manifested by changes in the skin, nervous system, bones, and endocrine glands. These changes include a variety of congenital anomalies, tumors, and hamartomas.
- *Diagnostic criteria for neurofibromatosis type I (NFI) (two or more of the following must be recent)*:
  - Six or more café-au-lait macules (>5 mm if prepubertal, >15 mm if postpubertal) **(Figs. 10A to D)**.
  - Two or more neurofibromas of any type or type 1 plexiform neurofibromas **(Figs. 11 and 12)**.
  - "Freckling" in the axillary or inguinal region.
  - Optic gliomas
  - Two or more Lisch nodules
  - Typical osseous lesions, e.g., sphenoid wing dysplasia, and thinning of long bone cortex
  - First-degree relative with NFI (parent, siblings, or offspring).
- *Course and prognosis*: Mortality rate is higher than normal population, principally because of the development of neurosarcoma in adult life.

TUBEROUS SCLEROSIS

- Incidence of approximately 1 in 10,000 births
- An autosomal dominant disease arising from a generally programed hyperplasia of ectodermal and mesodermal cells and manifested by a variety of

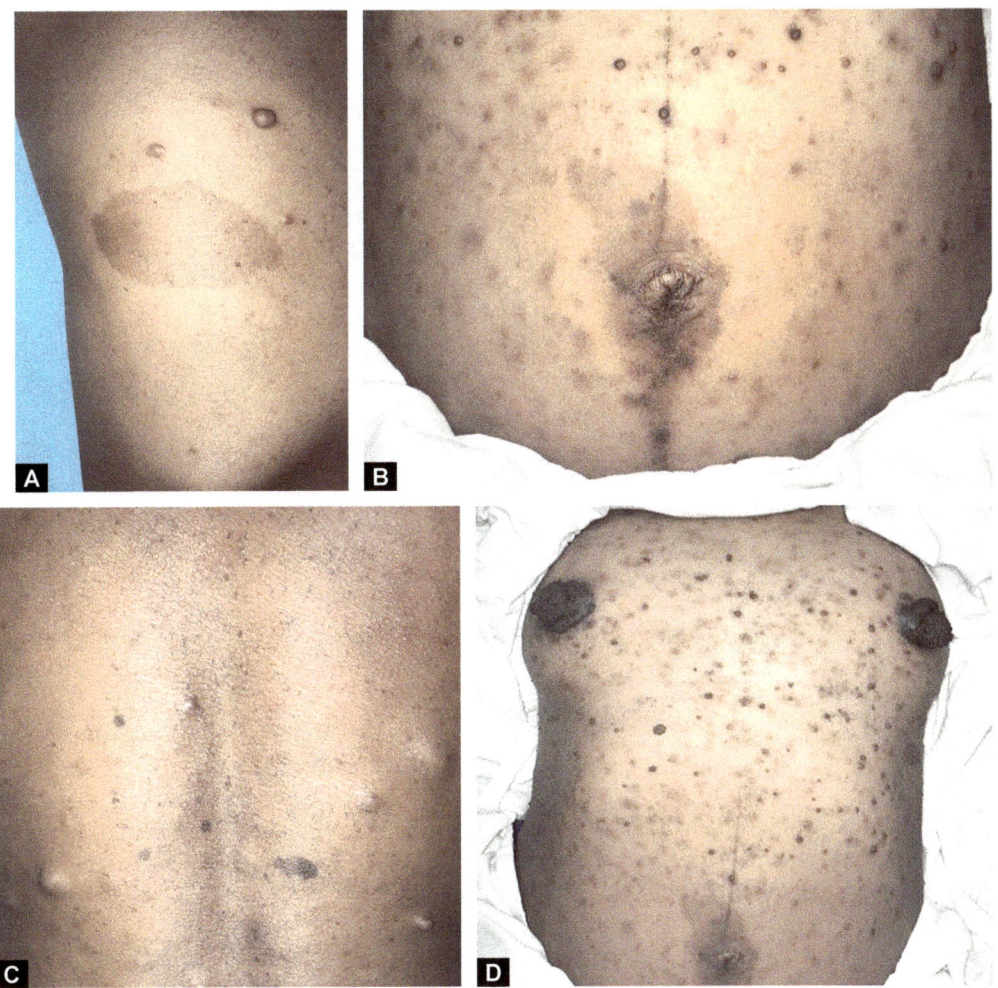

FIGS. 10A TO D: Café-au-lait macules and patches.

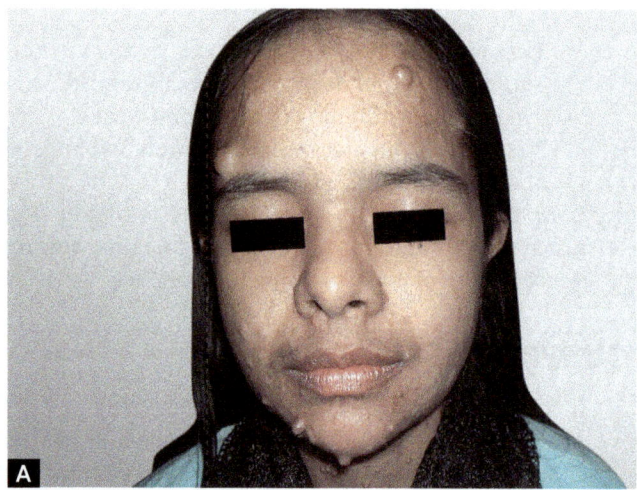
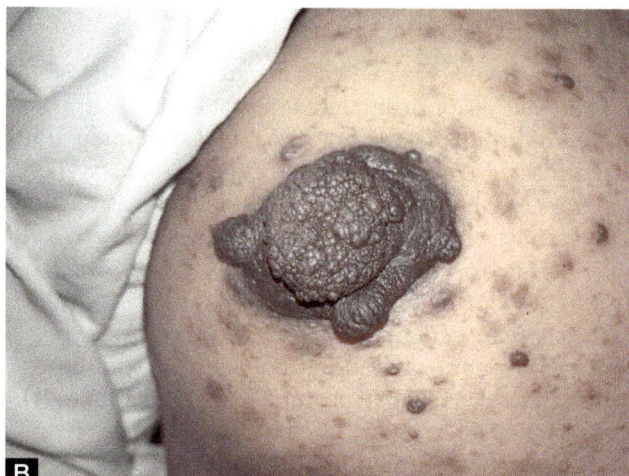

FIGS. 11A AND B: Neurofibromatosis.

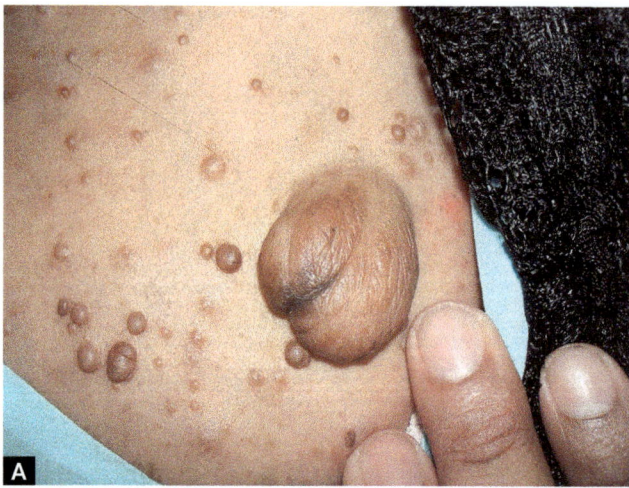
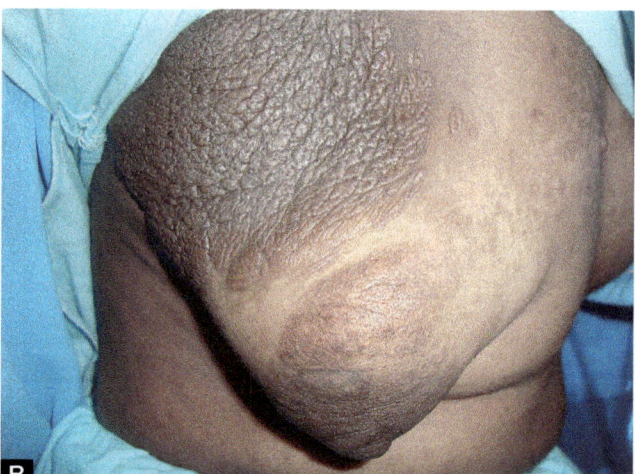

FIGS. 12A AND B: Plexiform neurofibroma.

lesions in the skin, central nervous system (CNS), heart, kidney, and other organs.
- *Central nervous system manifestations*:
  o Seizures
  o Mental retardation
  o Congenital white spots
- Hypopigmented macules—off-white ash leaf spots on trunk, upper and lower extremities, and neck.
- Facial angiofibromata are pathognomonic, but do not appear until third or fourth decade.
- "Shagreen" patch—plaque represents connective tissue nevi, periungual papules, or nodules **(Figs. 13A to D)**.
- Ungual fibromas (Koenen tumors) represent in 22% of individuals.
- *Course and prognosis*:
  o Up to 30% die before the 5th year of life.
  o Up to 50–70% die before reaching adult age.

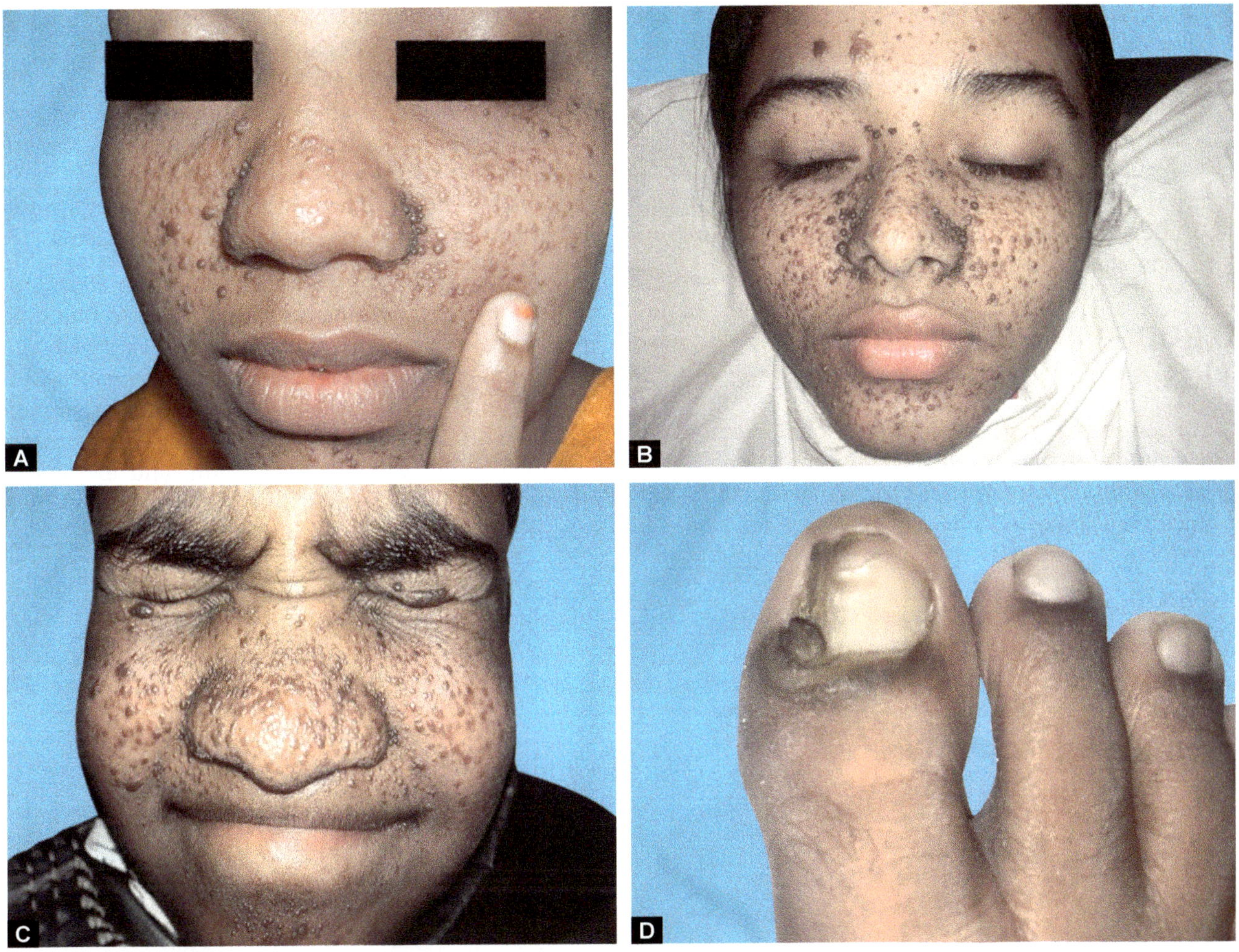

FIGS. 13A TO D: Angiofibroma and periungual fibromas.

PSEUDOXANTHOMA ELASTICUM (FIG. 14)

- Hereditary disorder of connective tissue that involves the elastic tissue in the skin, blood vessels, and eyes result in fragmented elastic fibers in the skin, eyes, and arteries.
- Grouped clusters of yellow papules in a reticular pattern resembling peau d'orange surface pattern on neck, axilla, and body folds.
- *Effects in the vascular system*:
  - Gastrointestinal tract (GIT) hemorrhage
  - Hypertension (HTN) in young persons
  - Retinal hemorrhage
  - Angioid streaks

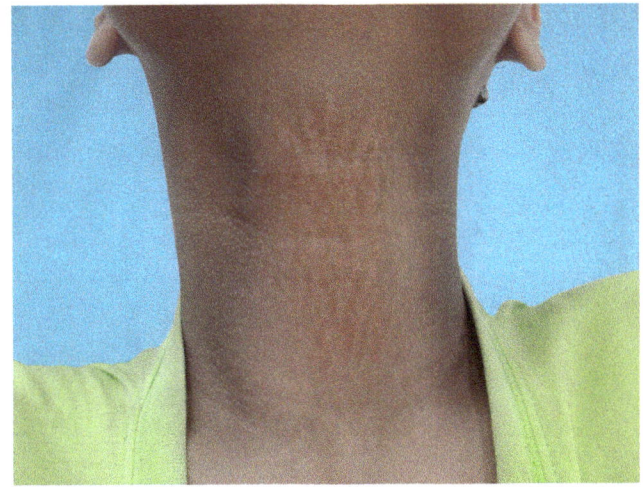

FIG. 14: Pseudoxanthoma elasticum.

- Cardinal physical findings of—hyperextensible, fragile skin, hypermobile joints, easy bruising, and "fish-mouth" wound from minor trauma that heal with widened and atrophic scars.
- *Treatment*:
  - Antioxidant and magnesium supplements
  - Moderate calcium intake
  - Regular exercise, weight control, avoidance of smoking, or excessive alcohol intake

XERODERMA PIGMENTOSUM (FIGS. 15A TO H)

- An autosomal recessive disorder characterized by extreme sun sensitivity, freckling, and skin cancer as a result of defective deoxyribonucleic acid (DNA) thymidine dimer excision repair.
- Sun sensitivity and lentigines are early skin findings onset before 2 years of age.
- Skin cancer usually before 10 years.
- Thousands of malignant foci—squamous cell carcinoma (SCC), basal cell carcinoma (BCC), and melanoma are present in a single individual.
- Ocular abnormalities are photophobia, ectropion, corneal opacity, blepharospasm, and neoplasms.

Note: Maternal cousins were married in year 2004. They came in my chamber one evening of 2009. At that time, Sumon was 4-year-old and Sumaiya was 3-year-old. Sumon was presented with giant SCC with metastasis in different internal organs. He got conservative treatment and died in 2012. Sumaiya underwent cryosurgery, carbon dioxide (CO_2) laser excision, and excision of different malignant tumors in different times with acitretin treatment coverage and died in 2016.

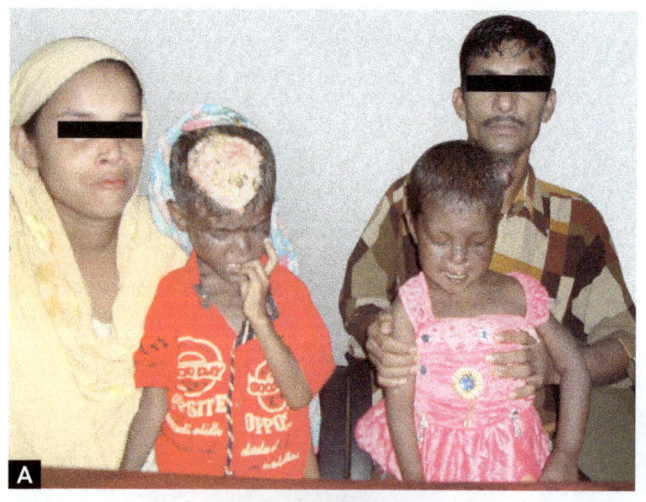
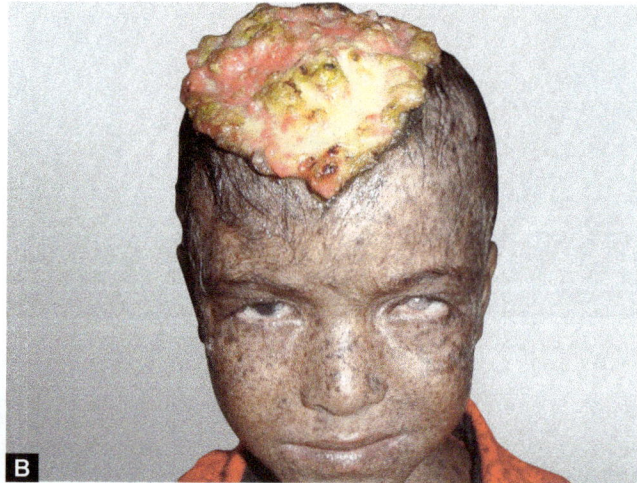
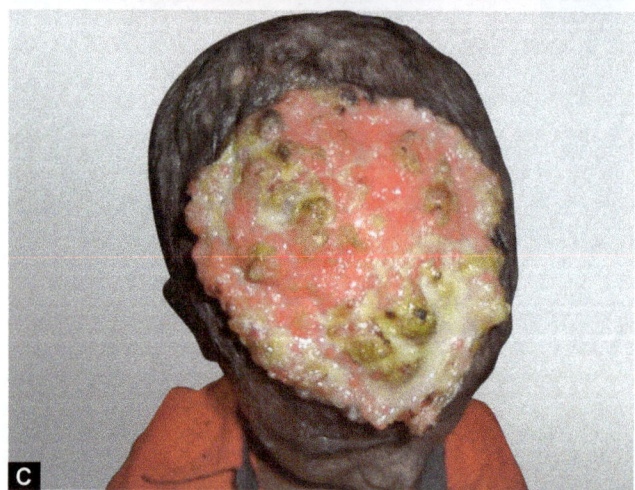
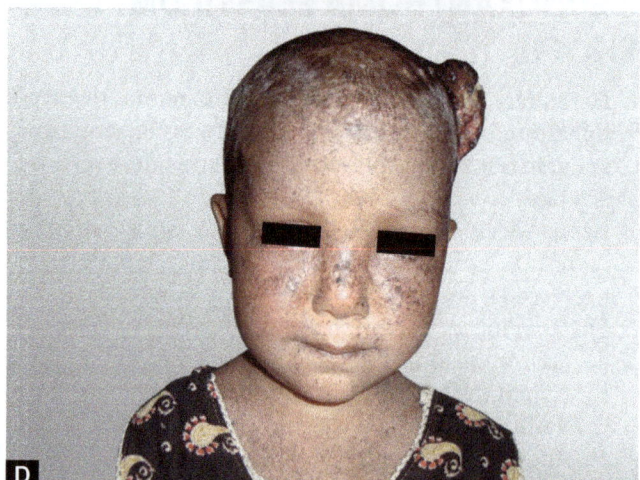

FIGS. 15A TO H: *Continued*

Continued

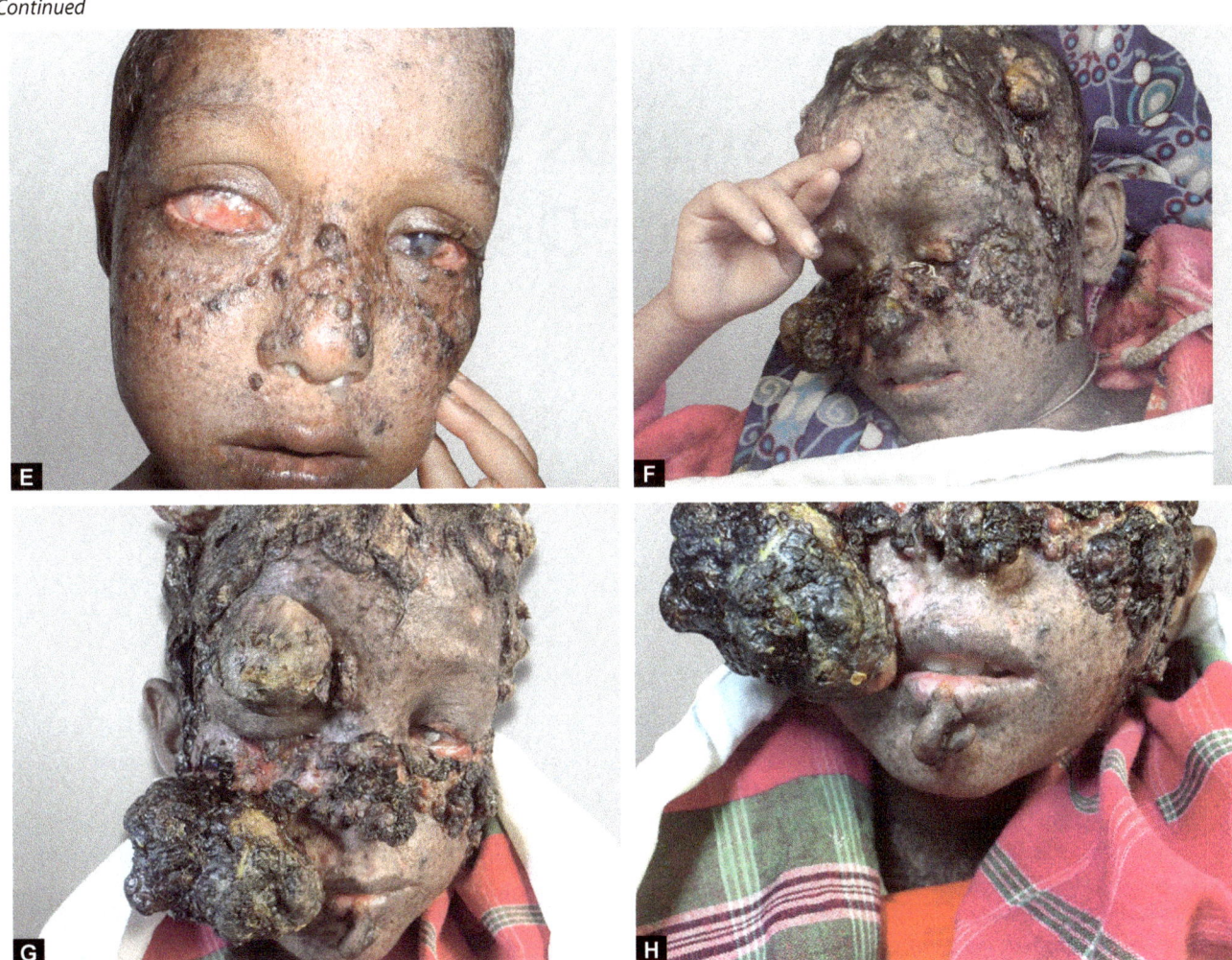

FIGS. 15A TO H: Xeroderma pigmentosum.

CHAPTER 11
Cutaneous Signs of Systemic Disease

CUTANEOUS GASTROINTESTINAL

- *Cutaneous disease associated with gastrointestinal abnormalities:*
  - Gastrointestinal hemorrhage
  - Pseudoxanthoma elasticum
  - Progressive calcification of tissue rich in elastic fibers including skin, retina, and blood vessels
  - Diffuse superficial erosions rather than focal bleeding found
  - *Skin findings: Yellowish papules coalescence on the neck, axilla, and groin which may give a pseudo-orange appearance.*
- *Hereditary hemorrhagic telangiectasis:*
  - Autosomal dominant trait characterized by multi system vascular dysplasia.
  - Telangiectasis begins from the mucous membrane of the nose and mouth during early childhood.
  - Recurrent epistaxis is a common complaint in the first two decades and severity increases with age.
  - Involvement with telangiectasia extends to the face, upper extremities, palm, and sole
  - Lesions are prone to hemorrhage with little or no trauma.
  - It is potentially fatal with gastrointestinal bleeding.
- Acrodermatitis enteropathica
- Dermatitis herpetiformis
- *Inflammatory bowel disease:*
  - Specific lesion:
    - Fissure and fistula
    - Metastatic Crohn disease
    - Mucosal lesions
  - Reactive lesion:
    - Aphthous ulcer
    - Pustular vasculitis
    - Erythema nodosum
    - Pyoderma gangrenosum
    - Vasculitis
    - Urticaria
    - Sweet syndrome
- *Other associations:*
  - Epidermolysis bullosa acquisita
  - Vitiligo
  - Fingernail clubbing

CUTANEOUS HEPATOLOGY

■ Cirrhosis

Changes in the skin, nail, and hair occur.

Skin

- Vascular lesions due to portal hypertension
- Spider angiomas
- Palmar erythema
- Dilated abdominal veins

Nails (Not Specific to Liver Disease)

- Classic white nail of Terry (opaque white nail except distal portion)
- Transverse white band (Muehrcke's nail)
- Clubbed nail
- Koilonychia (spoon-shaped nails)

Hair

Axillary, pubic, and pectoral hair is usually sparse, but thinning of all body hair is also common.

Primary Biliary Cirrhosis

- Pruritus
- Jaundice
- Hyperpigmentation
- Xanthema

Hemochromatosis

Also known as bronze diabetes, an autosomal recessive disorder characterized by:
- *Cutaneous hyperpigmentation-generalized accentuation in exposed areas. Oral mucosa may involve*:
  - Cirrhosis of liver
  - Diabetes mellitus

Basic defect is iron metabolism, results in increased absorption of iron from intestine and deposition of iron in venous tissue, especially the skin, liver, heart, pancreas, and endocrine glands.

Secondary forms of hemochromatosis result in:
- Excess oral intake of iron
- Repeated transfusion
- Congenital transferrin deficiency

Cutaneous Disease associated with Viral Hepatitis

- *Hepatitis B virus—associated with reactive erythema*: Urticaria, vasculitis, Gianotti-Crosti syndrome.
- *Hepatitis C virus*:
  - Serum sickness like prodrome
  - Porphyria cutanea tarda (PCT)
  - Livedo reticularis
  - Vitiligo
  - Pyoderma gangrenosum
  - Polyarteritis nodosa
  - Alopecia areata
  - Lichen planus

Pancreatic Disease

Cutaneous changes related to pancreatitis:
- Cutaneous hemorrhage
- Panniculitis
- Livedo reticularis

Related to pancreatic carcinoma:
- Metastatic nodule epically to umbilicus
- Panniculitis
- Migratory thrombophlebitis

CHAPTER 12: Cutaneous Manifestation of Bacterial, Viral, Protozoal, Worm, Fungal Infection, and Other Infections/Infestation

BACTERIAL INFECTIONS

Name of bacterial infections by depth and extent of skin involvement are given in **Figure 1**.

Gram-positive Cocci (Staphylococcal and Streptococcal Infections)

An intact stratum corneum is the most important defense against invasion of pathogenic bacteria.

Impetigo

- Major organisms are *Staphylococcus aureus* (*S. aureus*) and *Streptococcus pyogenes* (group A). Group A β-hemolytic streptococcal infection is sometimes followed by acute glomerulonephritis (AGN). Nephritogenic streptococci (types 49, 55, 57, 60, and M—type 2) are generally associated with impetigo rather than with upper respiratory tract infections.
- Very common, highly contagious bacterial infection among children, commonly seen in exposed part of body (face, extremity). Usually, the skin is eroded with overlying "honey-colored" crusts. On the other hand, bullous variant is seen where bullae formation due to *S. aureus* can be explained by local release of an exfoliative toxin that binds to desmoglein-1 and leads to dissolution (acantholysis) of the upper epidermis **(Figs. 2A to M)**.
- Differential diagnosis of eroded lesions—insect bites, prurigo simplex, atopic dermatitis, and scabies.
- Differential diagnosis of vesiculobullous lesions—insect bites, herpes simplex virus (HSV) infection, and chronic bullous disease of childhood (CBDC).
- Medical prescription—oral and topical antibiotics.

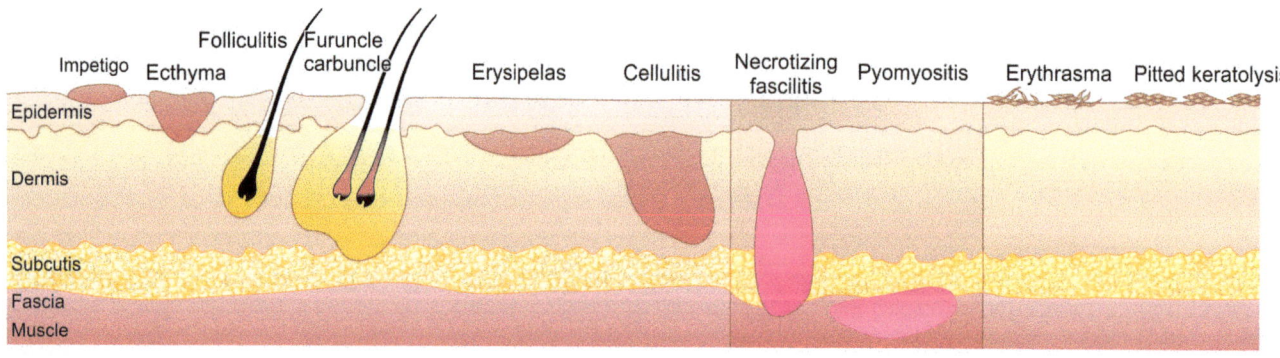

FIG. 1: Various bacterial infections by depth and extent of skin involvement.

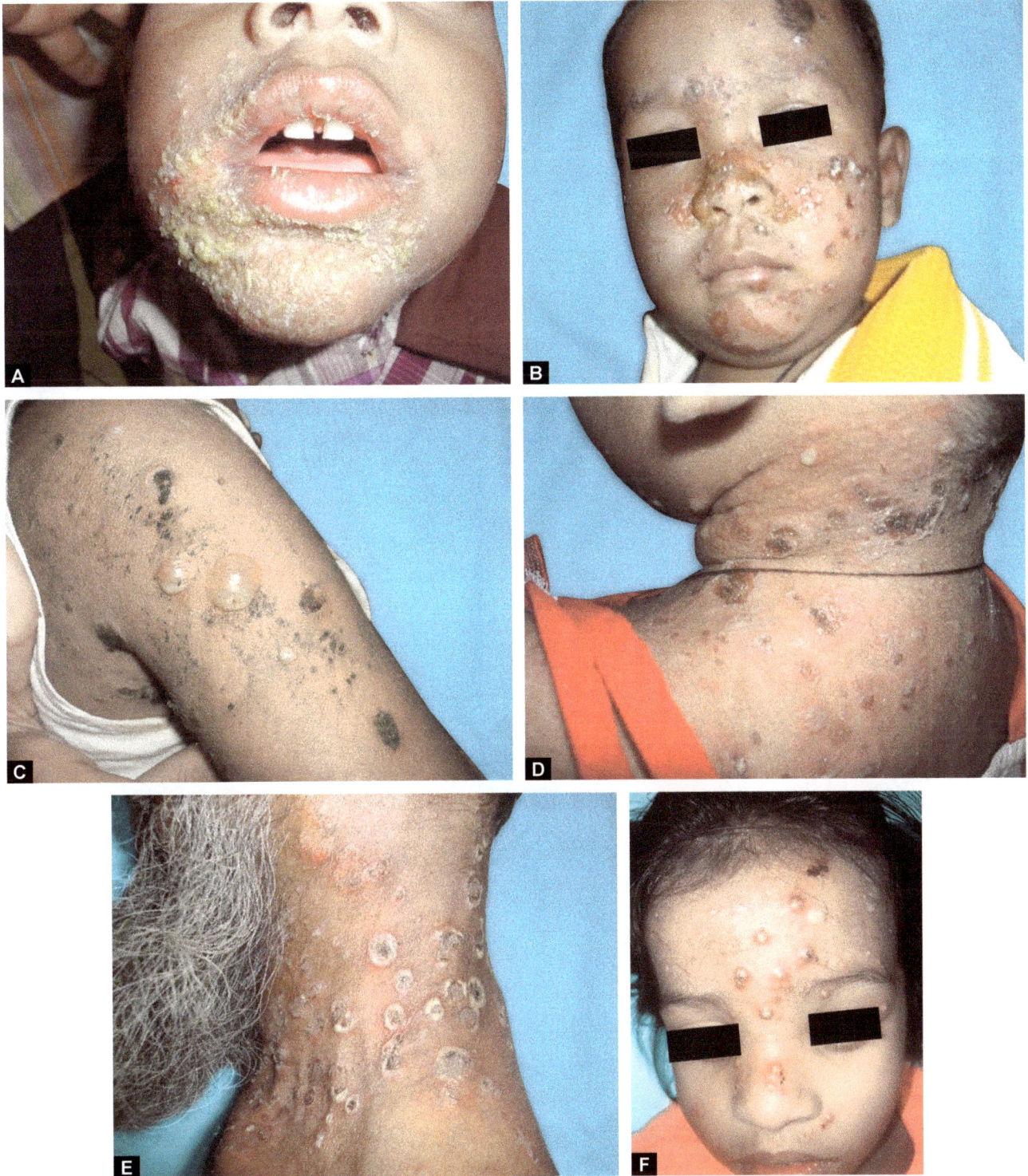

FIGS. 2A TO M: *Continued*

Continued

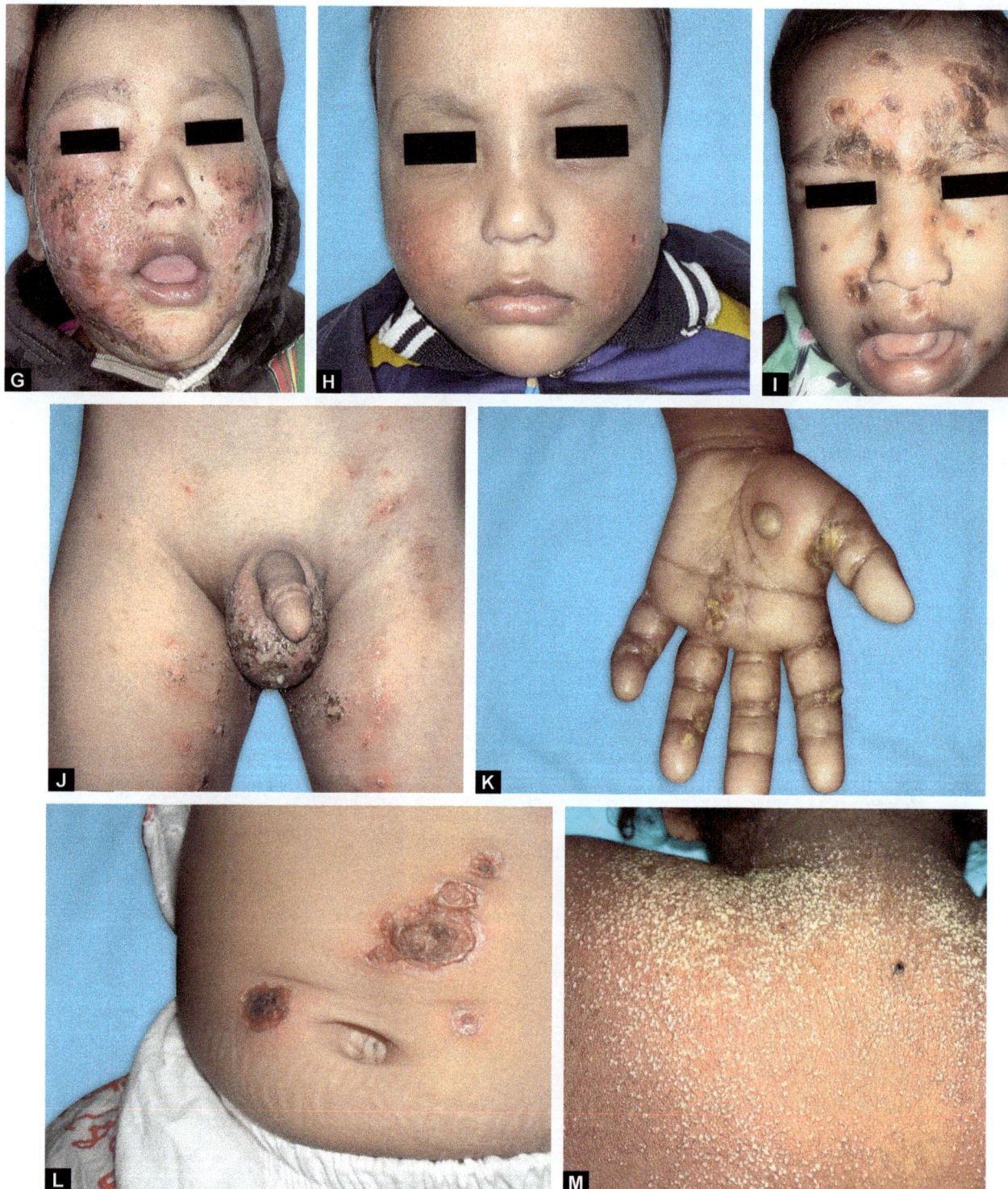

FIGS. 2A TO M: Bullous and nonbullous impetigo; edema, crust, boil, and pustule at different sites due to *Staphylococcus* or streptococcal infections.

Ecthyma

Ecthyma is an ulcerative streptococcal or less commonly staphylococcal pyoderma and healing by scarring (Figs. 3A and B).

Folliculitis (Figs. 4A to D)

- This is the infection of hair follicles caused by mainly *S. aureus*, followed by gram-negative bacteria.
- Usually superficial, but occasionally deep infection referred to as sycosis centered on hair follicles. Here, tender erythematous papulonodule often with a center pustule is seen.

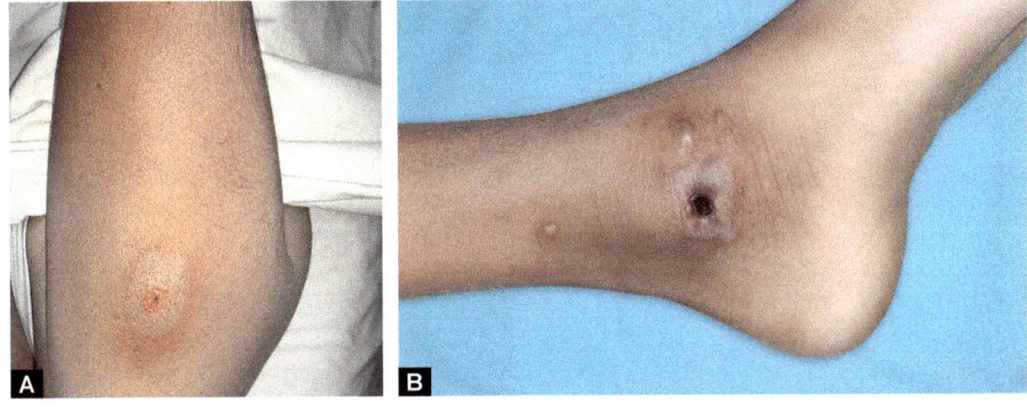

FIGS. 3A AND B: Ulcerative pyoderma—ecthyma.

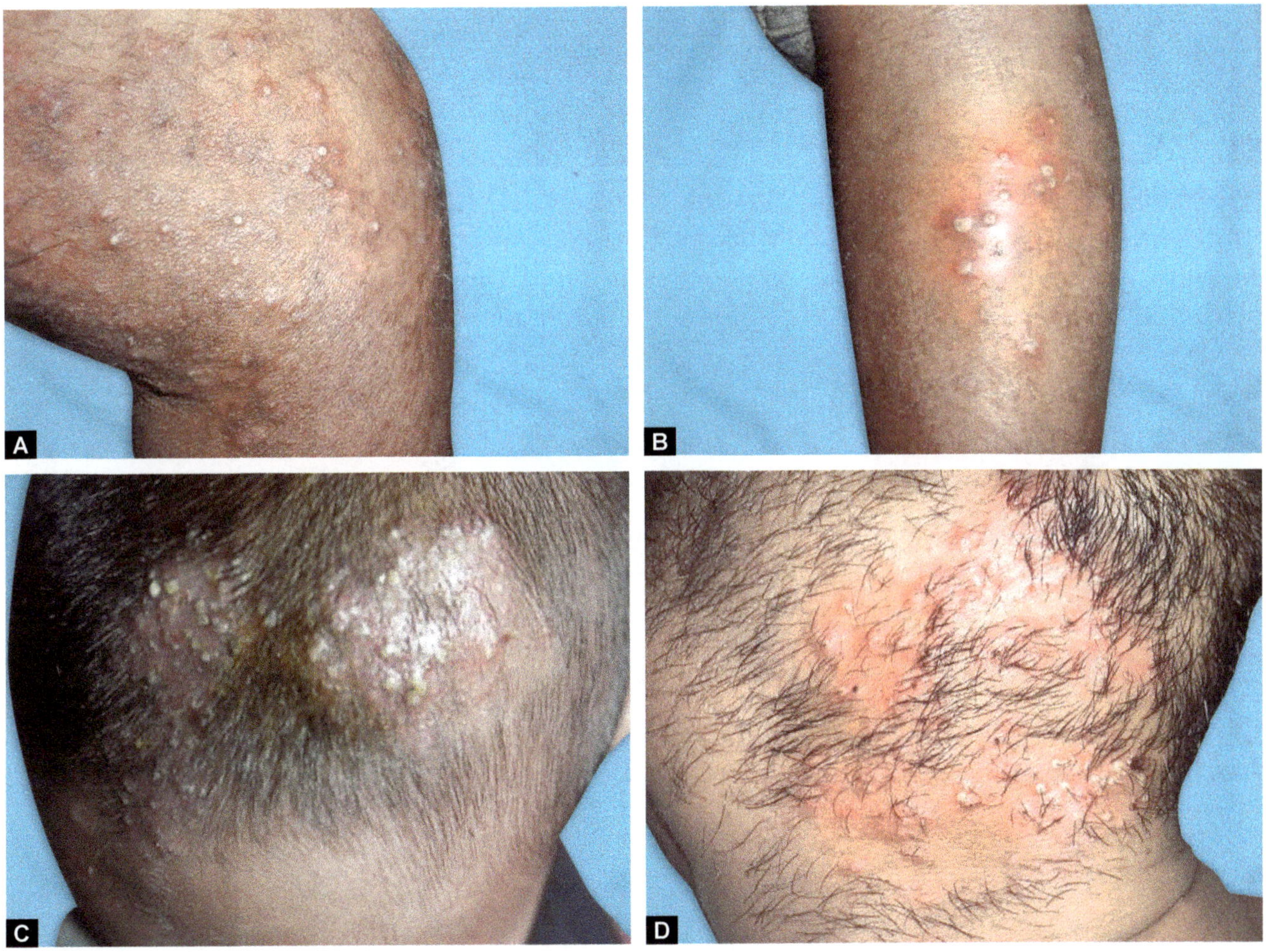

FIGS. 4A TO D: Infection of hair follicle resulted in folliculitis.

Medical Prescription

Topical and systemic antibacterial with or without topical corticosteroid (as an anti-inflammatory). Treatment of primary cause, if exists.

Furuncles (Figs. 5A and B)

An acute, round, circumscribed, and perifollicular (single hair follicle) staphylococcal abscess that generally ends in central suppuration.

Carbuncles

Multiple, acute, rounded, circumscribed, and group of perifollicular (multiple hair follicles) staphylococcal abscess with involvement of multiple and adjacent follicles **(Figs. 6A and B)**.

Abscess

An abscess is a localized collection of pus in tissue, organ, or confined spaces usually because of infection **(Figs. 7 to 9)**.

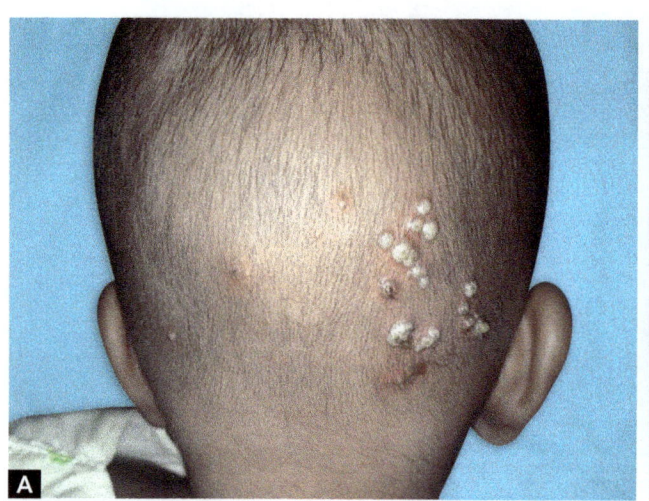

FIGS. 5A AND B: Furuncles.

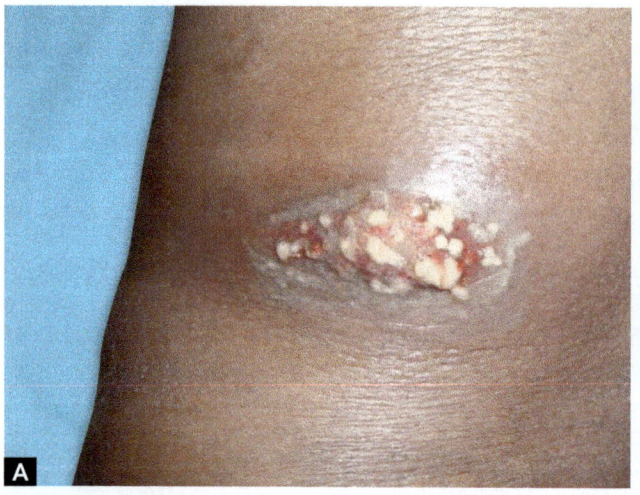
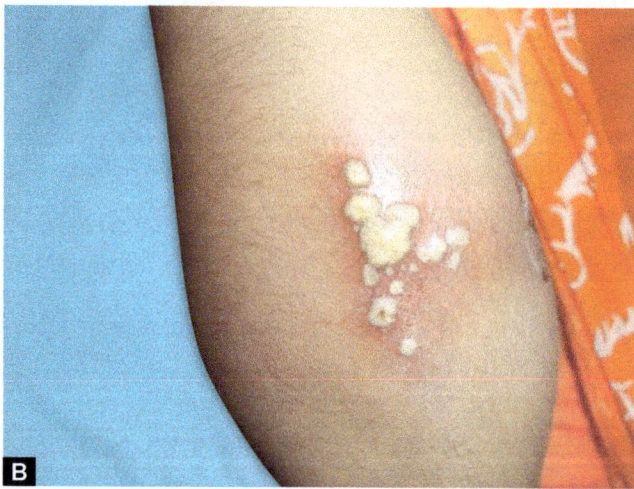

FIGS. 6A AND B: Multiple groups of perifollicular abscesses.

CHAPTER 12 Cutaneous Manifestation of Bacterial, Viral, Protozoal, Worm, Fungal Infection, and Other...

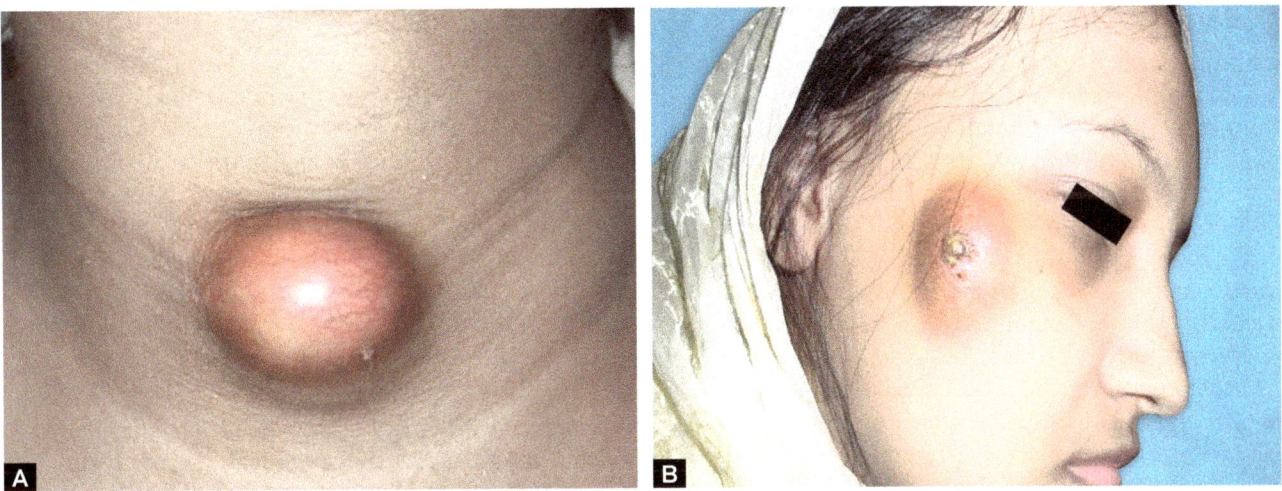

FIGS. 7A AND B: Tuberculous (TB) abscess and sterile abscess (cystic acne).

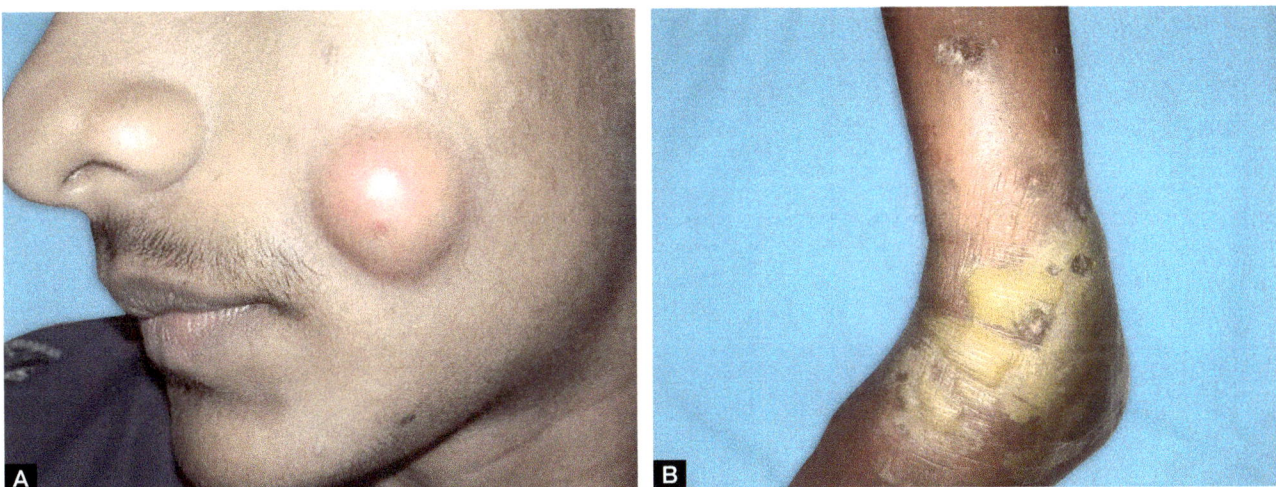

FIGS. 8A AND B: Sterile abscess (acne) and *Staphylococcus* abscess.

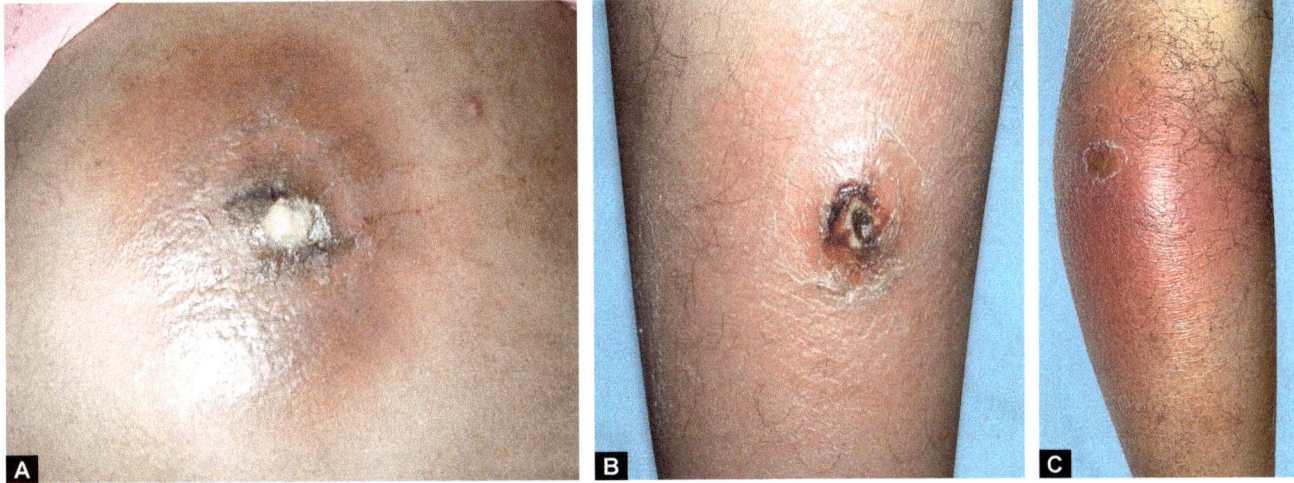

FIGS. 9A TO C: Staphylococcal cellulitis, abscess and ulcer.

Pyogenic Paronychia

Acute or chronic tender and painful swelling of the tissues around the nail that at first will be red and pustular, caused by an abscess in the nailfold and in chronic or recurrent cases, horizontal ridges with nail growth retardation occurs **(Figs. 10 and 11)**.

Mechanical damages of nailfold area (separation of the eponychium/cuticle from the nail plate) are the primary predisposing factor for these cases. It may be due to external or internal injury (by nail plate) of nailfold.

Streptococcus aureus, Streptococcus pyogenes, Pseudomonas species, *Proteus* species, and anaerobes, or *Candida albicans* cause infection in an open area resulting in acute abscess formation or erythema or chronic swelling.

Medical Prescription

- Protection against trauma. For this, work with precautions. Rapidness of work should be avoided.
- Rubber or plastic gloves over cotton gloves should be used when hands are placed in water.
- Acute inflamed pyogenic abscess should be incised and drained.
- A broad-spectrum antibiotic, if possible, according to culture and sensitivity report should be preferred.
- Oral antifungal, if associated with *Candida* infection.

Erysipelas (Figs. 12 and 13)

It is an acute β-hemolytic group A streptococcal infection of the skin involving the superficial dermal lymphatics. Group B *Streptococcus* is often responsible in the newborn

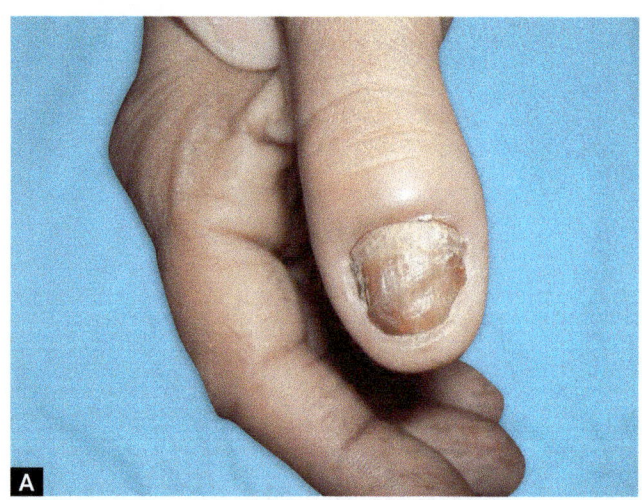 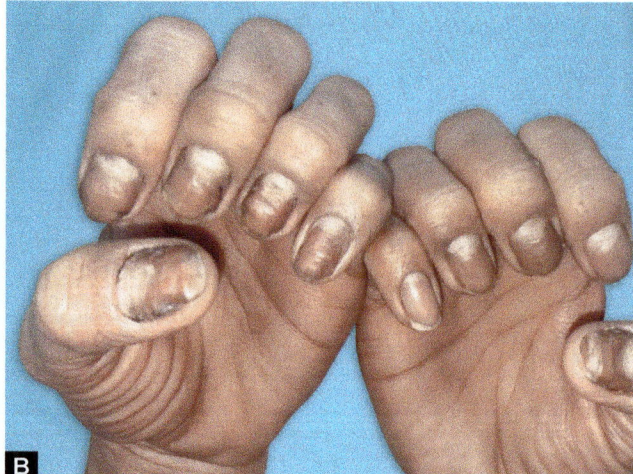

FIGS. 10A AND B: Chronic paronychia due to repeat injury of nailfold with defective nail.

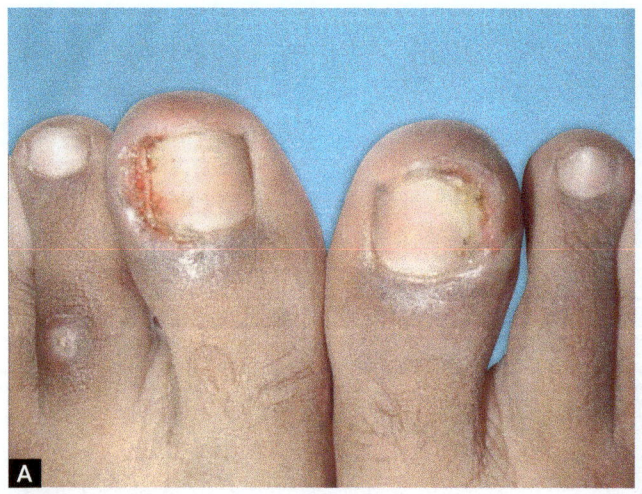 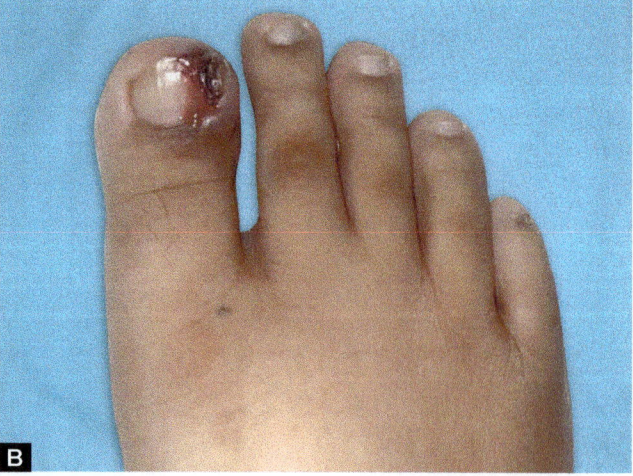

FIGS. 11A AND B: Acute paronychia.

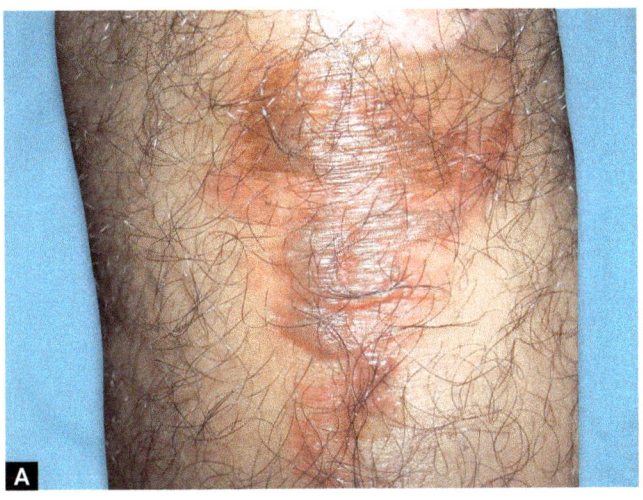
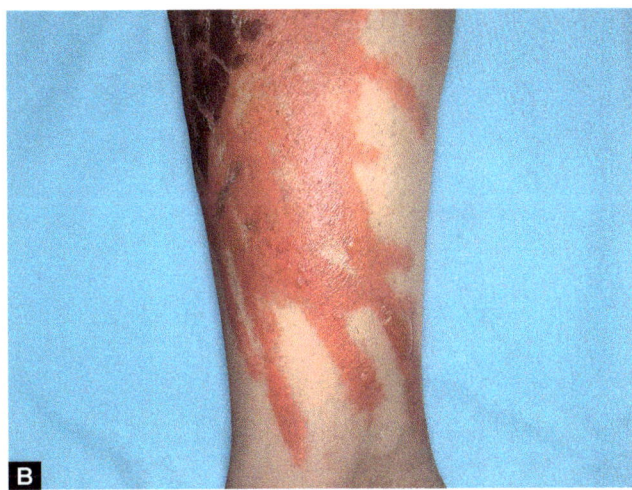

FIGS. 12A AND B: Erysipelas.

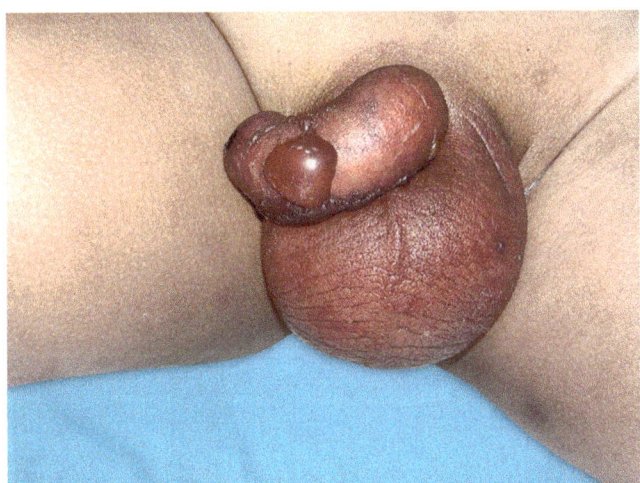

FIG. 13: Erysipelas.

and may be the cause of abdominal or perineal erysipelas in postpartum women.

The skin lesions may vary from transient hyperemia followed by slight desquamation to intense inflammation with vesicles or bullae.

Systemic penicillin is rapidly effective and improvement occurs usually in 24–48 hours, but resolution of the lesion may require several days. Vigorous treatment with antibiotics should be continued for at least 10 days.

Cellulitis (Figs. 14A and B)

It refers to infection of deep dermis and subcutaneous fat. On the leg, xerosis cutis, tinea pedis, and trauma are the common portal of entry.

Mild local erythema and tenderness, malaise, fever, and chills may be present. The erythema rapidly becomes intense and spreads. The area may be infiltrated and pit on pressure. The central part may become nodular and surrounded by vesicle that ruptures and discharges pus and necrotic materials. Lymphatic spread, gangrene, metastatic abscesses, and severe sepsis may follow.

Necrotizing Fasciitis (Figs. 15A to D)

- Necrotizing fasciitis is acute necrotizing infection involving the fascia. Redness, pain, and edema quickly progress to central patches of dusky blue discoloration, with or without serosanguineous blisters usually followed by surgery or perforating trauma or may occur de novo. Anesthesia of the involved skin is characteristic. By the 4th or 5th day, these purple areas become gangrenous.
- Causative species include β-hemolytic streptococci, hemolytic *Staphylococcus*, coliform, enterococci, *Pseudomonas*, and bacteroides.
- Both aerobic and anaerobic bacteria should be taken.

Medical Prescription

- Early surgical debridement
- Appropriate intravenous antibiotic with full coverage or according to culture sensitivity report
- Poor prognostic factors—over 50 years, diabetes mellitus (DM), atherosclerosis, delay in diagnosis >7 days, infection near to trunk, and on surgical intervention

Erythrasma (Figs. 16A and B)

- Sharply delineated, dry, brown, and slightly scaling patches occurring in the intertriginous areas, especially axillae, genitocrural creases and webs between third and fourth or fourth and fifth toe, intergluteal cleft, perianal skin, and inframammary areas. Vulvar mucosa may also be affected.

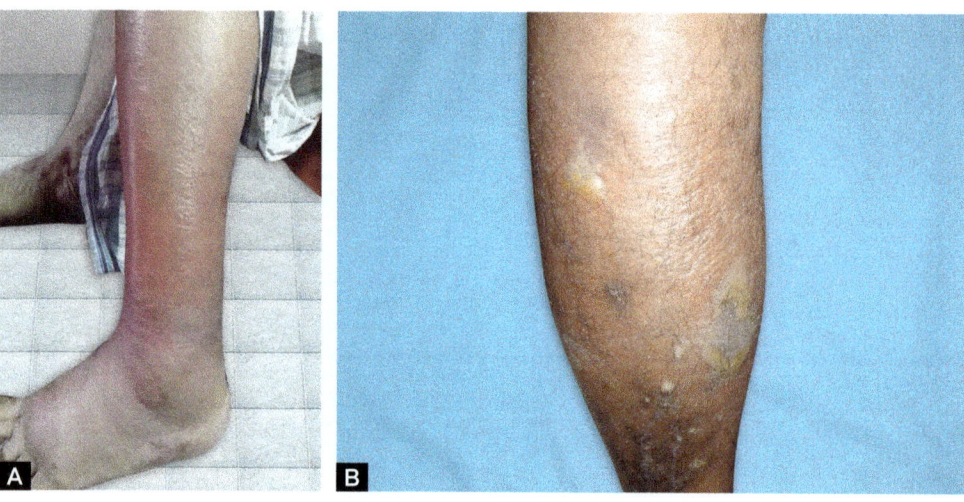

FIGS. 14A AND B: Cellulitis.

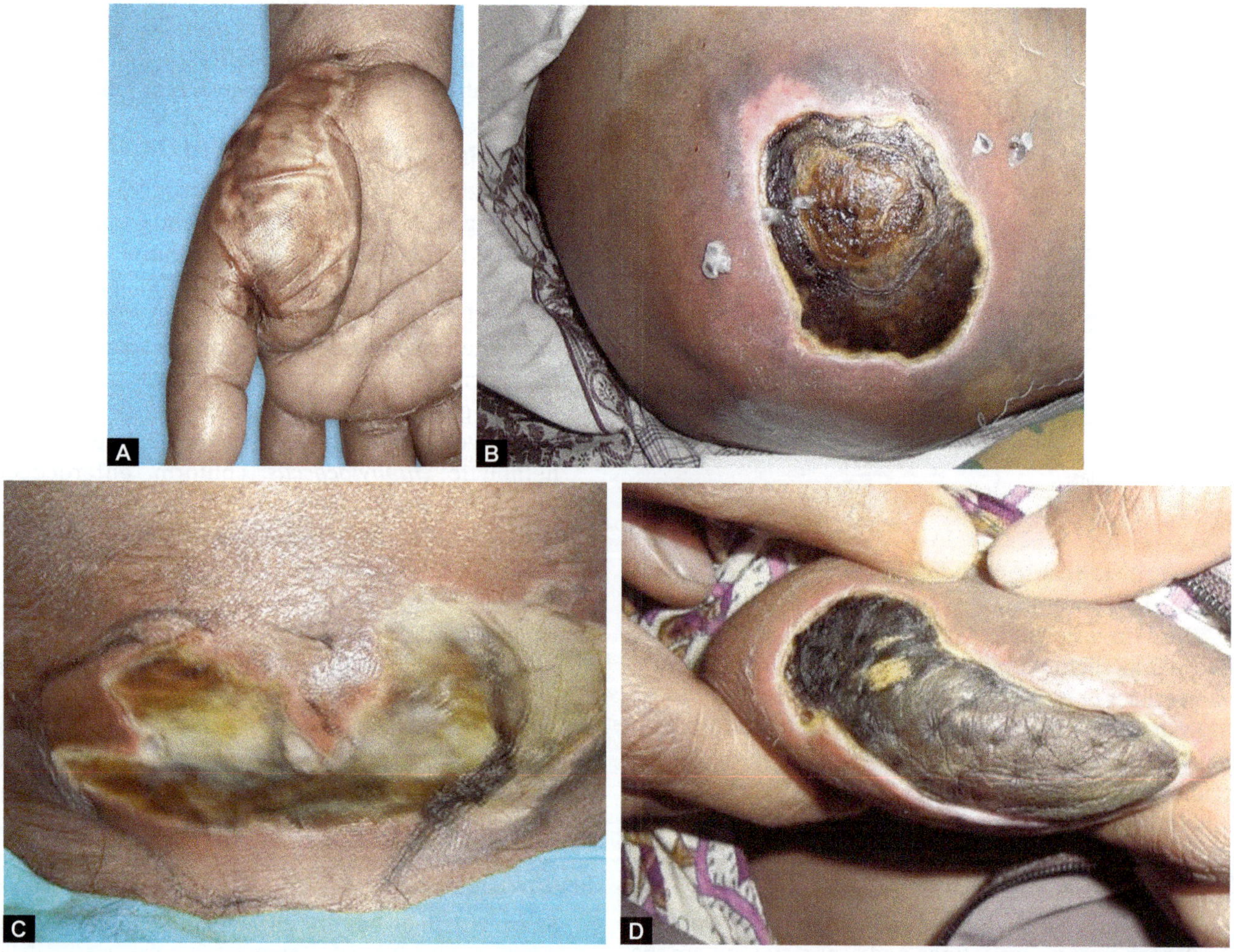

FIGS. 15A TO D: Necrotizing fasciitis.

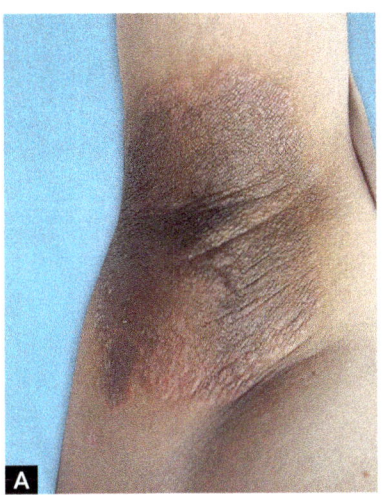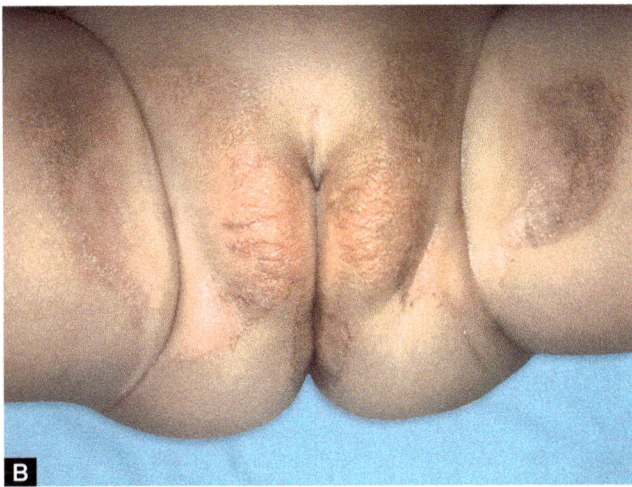

FIGS. 16A AND B: Erythrasma.

- It is caused by the diphtheroid *Corynebacterium minutissimum*.
- Under Wood's lamp, affected areas show a coral red fluorescence due to presence of porphyrin which is diagnostic.

Medical Prescription
- Topical erythromycin or clindamycin.
- Plus oral erythromycin 250 mg 6 hourly for 14 days or single dose of clarithromycin 1 g is equally effective.

Perianal Dermatitis (Fig. 17)
- Superficial, perianal, and well-demarcated rim of erythema, sometimes fissuring may also be seen. Tender on touch and pain during defecation may lead to fecal retention in affected individuals. It may affect vulvar or penile tissue.
- Group A streptococci are the most common cause; however, *S. aureus* may be the culprit sometimes.

Intertrigo (Figs. 18A to F)
It refers to superficial inflammatory dermatitis in apposition skin surfaces. As a result of friction, sweat, and heat, the affected fold becomes erythematous, macerated, and secondarily infected. There may be erosions, exudation, and fissuring with symptoms of burning and itching. These are most frequently seen in humid weather in obese individuals. Involvement in retroauricular area, folds of upper eyelids, creases of neck, axillae, antecubital area, finger webs, inframammary area, umbilicus, inguinal, perineal, intragluteal areas, toe webs, and popliteal spaces.

Here, secondary infection by bacteria or fungus or both.

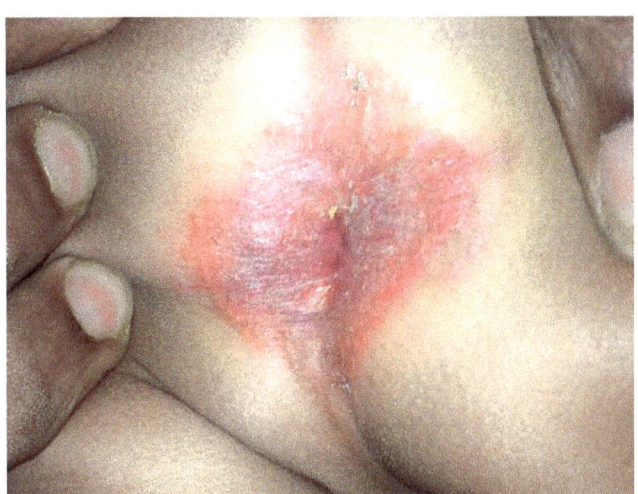

FIG. 17: Perianal dermatitis.

Differential Diagnosis
Seborrheic dermatitis, inverse psoriasis, and erythrasma.

Medical Prescription
Treatment of primary and secondary causes.

Pitted Keratosis (Figs. 19A to D)
- Bacterial infection (*Kytococcus sedentarius*) of the plantar stratum corneum. Weight-bearing part of sole becomes shallow pitted which is asymptomatic.
- Occupation and causes of hyperhidrosis should be noticed.

Medical Prescription
- Topical erythromycin, mupirocin, or clindamycin first-line therapy.

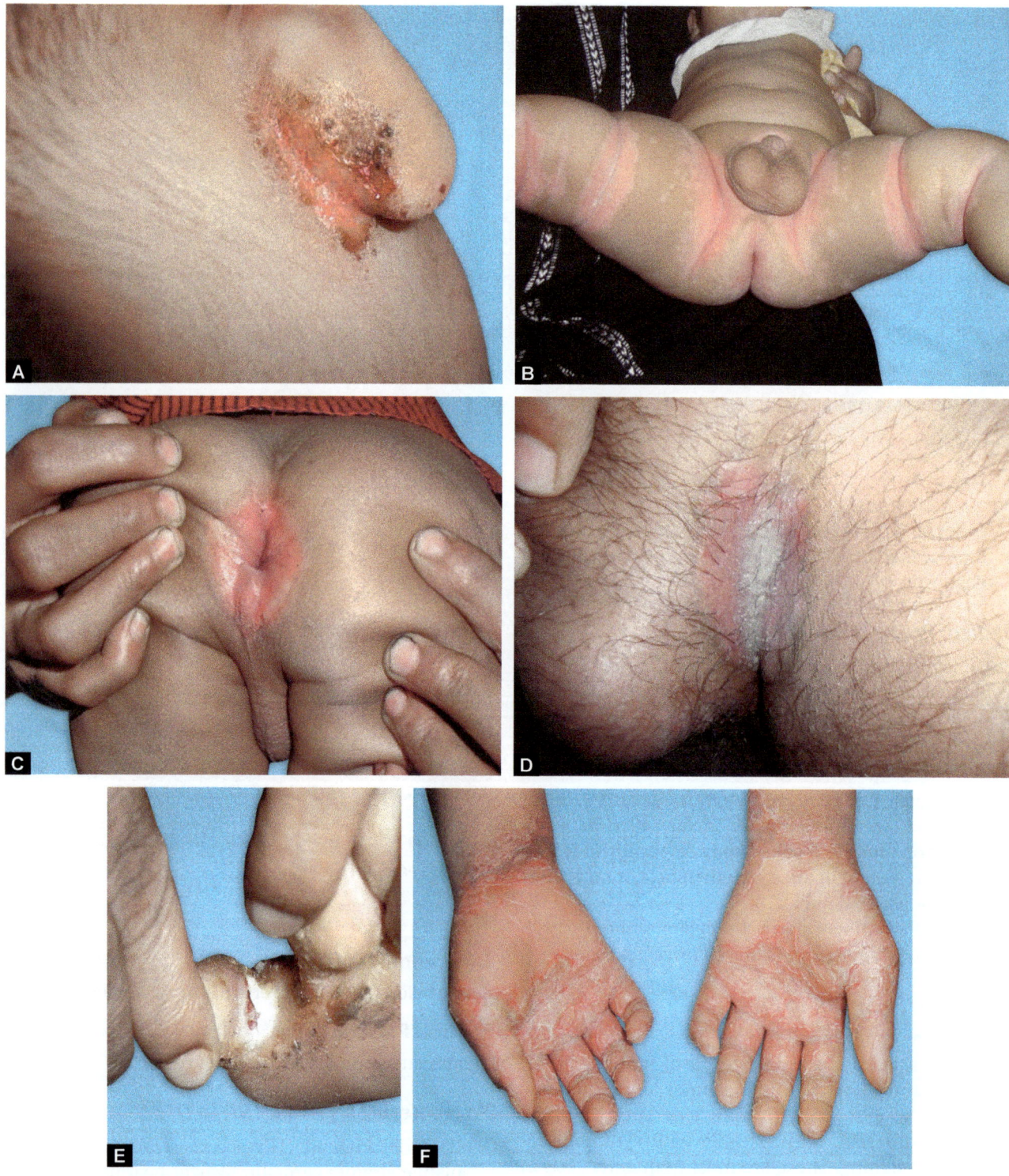

FIGS. 18A TO F: Intertrigo.

- Miconazole, clotrimazole, and Whitfield's ointment are effective alternative.
- Iontophoresis in hyperhidrotic cases is good response with topical medication.
- Botulinum toxin for recurrent cases with hyperhidrosis.

Ecthyma Gangrenosum (Figs. 20A and B)

- *Pseudomonas* (*Pseudomonas aeruginosa*) infection of debilitated persons who may be suffering from leukemia, burned patient, patient developing

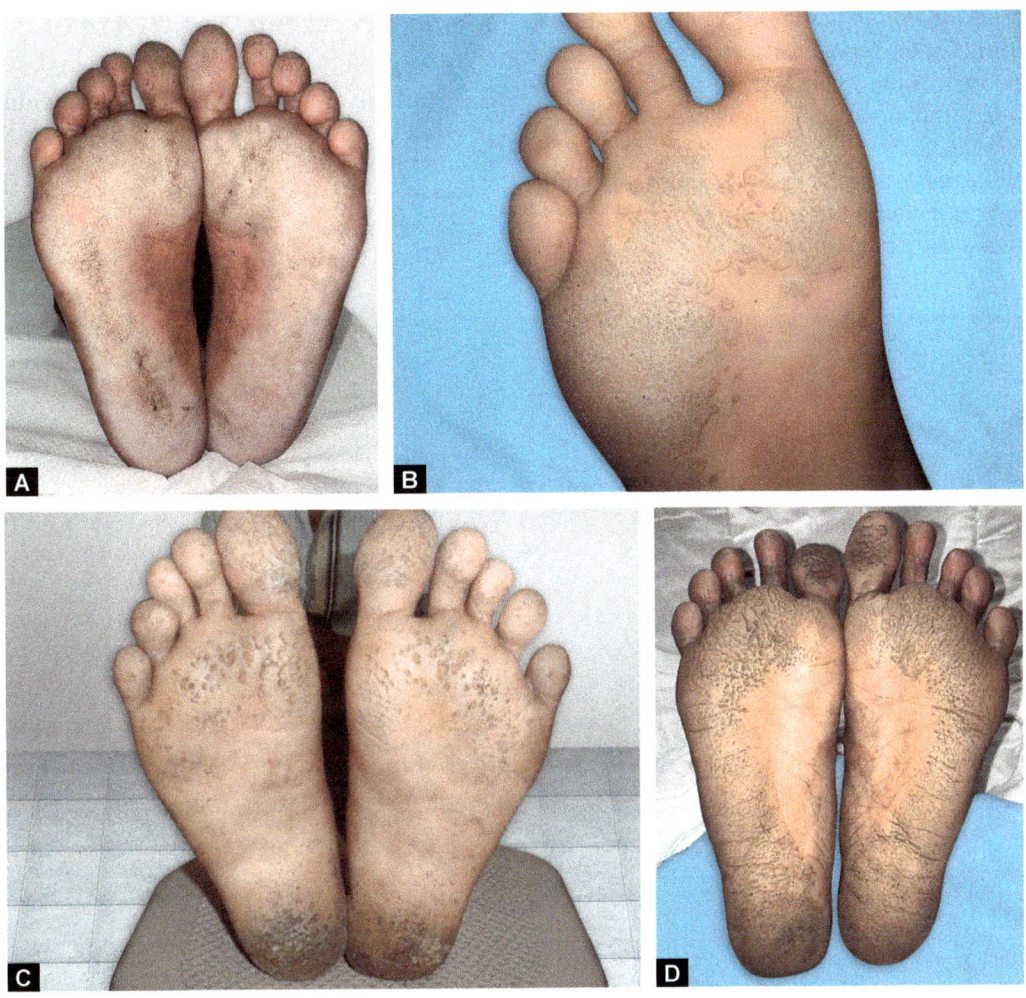

FIGS. 19A TO D: Pitted keratolysis.

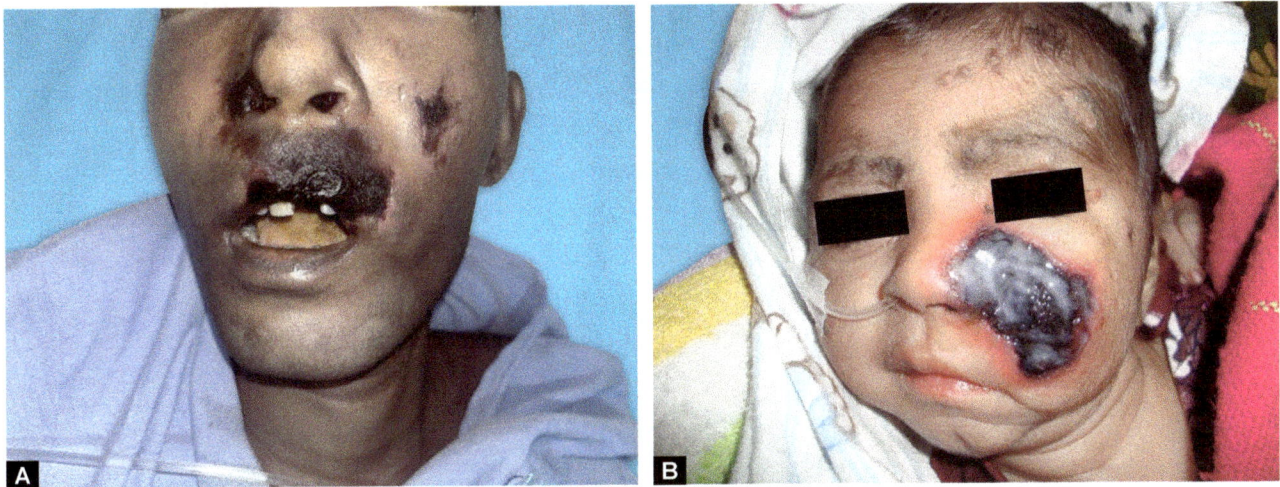

FIGS. 20A AND B: Ecthyma gangrenosum.

pancytopenia or neutropenia, terminal carcinoma, human immunodeficiency virus-acquired immunodeficiency syndrome (HIV-AIDS) patient, rarely healthy individual, and other severe chronic disease patients.

- Opalescent, tense vesicles or pustules quickly become hemorrhagic and violaceous and rupture and become round ulcers with necrotic black center.

Meningococcemia (Figs. 21A to G)

- Fever, chills, hypotension, and meningitis are the common presentation of acute meningococcemia. Half to two-thirds of patients develop petechial eruption, most frequently on extremities and trunk which may progress to ecchymosis, bullous hemorrhagic lesions, and ischemic necrosis **(Fig. 22)**. Oral and conjunctival mucous membrane may be affected.

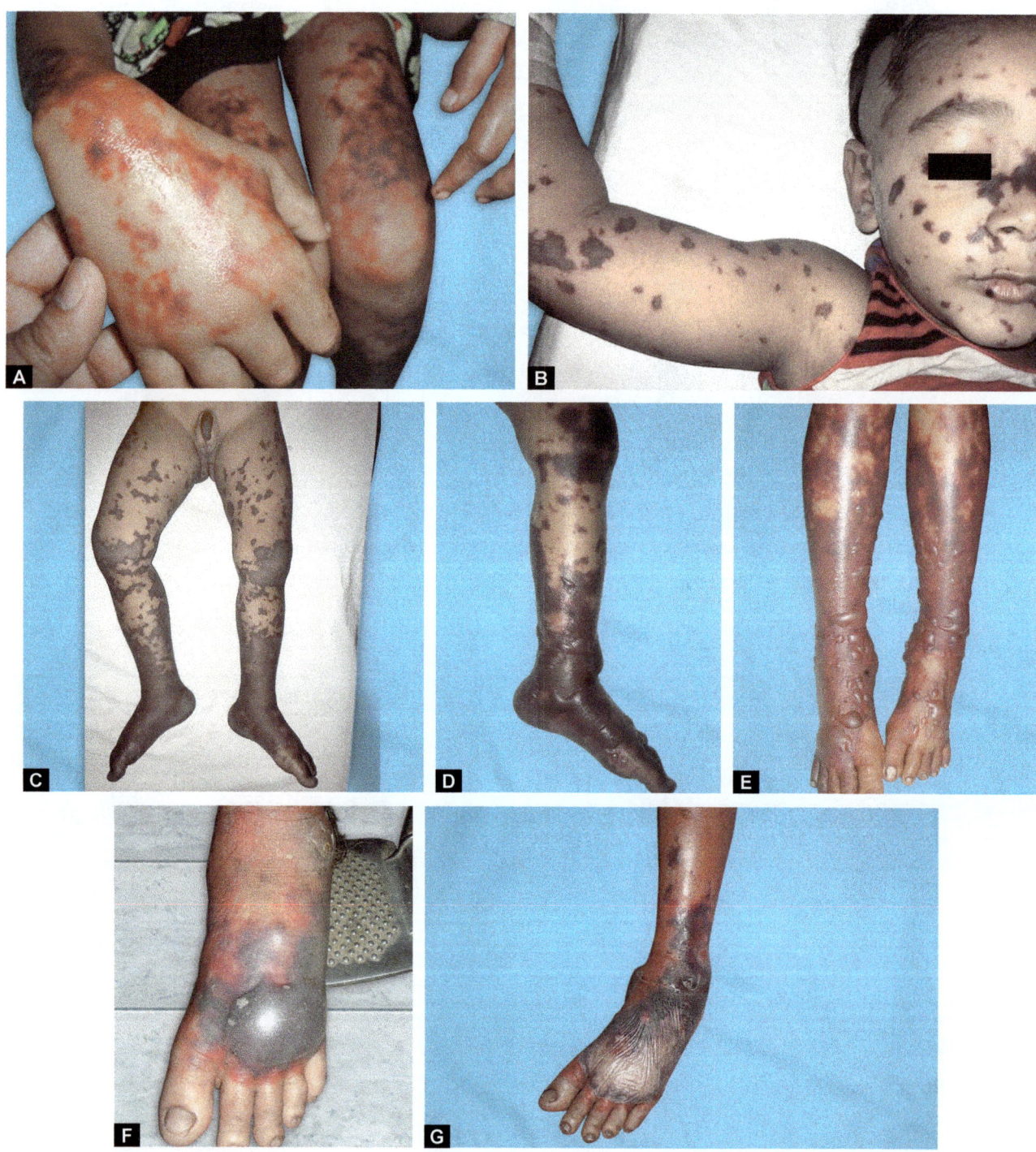

FIGS. 21A TO G: Meningococcemia.

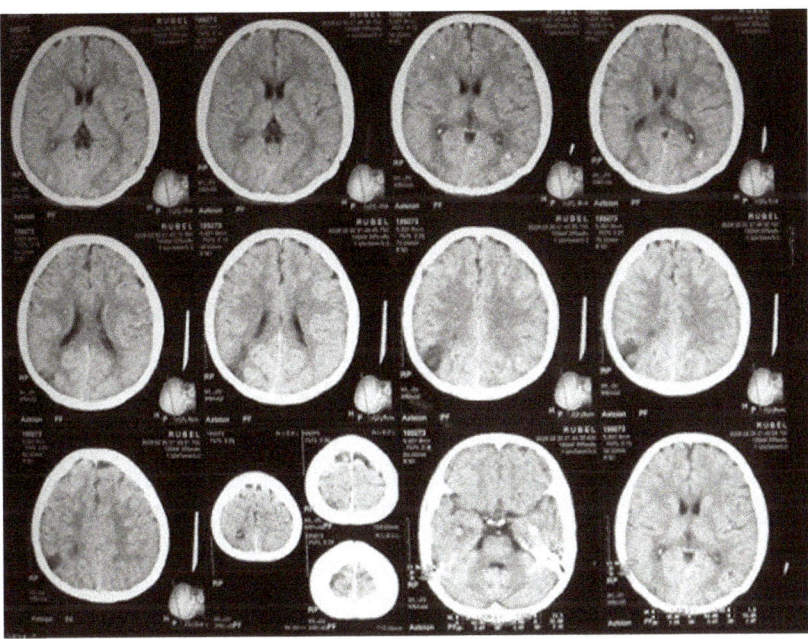

FIG. 22: Infarction on computed tomography (CT) of brain.

- Caused by gram-negative diplococcus *Neisseria meningitidis*.
- Intravenous (IV) ceftriaxone 2 g twice daily for 7 days is the treatment of choice. One dose of ciprofloxacin 500 mg is given after initial course of antibiotic to clear nasal carriage.

Staphylococcal Scalded Skin Syndrome (Figs. 23A to D)

- Staphylococcal scalded skin syndrome (SSSS) is a generalized, confluent, and superficially exfoliative disease, occurring most frequently in neonates and children under 5 years. It may occur in adults with immunosuppression.
- Usually begins with skin redness and tenderness initially in periorificial area, intertriginous areas such as neck, groin, axillae, and inguinal folds.
- Fever is variable. Peeling usually starts from around mouth, eye, and nose then gradually other areas' involvement occur. The areas of red eventually slough with large sheets sparing palms, soles, and mucous membrane.
- Nikolsky sign is positive.
- Group 2 *S. aureus* (type 71 or 55) is the causative agent in most cases. Exfoliative toxins such as A, B, and D cleave desmoglein-1, thus produces this type of cleavage in skin-sparing mucous membrane.

Chancroid (Figs. 24A and B)

- Sexually transmitted infection caused by the gram-negative bacillus *Haemophilus ducreyi* (the Ducrey's bacillus). One or more tender ulcers on the genitalia and painful inguinal lymphadenitis that may be suppurate.
- An inflammatory macule or pustule lasting 1–5 days or rarely as long as 2 weeks after sexual intercourse on distal penis, perianal area in men, and on vulva, cervix, and perianal area on female.
- Pustule ruptures with formation of a ragged ulcer that is soft and becomes punched out and covered by purulent dirty exudates. The ulcers bleed easily and are very tender.
- Diagnosis is made by exclusion of differential diagnosis such as chancre, herpes progenitalis, fixed drug eruption, and granuloma inguinale (GI).
- Smear and culture may be done for identification of organisms.

Medical Prescription

- The treatment of choice is azithromycin 1 g orally single dose or ceftriaxone 250 mg intramuscular single dose.
- Erythromycin 500 mg four times a day or ciprofloxacin 500 mg twice a day for 3 days is also recommended.

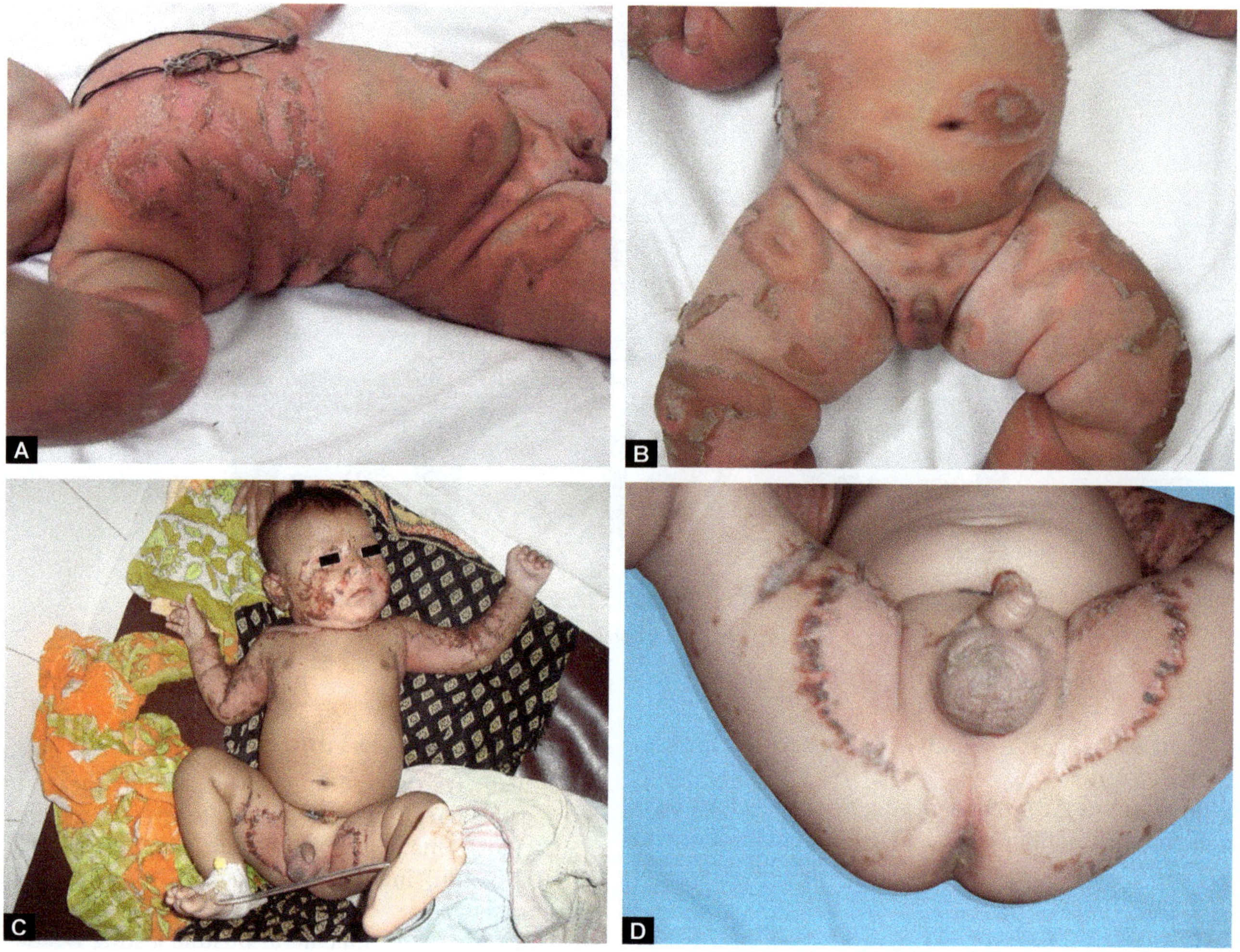

110 | CHAPTER 12 Cutaneous Manifestation of Bacterial, Viral, Protozoal, Worm, Fungal Infection, and Other...

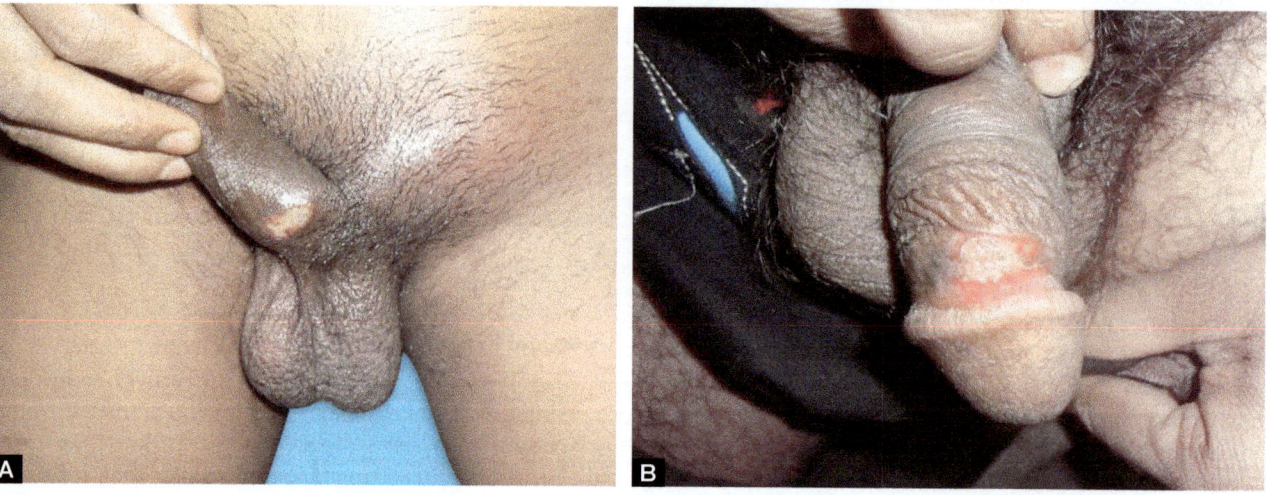

FIGS. 23A TO D: Staphylococcal scalded skin syndrome (SSSS).

FIGS. 24A AND B: Chancroid.

Gonorrhea (Figs. 25A to D)

- *Gonococcus* (*Neisseria gonorrhoeae*) infects mucous membrane lined by columnar epithelium (lower genitourinary tract, anus, rectum, and pharynx).
- Acquired primarily by sexual contact.
- *Incubation period*: 2–5 days.

Clinical Features

- *Genitalia*:
  - *Men*: Acute urethritis in men characterized by purulent urethral discharge ranging from scanty, clear to purulent and copious with erythematous, edematous meatus.
  - *Women*: Periurethral edema and urethritis. Purulent discharge from cervix but scanty. In prepubescent females, vulvovaginitis and Bartholin gland abscess are seen. In neonates, vaginal discharge profuses due to vaginal columnar epithelial lining.
- *Anorectum*—proctitis with pain and purulent rectal discharge.
- *Pharynx*—due to orogenital sex, pharyngitis occurs.
- *Disseminated gonococcal infection (DGI)* **(Figs. 26A to D)**—hemorrhagic, painful pustules on erythematous base, macules, papules, and vesicles on palms, soles, trunk, limbs, and usually spare the face, scalp, and mouth.
- *Gonococcal arthritis*—usually monoarthritis. Knees and ankles involvement.
- *Neonates*—conjunctivitis, swollen eyelids, severe hyperemia, chemosis, and profuse purulent discharge. Corneal ulcer and perforation may occur. Genital discharge may present.

Doctor's Prescription

- Gram-stain—gram-negative intracellular diplococcus presents in polymorphonuclear (PMN) leukocytes.
- Culture—smear from urethra, rectum, cervix, oropharynx, and blood in case of DGI.
- In gonococcal selective media (chocolatized blood agar, Martin–Lewis media, and Thayer–Martin media).

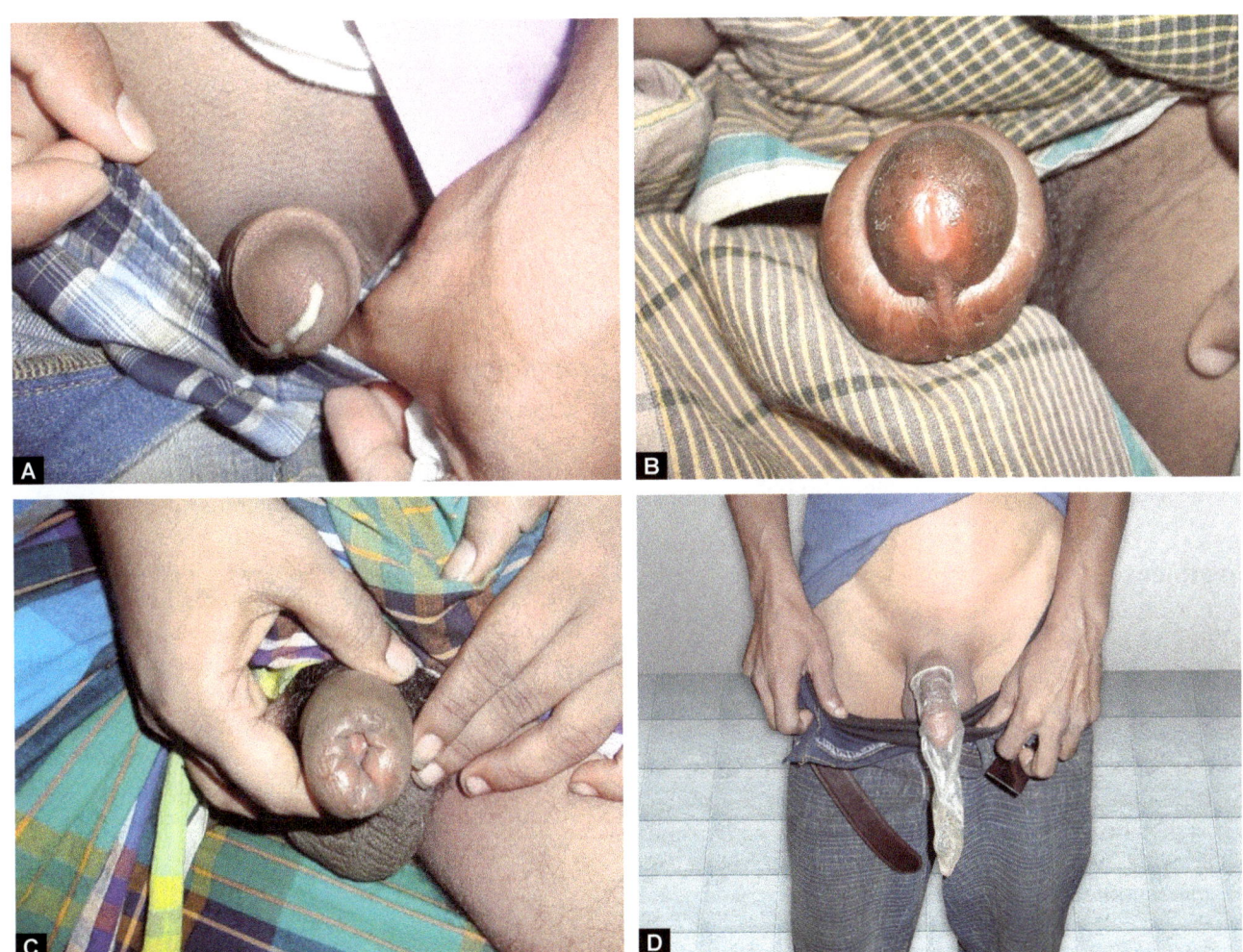

FIGS. 25A TO D: Gonorrhea.

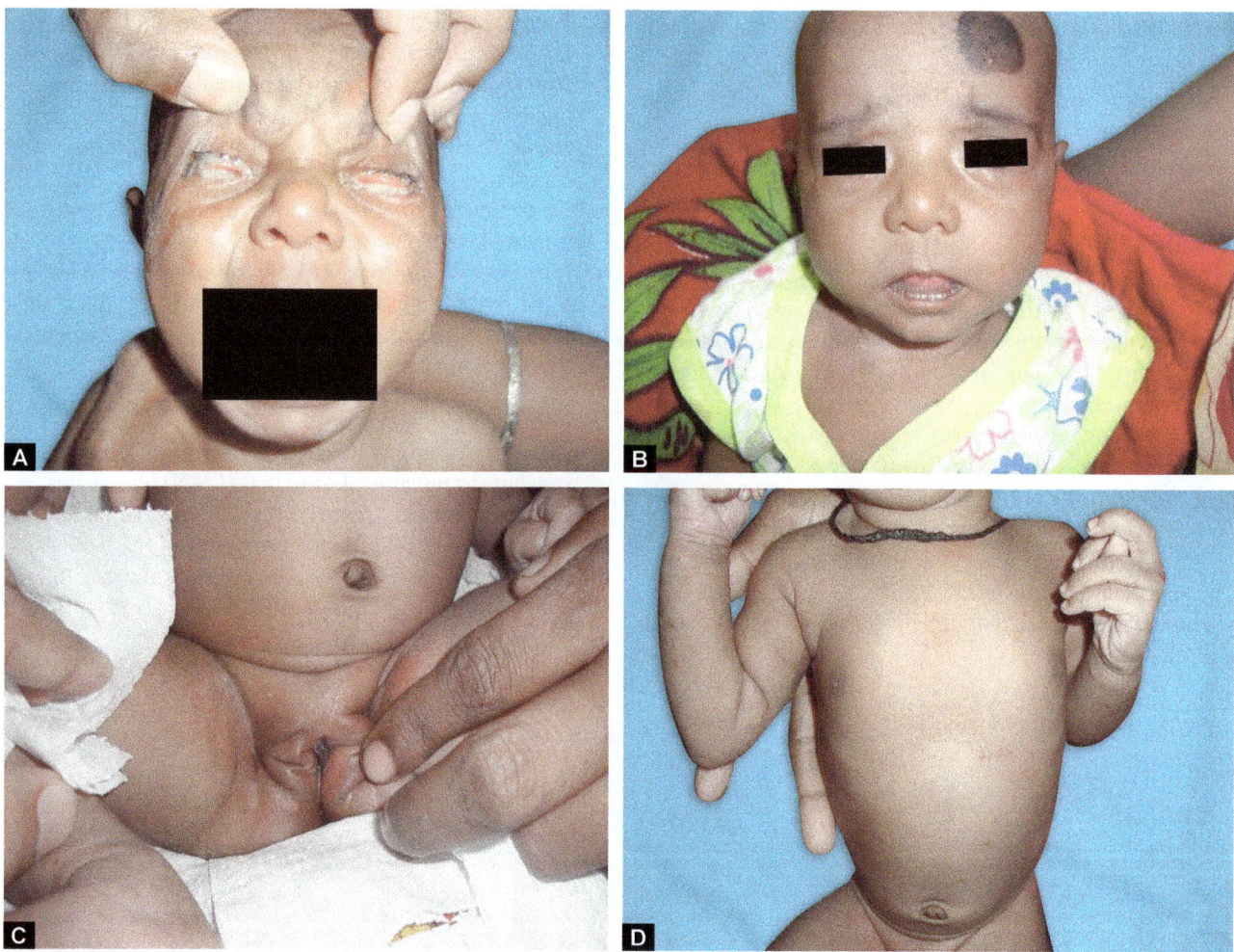

FIGS. 26A TO D: Ophthalmia neonatorum, vaginal discharge, and disseminated gonococcal infection (DGI).

Complications

- *In women*: Bartholin gland abscess, pelvic inflammatory disease (PID), tubal scarring, infertility, ectopic pregnancy, and DGI.
- *In men*: Urethral stricture, infertility, epididymorchitis, orchitis, prostatitis, and prostatic abscess.

Treatment

- *Localized uncomplicated gonorrhea*: Single dose intramuscular ceftriaxone 500 mg plus azithromycin 1 g or oral cefixime 400 mg or oral ofloxacin 400 mg or intramuscular cefotaxime 500 mg or intramuscular cefoxitin 2 g plus oral probenecid 1 g.
- *Penicillin allergy*: Intramuscular spectinomycin 2 g.
- Disseminated gonococcal infection—intramuscular or IV ceftriaxone 1 g daily for 7 days or IV cefotaxime or ceftizone 1 g 8 hourly for 7 days or intramuscular spectinomycin 2 g daily for 7 days.

Granuloma Inguinale (Figs. 27A and B)

- Granuloma inguinale (GI) is mildly contagious, sexually transmitted chronic, granulomatous, and locally destructive disease characterized by progressive, indolent serpiginous ulceration of the groins, pubis, genitalia, and anus.
- Granuloma inguinale begins as a single or multiple subcutaneous nodules which erode through the skin to produce clean, sharply defined painless lesion.
- More than 80% cases show hypertrophic, vegetative granulation tissue, which is soft and bleeds easily.
- Caused by the gram-negative bacterium *Klebsiella granulomatis*.
- Diagnosis is made by clinical findings and exclusion of differential diagnosis—chancre, chancroid, and lymphogranuloma venereum.

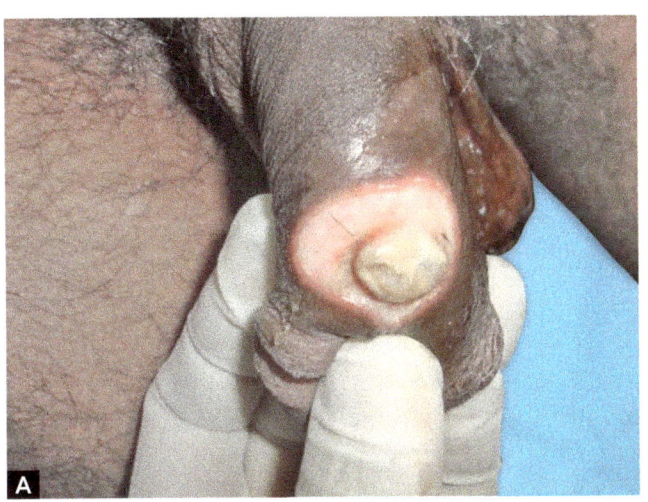
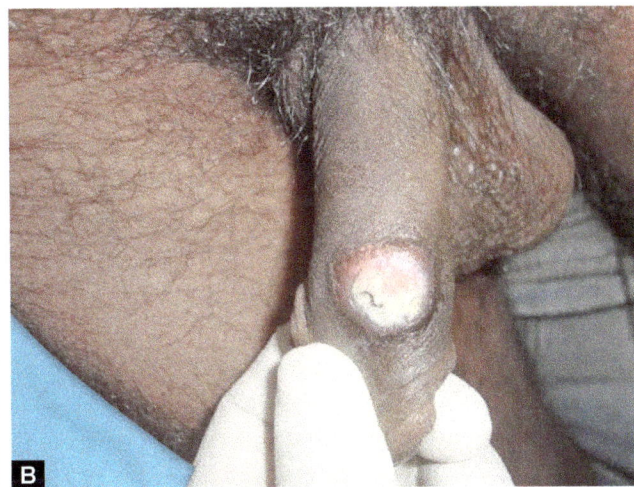

FIGS. 27A AND B: Granuloma inguinale.

Medical Prescription

- Azithromycin 1 g once weekly for 3 weeks is the recommended regimen.
- Doxicap 100 mg, ciprofloxacin 750 mg twice daily, or erythromycin 500 mg four times daily for 21 days is the alternate regimen.

Mycobacterial Diseases

Tuberculosis Verrucosa Cutis (Figs. 28A to F)

- Exogenous inoculation of TB bacilli into the skin of previously sensitized person with strong immunity against *Mycobacterium tuberculosis*.
- Tuberculin test here is strongly positive.
- Lesion begins as a small papule, which becomes hyperkeratotic, resembling a wart. Lesion enlarges by peripheral expansion, with or without central clearing, sometimes reaching several centimeters in diameter.

Doctor's Prescription

By biopsy for histopathological examination.

Medical Prescription

Six months anti-TB regimen.

Lupus Vulgaris (Figs. 29A to F)

- Lupus vulgaris may appear at the site of inoculation, in scrofuloderma scar, or most frequently at the site from the underlying foci by hematogenous dissemination.
- Typically started as a single plaque composed of grouped red-brown papules, which when blanched by diascopic pressure appear pale, brownish yellow, or apple jelly color. Atrophy, ulceration, destruction, scarring, or shrunken of structures such as nose, earlobes, and nasal septum, if involved.

■ Cutaneous Tuberculosis from Endogenous Source by Direct Extension

Scrofuloderma (Fig. 30)

It refers to the tuberculosis of skin by direct extension from an underlying focus of infection. This occurs most frequently over the cervical lymph nodes, but also may occur over bone, joint, and chest wall. Clinically begins as subcutaneous masses which enlarge to form nodules. Suppuration occurs centrally. Lesions may be erythematous or skin color or hyperpigmented. Lesions may drain, forming sinuses, and ulcerate with reddish granulation tissue at the base.

Periorificial Tuberculosis (Fig. 31)

- Cutaneous TB occurs at the mucocutaneous borders of nose, mouth, anus, urinary meatus, vagina, or tongue. It is usually caused by autoinoculation from visceral TB.
- Here, impaired cellular immunity is present.

Hansen's Disease

- Slowly progressive disease characterized by granuloma formation in nerves or skin caused by *Mycobacterium leprae*.
- Spread of leprosy depends on droplet/nasal source of an infected person, susceptible person, and close or intimate contact.
- Incubation period is 4–11 years.
- Degree of immunity is reflected in clinical findings and histological features; the latter range from macrophages containing numerous bacilli in lepromatous leprosy (LL) to granulomatous without organisms in tuberculoid leprosy.

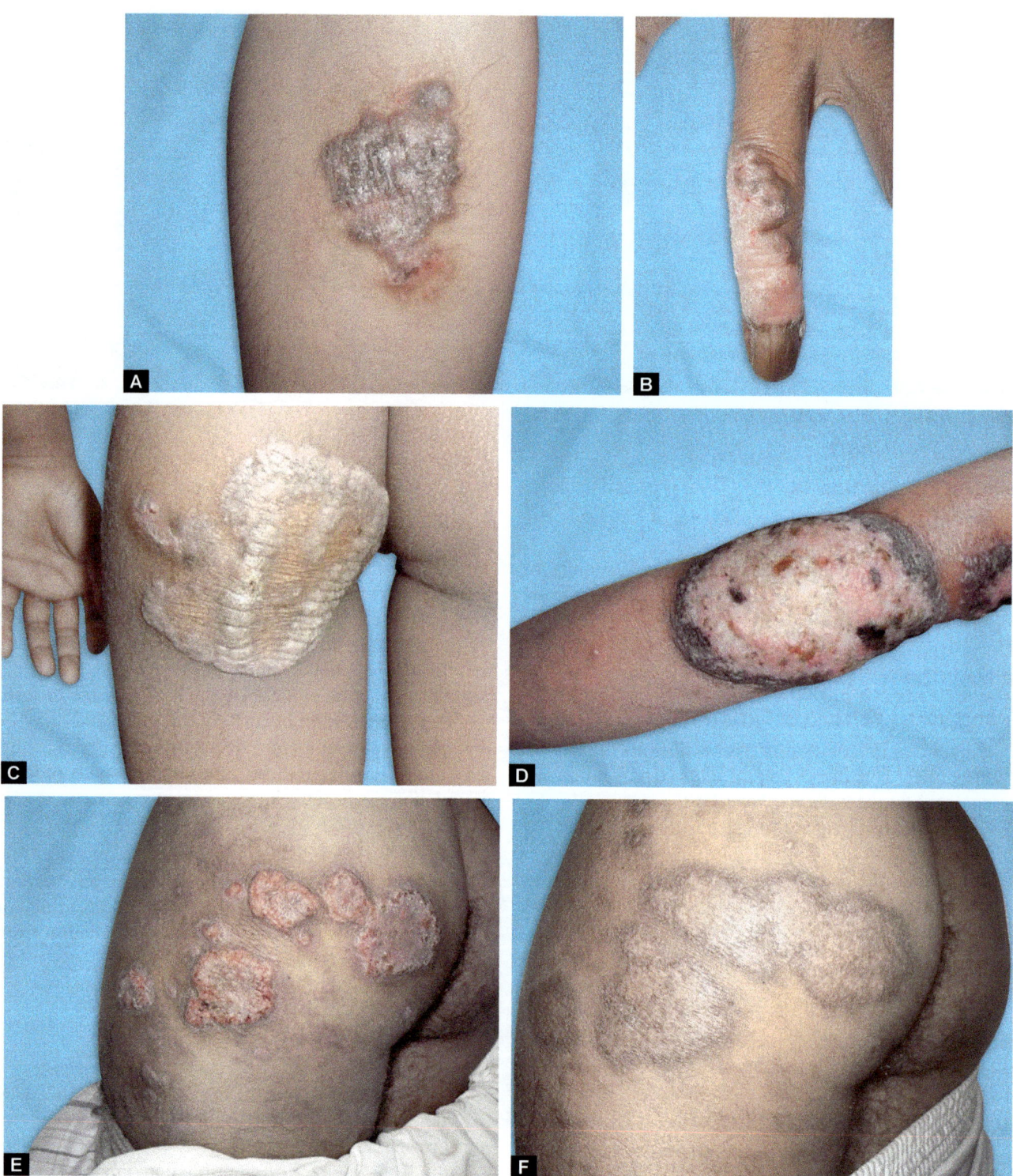

FIGS. 28A TO F: Tuberculosis verrucosa cutis.

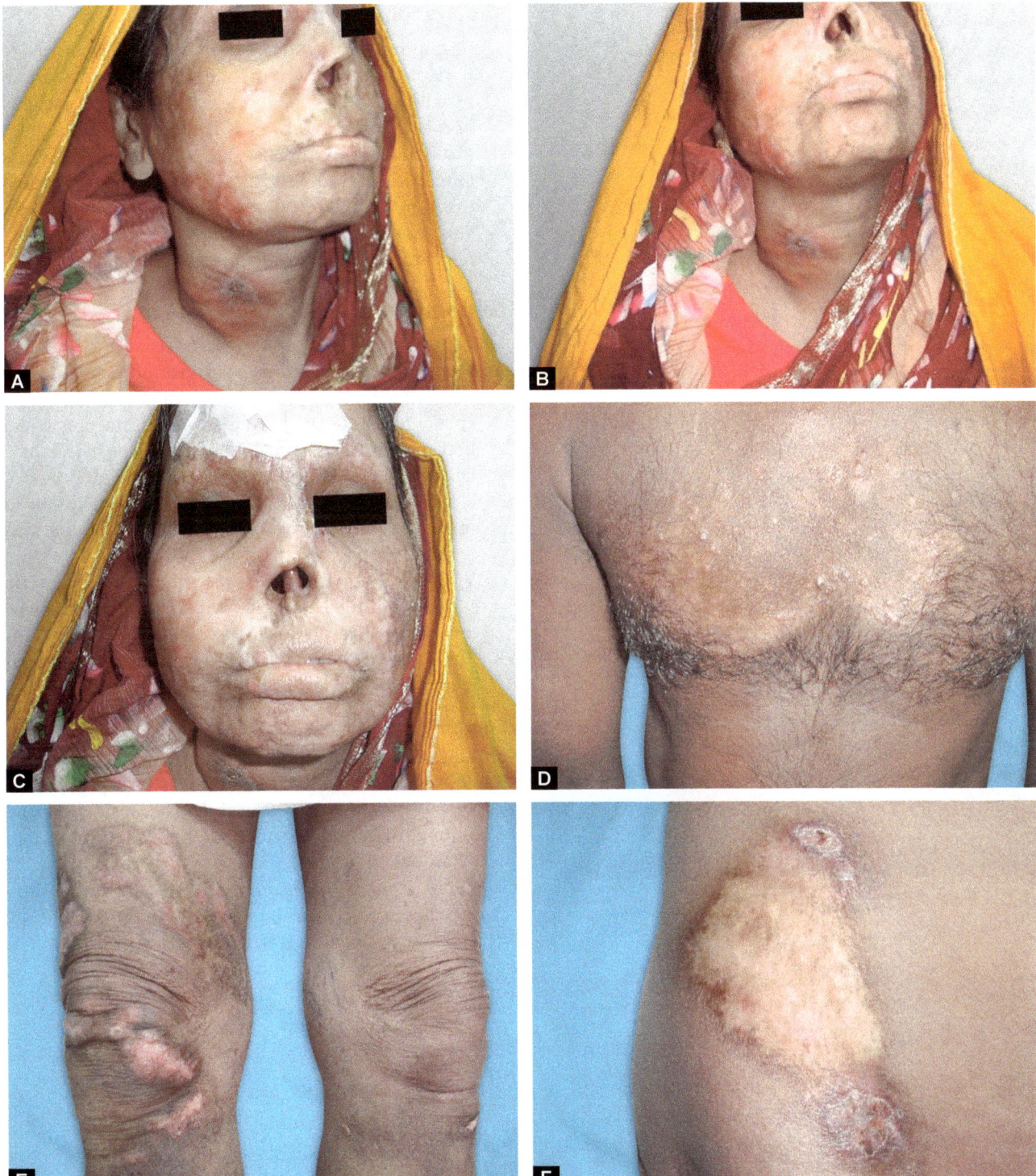

FIGS. 29A TO F: Lupus vulgaris.

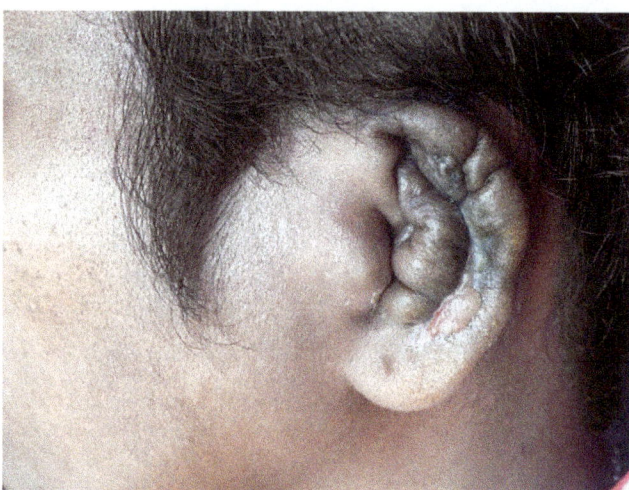

FIG. 30: Scrofuloderma.

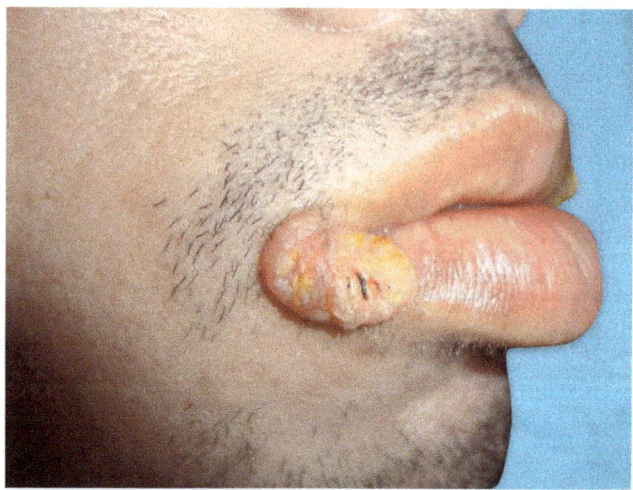

FIG. 31: Periorificial tuberculosis.

Tuberculoid Leprosy (Figs. 32A to F)

- Asymptomatic one to five lesions are characterized by hypopigmented or erythematous plaques which are usually dry, scaly, and hairless with a sharply elevated border that slopes down to a flattened atrophic center.
- A tuberculoid lesion is anesthetic or hypesthetic and anhidrotic and superficial peripheral nerves proximal to lesion are enlarge, tender, or both.
- The greater auricular nerve and superficial peroneal nerve may be visible and enlarged (**Figs. 33A and B**).

Lepromatous Leprosy (Figs. 34A to L)

- Lepromatous leprosy may begin as such or develop after indeterminate leprosy or from downgrading of borderline leprosy. Early presentations are ill-defined, small, and symmetrically distributed macules which become diffuse, plaque, and nodular type of lesions.
- Diffuse type is characterized by the development of a diffuse infiltration on face, especially the forehead, madarosis, and waxy shiny appearance of the skin. Sometimes, it is described as varnished.
- Visceral involvement is restricted mostly to the reticoendothelial system, which despite extensive involvement rarely produces symptoms or findings. Testicular atrophy with loss of androgens can result gynecomastia (**Fig. 35**) or premature osteoporosis.

Lepra Reactions

Immunologically mediated inflammatory states, occurring spontaneously or after initiation of antileprosy drugs.
- *Lepra Type 1 reactions*: Preexisting skin lesions become acutely inflamed, associated with edema and pain (**Figs. 34C, E, and H**).
- *Lepra Type 2 reaction*: Painful skin red nodule (erythema nodosum leprosum) arising superficially and deeply (**Figs. 34A, B, G, I and K, and 36**).

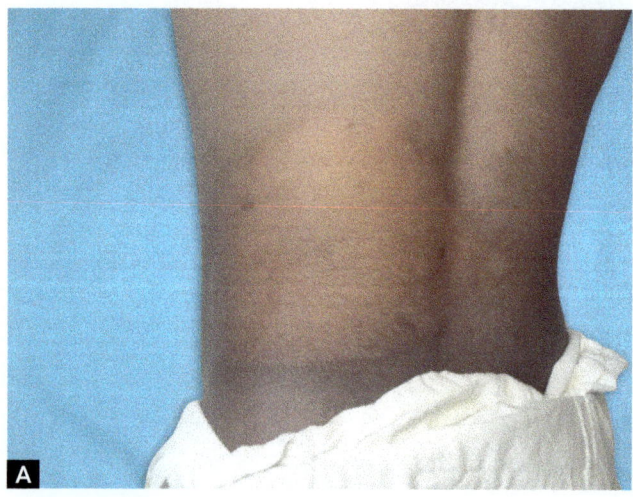

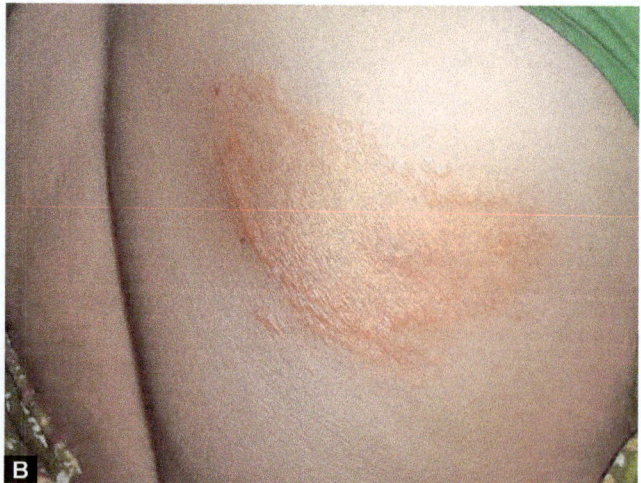

FIGS. 32A TO F: *Continued*

CHAPTER 12 Cutaneous Manifestation of Bacterial, Viral, Protozoal, Worm, Fungal Infection, and Other...

Continued

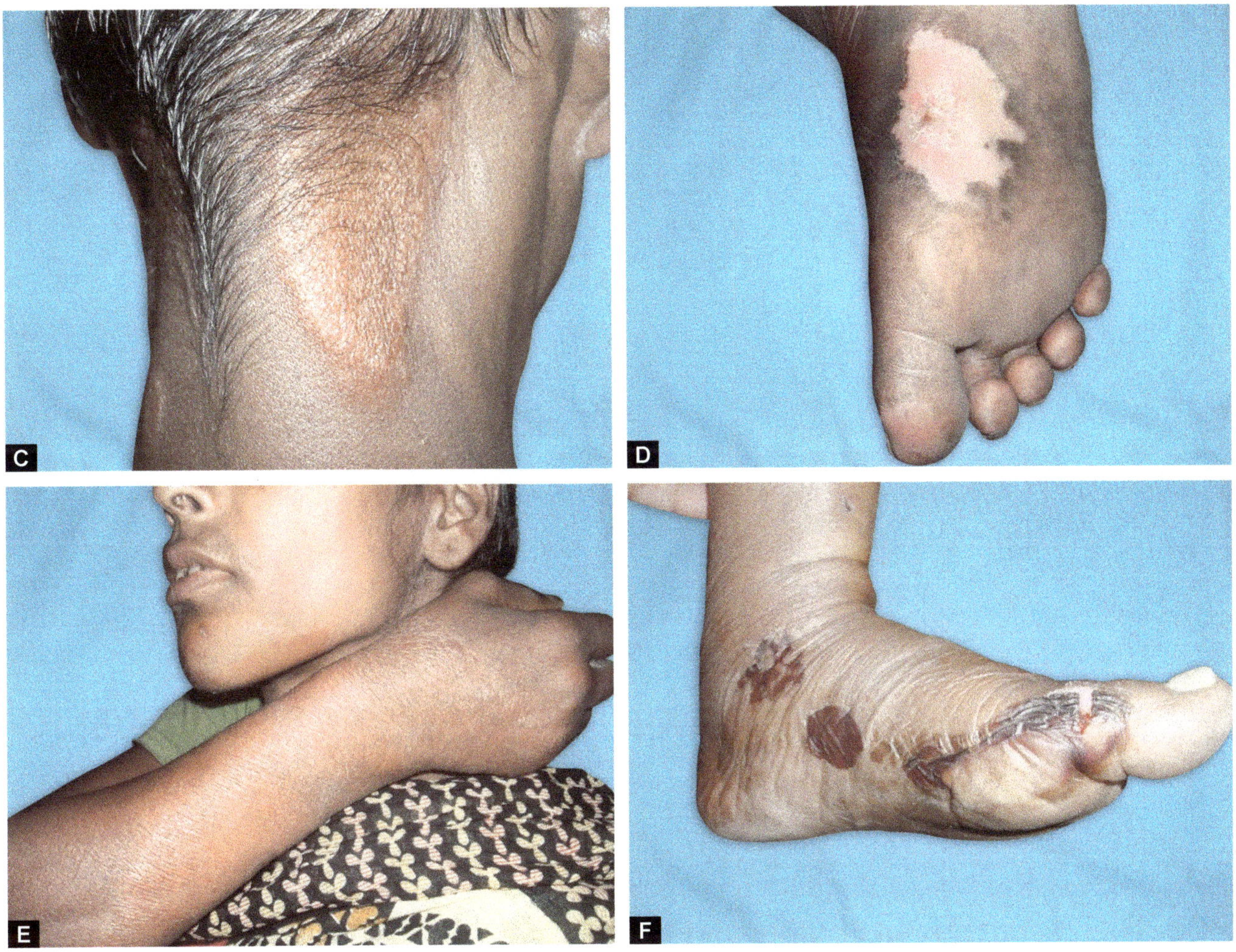

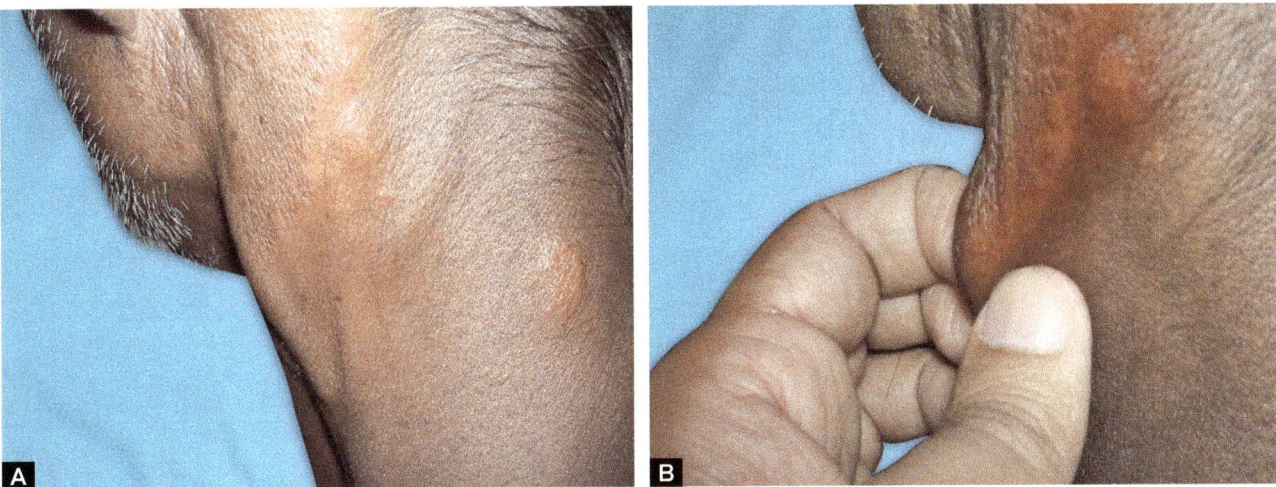

FIGS. 32A TO F: Tuberculoid leprosy.

FIGS. 33A AND B: Thick greater auricular nerve.

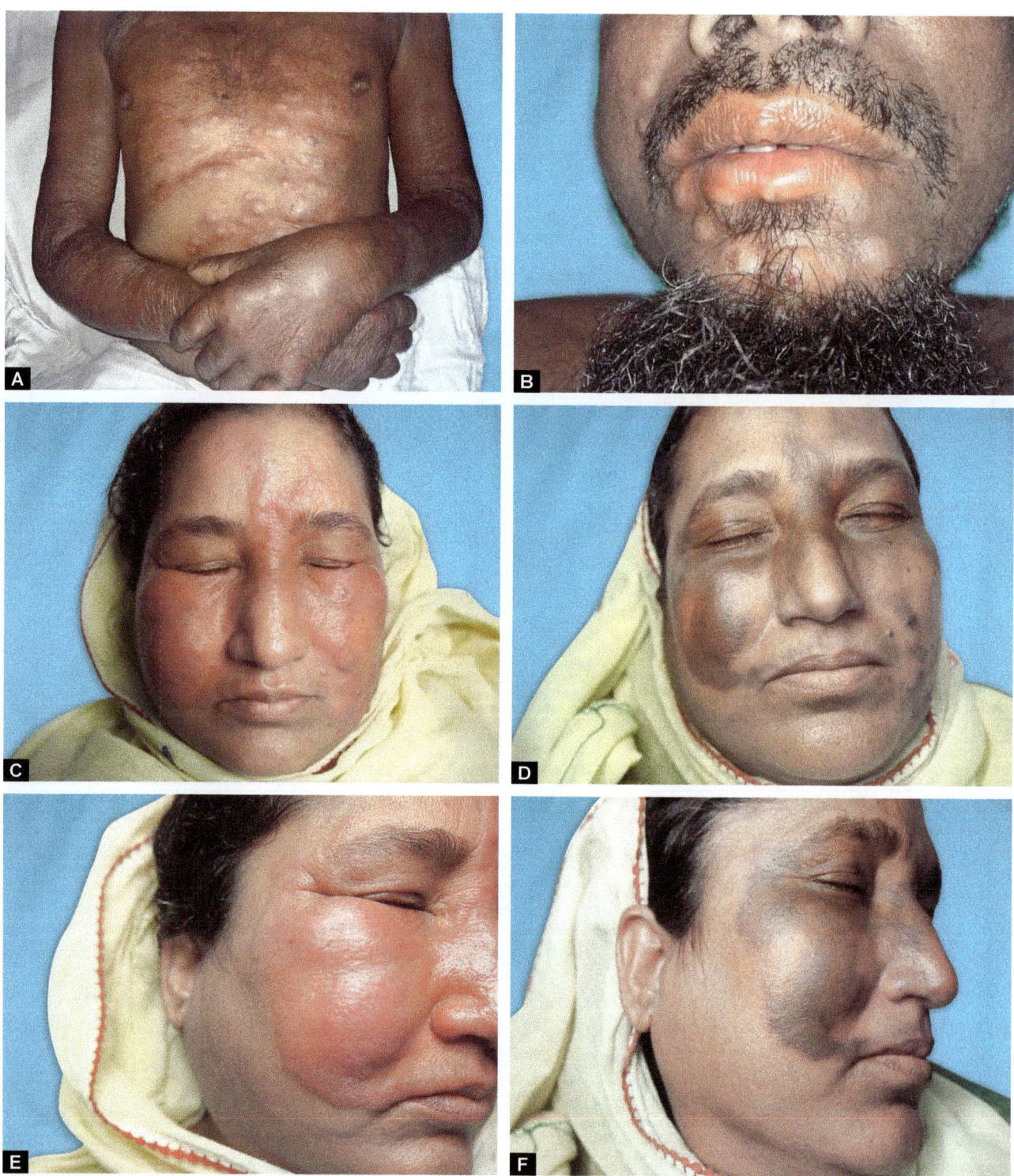

FIGS. 34A TO L: *Continued*

Continued

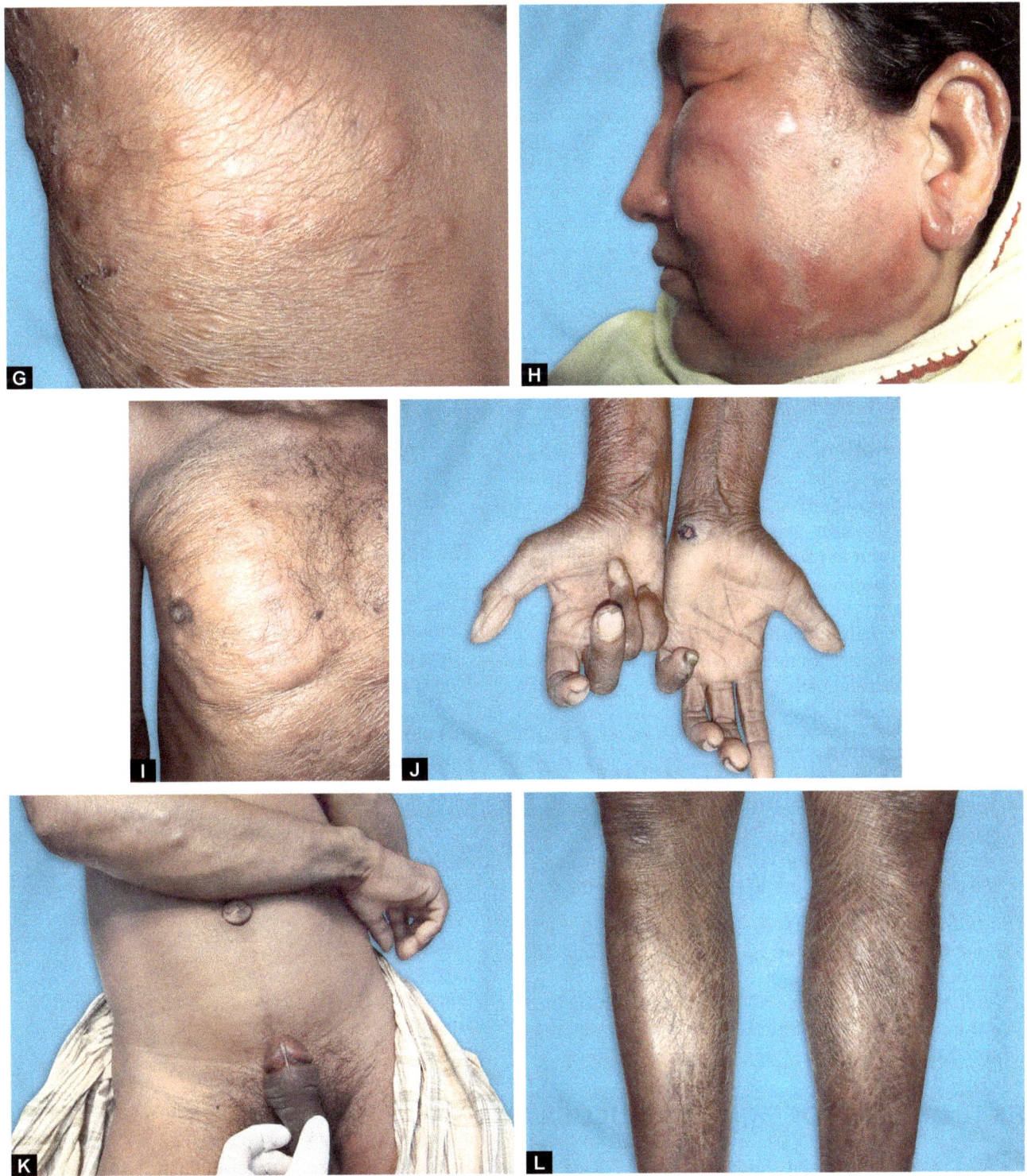

FIGS. 34A TO L: Lepromatous leprosy.

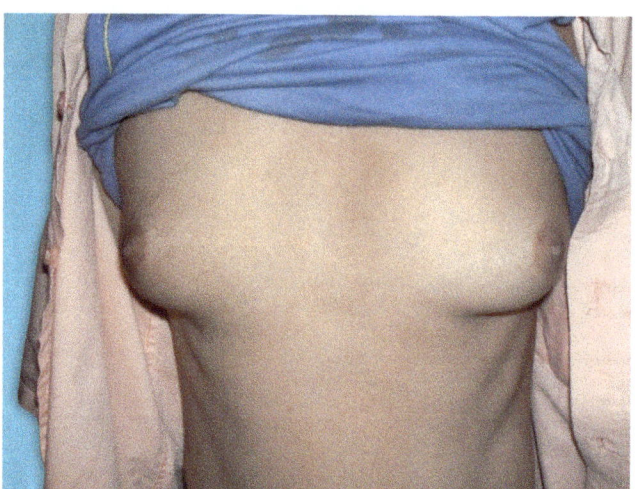

FIG. 35: Complication—gynecomastia.

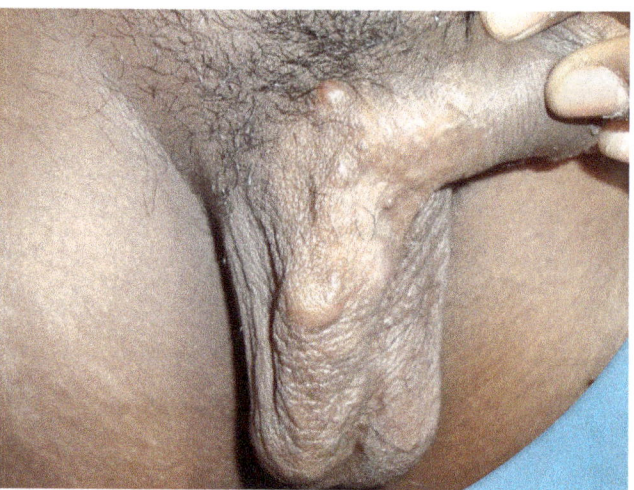

FIG. 36: Reaction type I.

Doctor's Prescription

- Slit-skin smear
- After collection of smear, it is made and examined under Ziehl–Neelsen staining. High bacterial index (BI) can be seen in LL and low or negative BI can be seen in paucibacillary cases.
- Culture
- Routine bacterial culture done for excludes secondary bacterial infection. No routine culture of *M. leprae* is done in mouse foot pad.
- Polymerase chain reaction (PCR)

Medical Prescription

US Health and Human Services guideline:
- *Paucibacillary*—Dapsone 100 mg/day + Rifampicin 600 mg/day—12 months.
- *Multibacillary*—Dapsone 100 mg/day + Rifampicin 600 mg/day + Clofazimine 50 mg/day—24 months.

World Health Organization (WHO) guideline:
- *Paucibacillary*—Dapsone 100 mg/day + Rifampicin 600 mg monthly—6 months.
- *Multibacillary*—Dapsone 100 mg/day + Rifampicin 600 mg monthly + Clofazimine 50 mg/day + 300 mg monthly—12 months.

VIRAL DISEASES OF SKIN AND MUCOSA

Measles (Rubeola)

- Caused by single-stranded ribonucleic acid (RNA) paramyxovirus.
- *Prodrome consists of*:
  - Fever (may exceed 104°F)
  - Cough
  - Coryza
  - Conjunctivitis
  - Photophobia
  - Myalgias

  And may lasts about 1 week.
- Classic exanthema consists of erythematous confluent macules and papules that are usually apparent at 2 weeks **(Figs. 37A and B)**.
- Cutaneous eruption spreads cephalocaudally over 3 days and resolves with fine desquamation and brown hyperpigmentation.
- Koplik spot—pathognomonic, 1-2 mm bluish macules on erythematous base (appears on buccal, labial, and gingival mucosa just prior to appearance of exanthem).
- Measles infection is usually benign and self-limited.

Complications

- Secondary bacterial infection
- Otitis media
- Pneumonia
- Laryngitis
- Encephalomyelitis
- Thrombocytopenic purpura

Rubella (German Measles)

- Common self-limited childhood infection by an RNA togavirus.
- Mild prodrome consists of malaise, anorexia, fever, headache, and coryza.
- Eruptions appear first on the forehead and rapidly spread inferiorly to involve the face, trunk, and extremities.
- Pink macules and papules become confluent, creating a scarlatiniform appearance **(Figs. 38A to D)**.

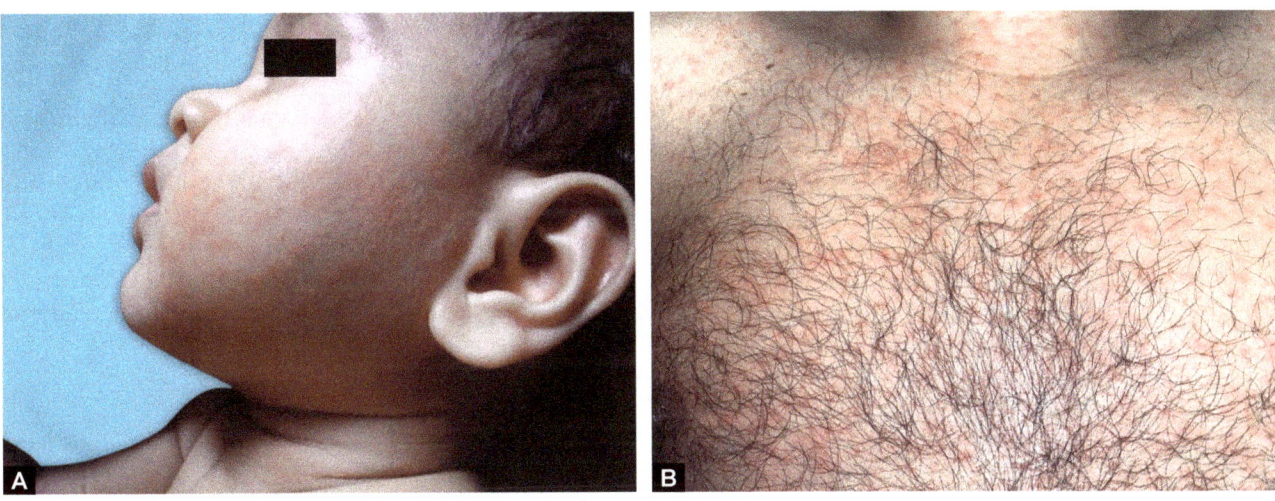

FIGS. 37A AND B: Erythematous confluent macules and papules.

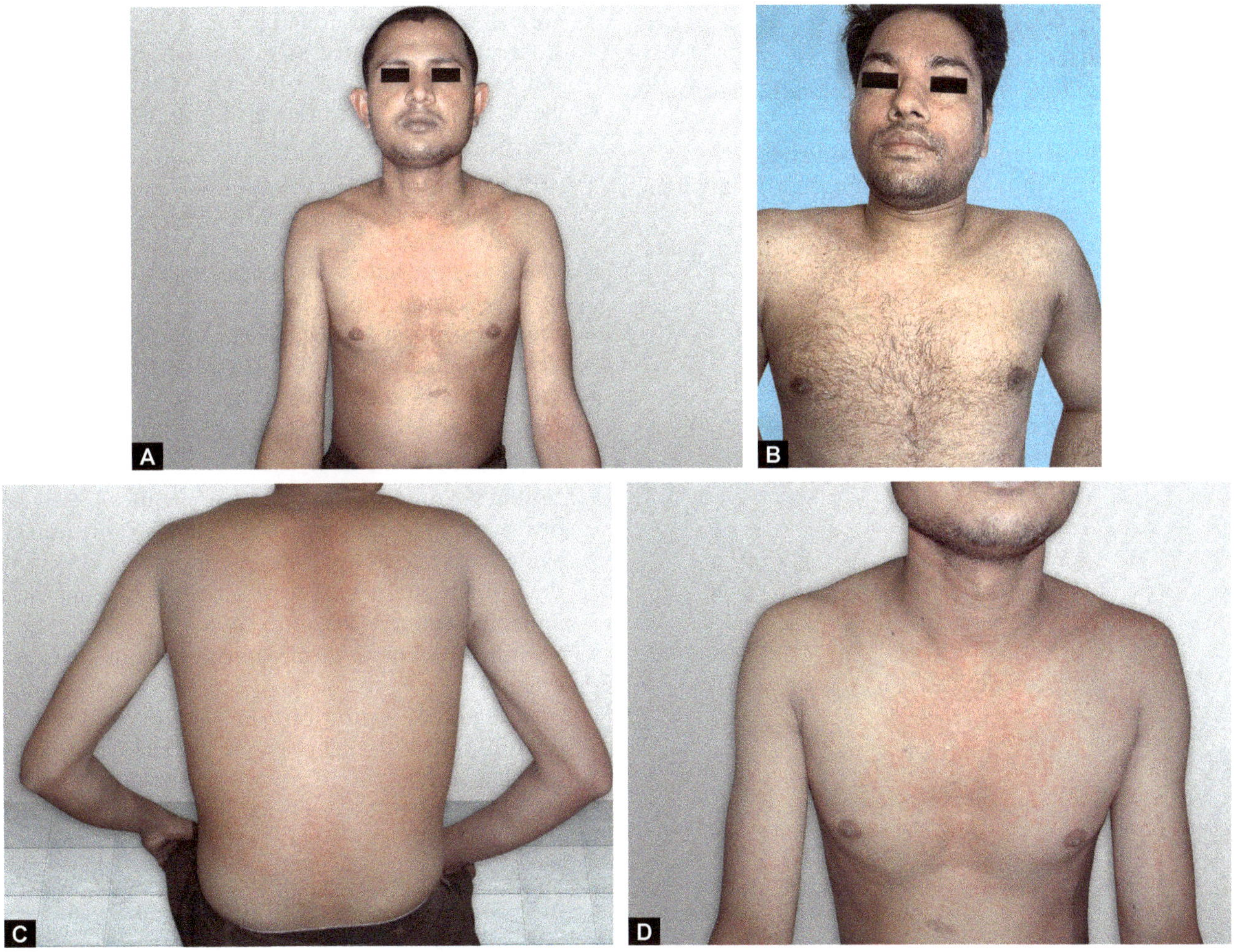

FIGS. 38A TO D: Pink macules and papules become confluent.

- Pruritus may be present.
- Time course of the rubella exanthem is 3 days.
- Exanthem of rubella does not desquamate.
- Petechiae of soft palate or Forchheimer spots may present.
- Arthritis and arthralgia are common complications, especially in female.
- Congenital rubella syndrome—maternal infection during the first 16 weeks of gestation results in a 65% risk for congenital rubella. Skin manifestations include extramedullary hematopoiesis (blueberry muffin body), thrombocytopenia, cataracts, deafness, and patent ductus arteriosus.
- Treatment is supportive.

Erythema Infectiosum (Fifth Disease, Slapped Cheek Disease)

- Childhood exanthem associated with primary human parvovirus B19 infection
- Edematous erythematous plaques on the cheeks (slapped cheeks) **(Fig. 39)**
- Edematous erythematous plaques on the trunk and extremities
- Mild prodrome of low-grade fever and headache
- May be accompanied by pharyngitis, myalgia, diarrhea, nausea, or conjunctivitis.
- Complications are arthritis, hemolytic anemia, encephalopathy, and aplastic crisis.
- Treatment is supportive.

Hand, Foot, and Mouth Disease (Figs. 40A and B)

- Coxsackievirus, enterovirus, and intestinal virus can cause the eruption.
- Characterized by painful ulcerative oral lesion, vesicular eruption on the distal extremities shortly after oral lesion.
- Mild constitutional syndrome
- Onset <10 years but young and middle-age adults are also affected.
- *Transmission*:
  - Highly contagious
  - Spread from person to person by oral and fecal-oral route.
- Symptomatic treatment

Varicella/Chickenpox (Figs. 41A to D)

- Highly contagious primary infection caused by varicella-zoster virus (VZV)
- Characterized by successive crops of pruritic vessels that evolve to pustules, crusts, and at times, scars.
- This infection is often accompanied by mild constitutional symptoms.
- *Transmission*:
  - Airborne droplets as well as direct contact.
  - Indirect contact.
- Patients are infectious for 5 days before the appearance of the eruptions. Infectivity ceases 5-6 days after no eruptions appear in most cases.
- Crusts are noninfectious.
- Incubation period is 14 days (range 10-23 days).

Skin Lesions

- In that lesions are erythematous papules (often not observed) that may appear as wheel and quickly evolve to vesicles and initially appear as small one drop of water or dew drop on a rose petal. Superficial and thin-walled vesicle.
- Within 8-12 hours, vesicles evolve to pustules and crusts.
- All stages of evolution (i.e., papules, vesicles, pustules, crusts, and polymorphic) may be noted simultaneously.
- Crusts fall off in 1-3 weeks leaving a pink, somewhat depressed base.
- Characteristic punched-out scar may persist.
- Mucous membrane may involve—vesicles and subsequent shallow erosion—palate, conjunctivae, pharynx, larynx, trachea, gastrointestinal (GI) tract, urinary tract, and vagina.

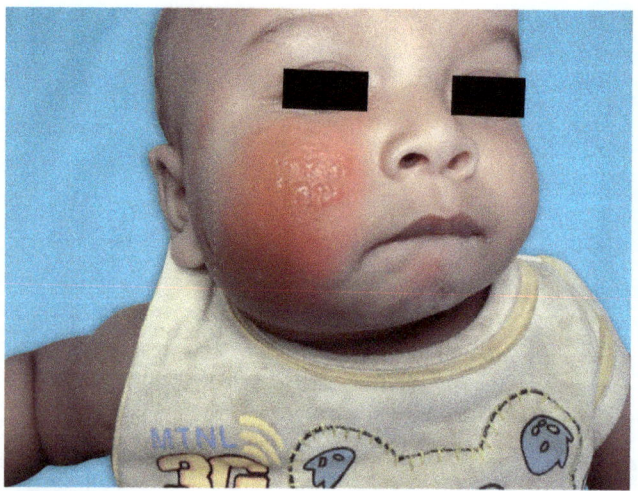

FIG. 39: Edematous erythematous plaques on the right cheek.

CHAPTER 12 Cutaneous Manifestation of Bacterial, Viral, Protozoal, Worm, Fungal Infection, and Other...

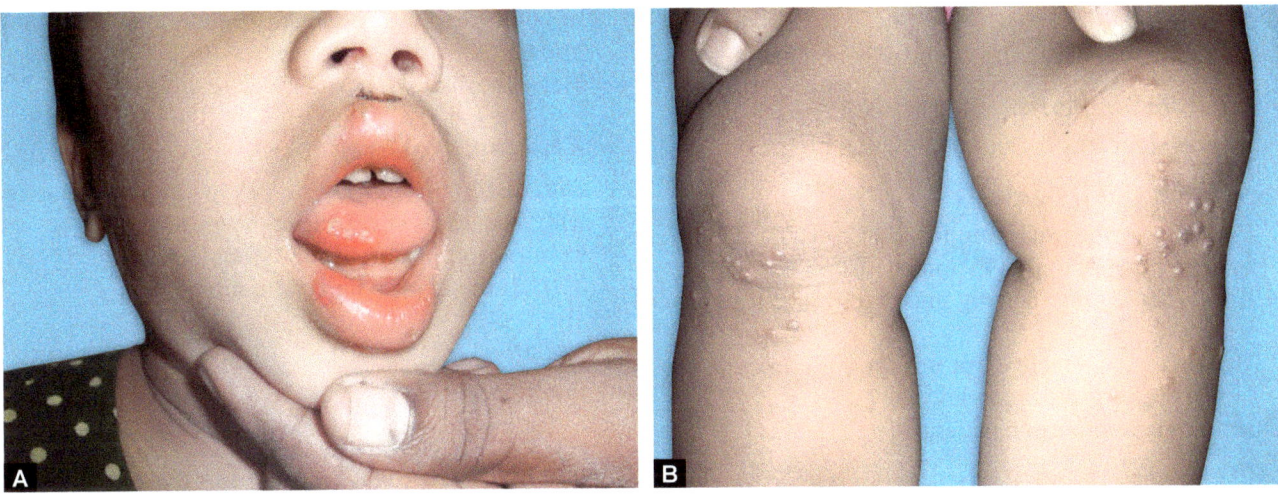

FIGS. 40A AND B: Hand, foot, and mouth disease.

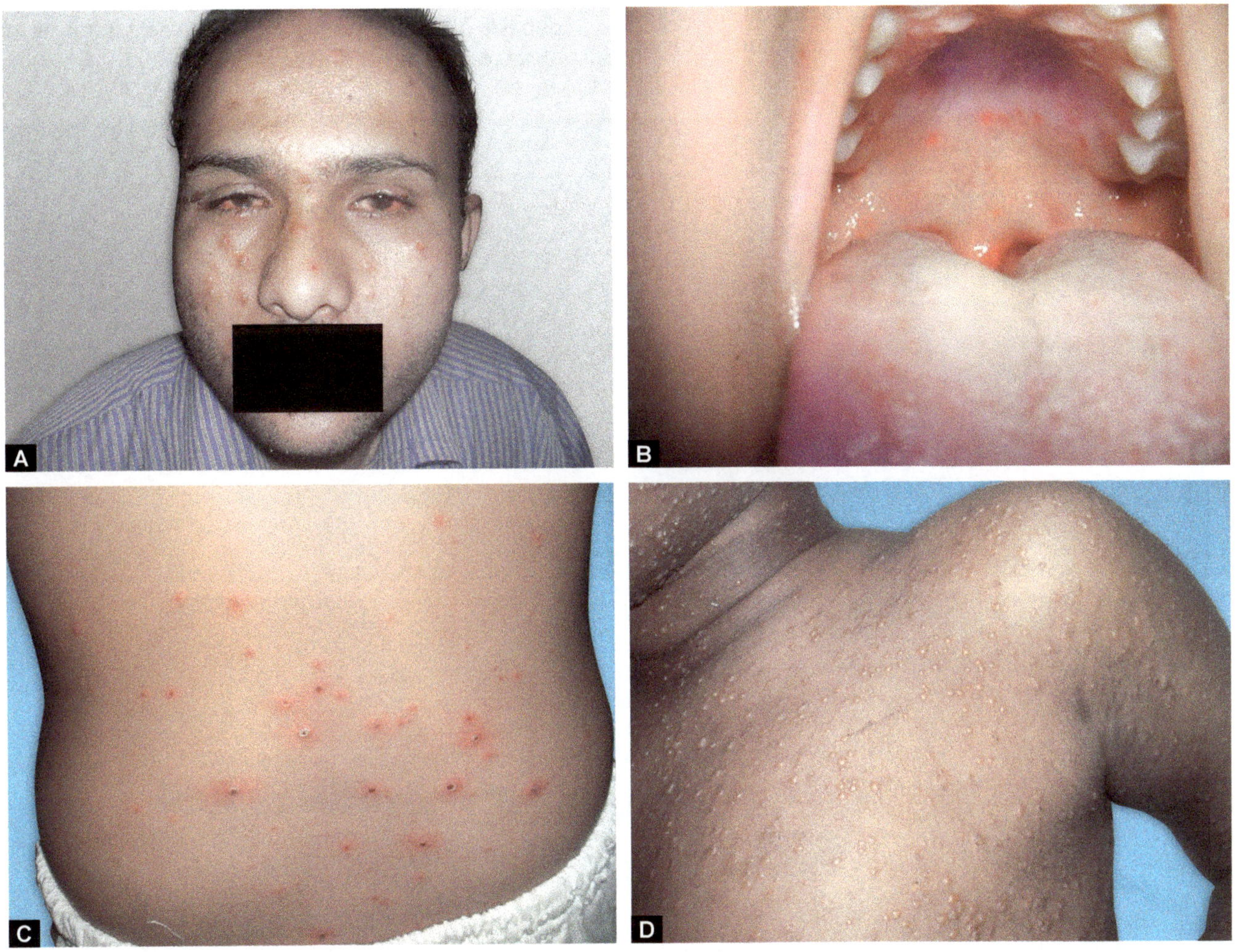

FIGS. 41A TO D: Varicella.

Complications
Pneumonitis, cerebellar ataxia, and encephalitis.

Differential Diagnosis
Usually on clinical background.

Prevention and Treatment
- Varicella-zoster virus immunization and 80% effective in preventing primary VZV infections.
- Acyclovir—20 mg (800 mg maximum) four times for 5 days.
- Valacyclovir—effective but not for an approved use (1,000 mg PO three times daily for 7 days).
- Immunocompromised patients.

▰ Herpes Zoster (Figs. 42A to F)
- An acute dermatomal infection associated with reactivation of VZV.
- Characterized by—painful unilateral lesion, vesicular or bullous eruptions limited to dermatome involved by a corresponding sensory ganglion (**Figs. 43A and B**).
- Major morbidity is postherpetic neuralgia (PHN).

Risk Factors
- Diminishing immunity to VZV with advancing age with most cases occurring in those ≥55 years.
- Immunocompromised conditions—malignancy, HIV/AIDS, radiotherapy, and chemotherapy.

Symptoms
- Prodromal stage
- Neuritic pain or paresthesia precedes for 2–3 weeks.

Signs
- Acute vesiculation is 3–5 days.
- Crust—2–3 weeks.
- Postherpetic neuralgia—months to years (if patient persists after the lesion heal or 4 weeks after lesion onset, regardless of degree of healing).

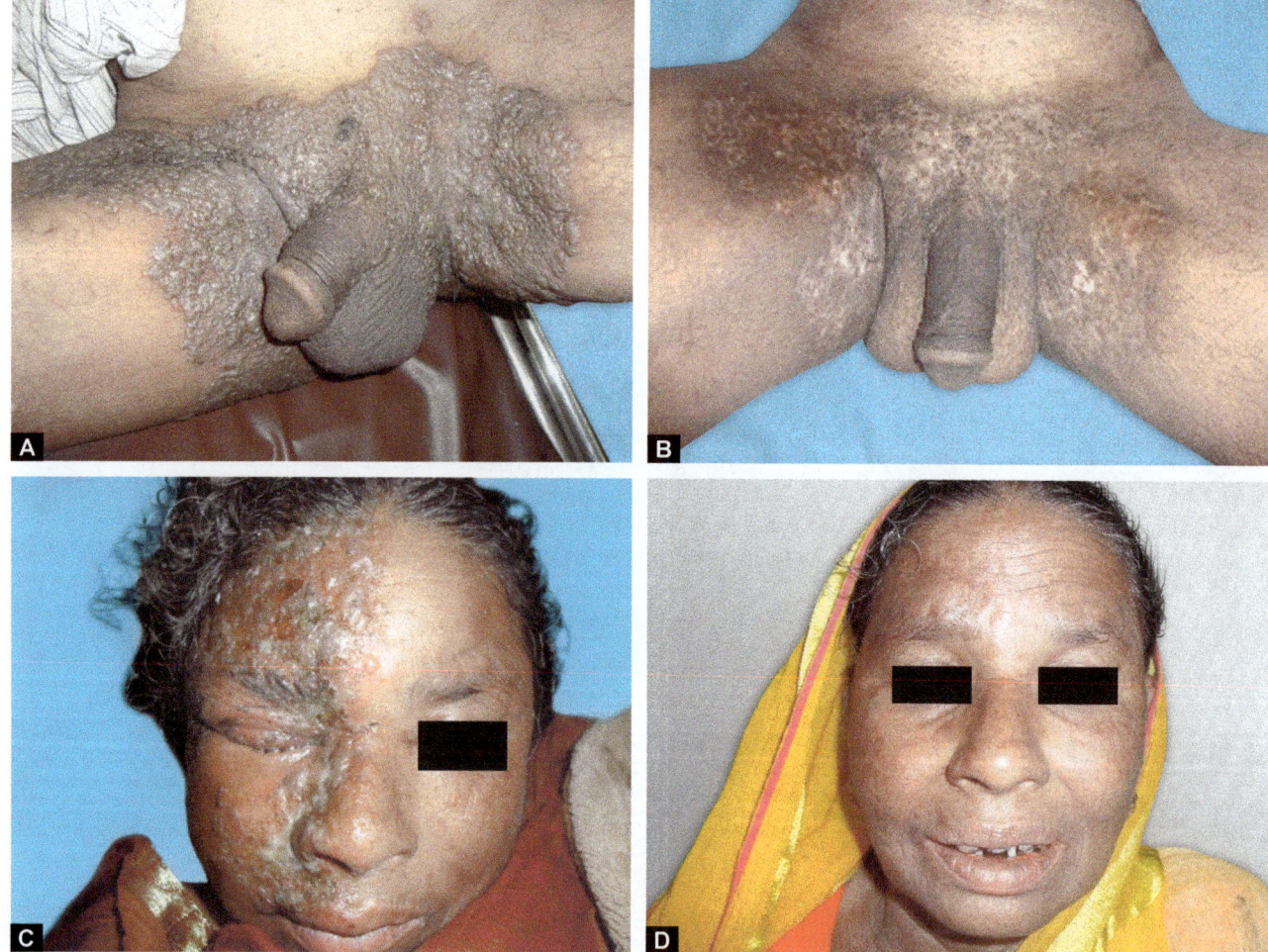

FIGS. 42A TO F: *Continued*

Continued

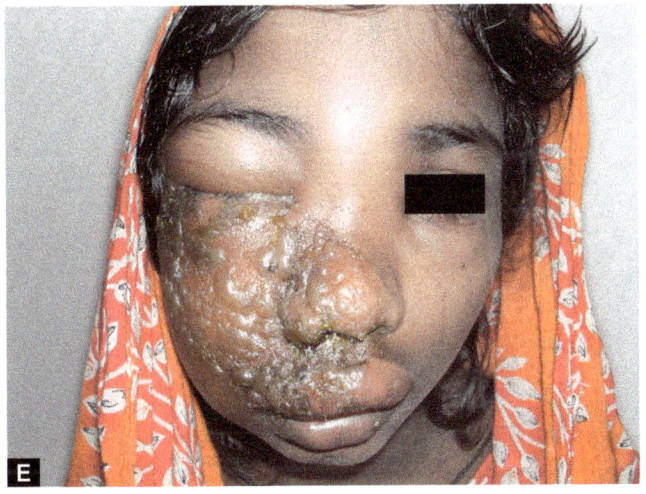
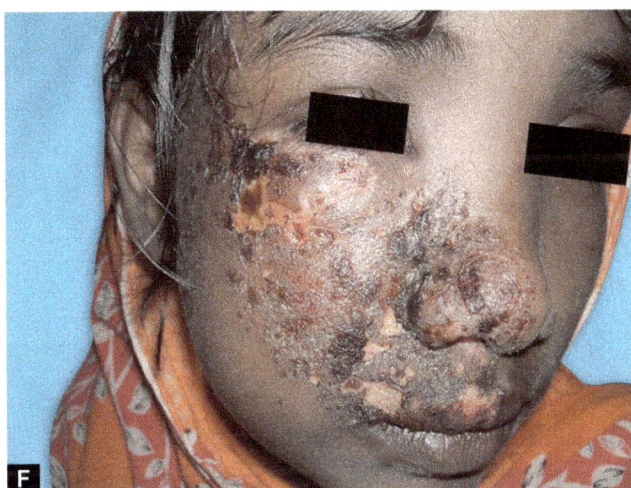

FIGS. 42A TO F: Herpes zoster before and after treatment.

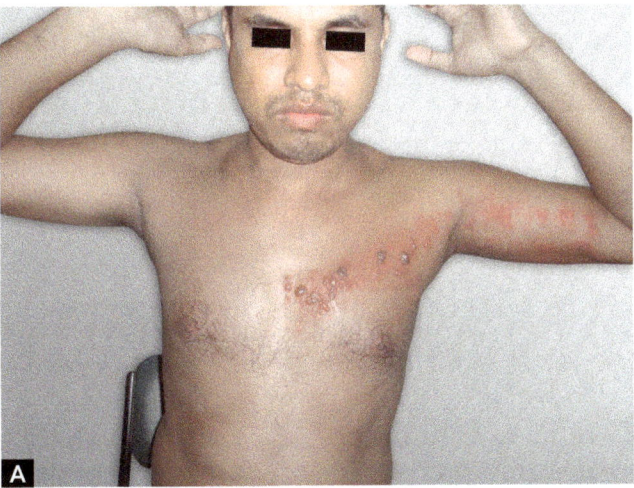
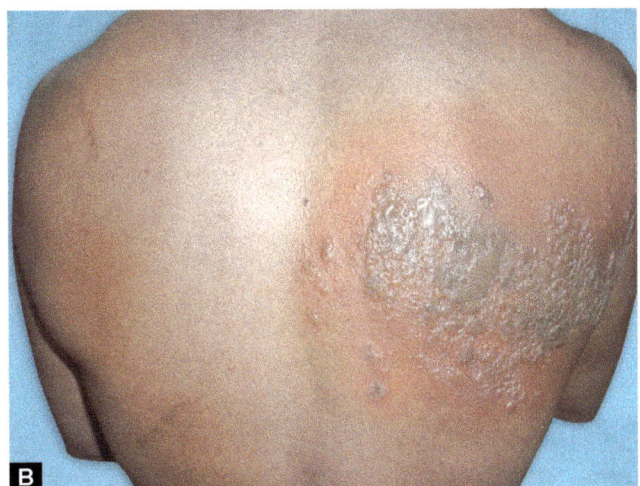

FIGS. 43A AND B: Typical dermatomal vesiculobullous eruption.

Complications of Herpes Zoster

- *Disseminated zoster*:
  - Defined as >20 vesicles outside the area of primary or adjacent dermatome that implies viremia and increased risk of visual or central nervous system (CNS) involvement.
  - Requires intravenous acyclovir.
- Postherpetic neuralgia and postherpetic itch (PHI) affect 10–15% of patients; incidence and severity increase with age.
- Treatment—gabapentin, amitriptyline, nortriptyline, etc.
- Scarring (keloid or hypertrophic scar) **(Figs. 44A and B)**.

Treatment

Same as varicella.

Herpes Simplex Viruses (HSV-1/HSV-2)

- Produce primarily orolabial (HSV-1/HSV-2) and genital infections (HSV-2 > HSV-1) characterized by recurrent vesicular eruptions **(Figs. 45A to L)**.
- Transmission can occur during both symptomatic and asymptomatic periods of viral shedding.
- Reactivations can occur either spontaneously or due to some stimulus [e.g., stress, trauma, ultraviolet radiation (UVR), fever, common cold, altered immune status, contact irritation, or sex].

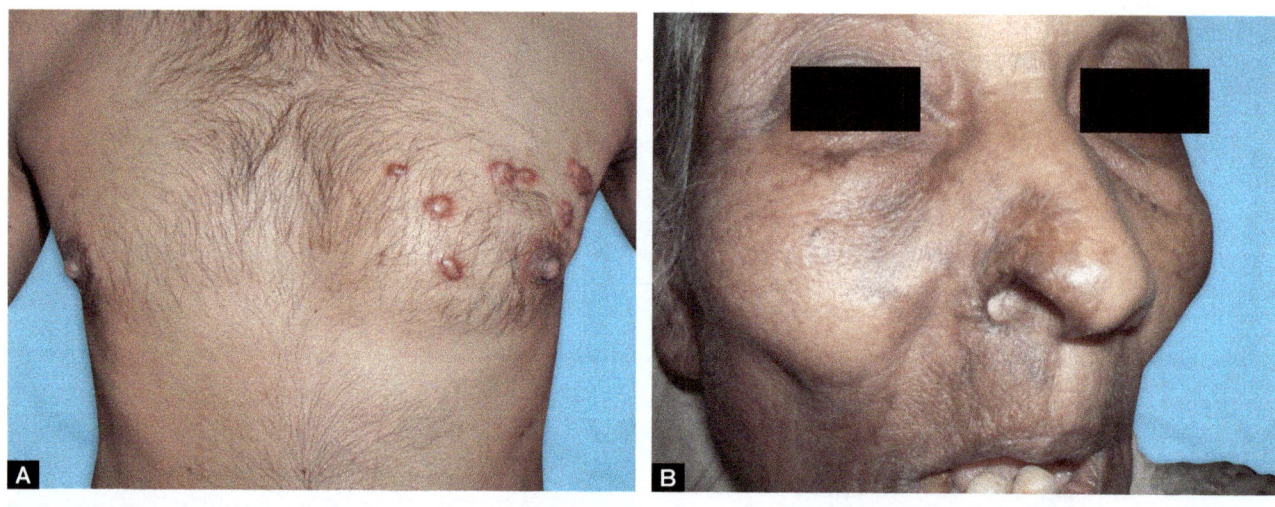

FIGS. 44A AND B: Complications—hypertrophic scar and atrophy.

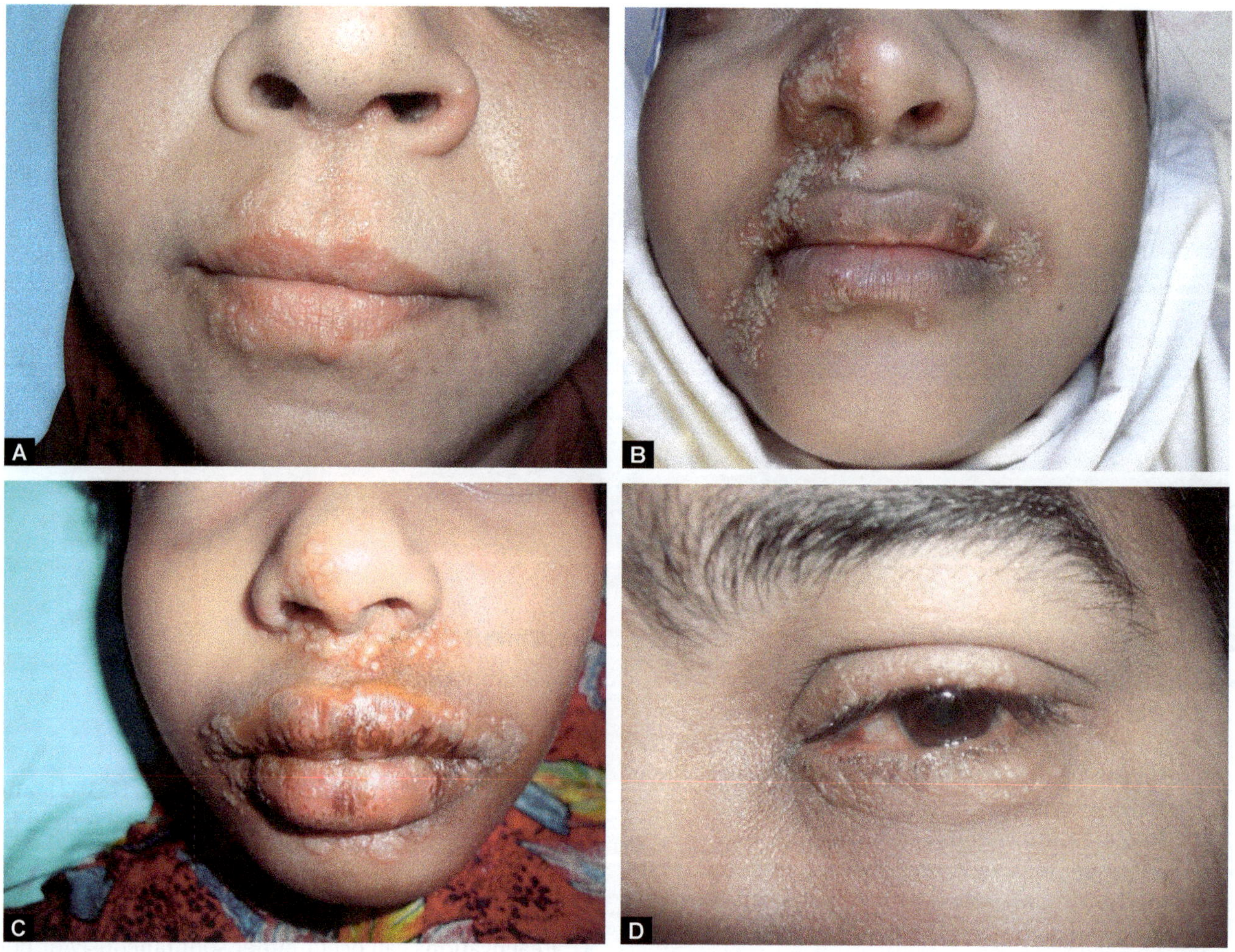

FIGS. 45A TO L: *Continued*

Continued

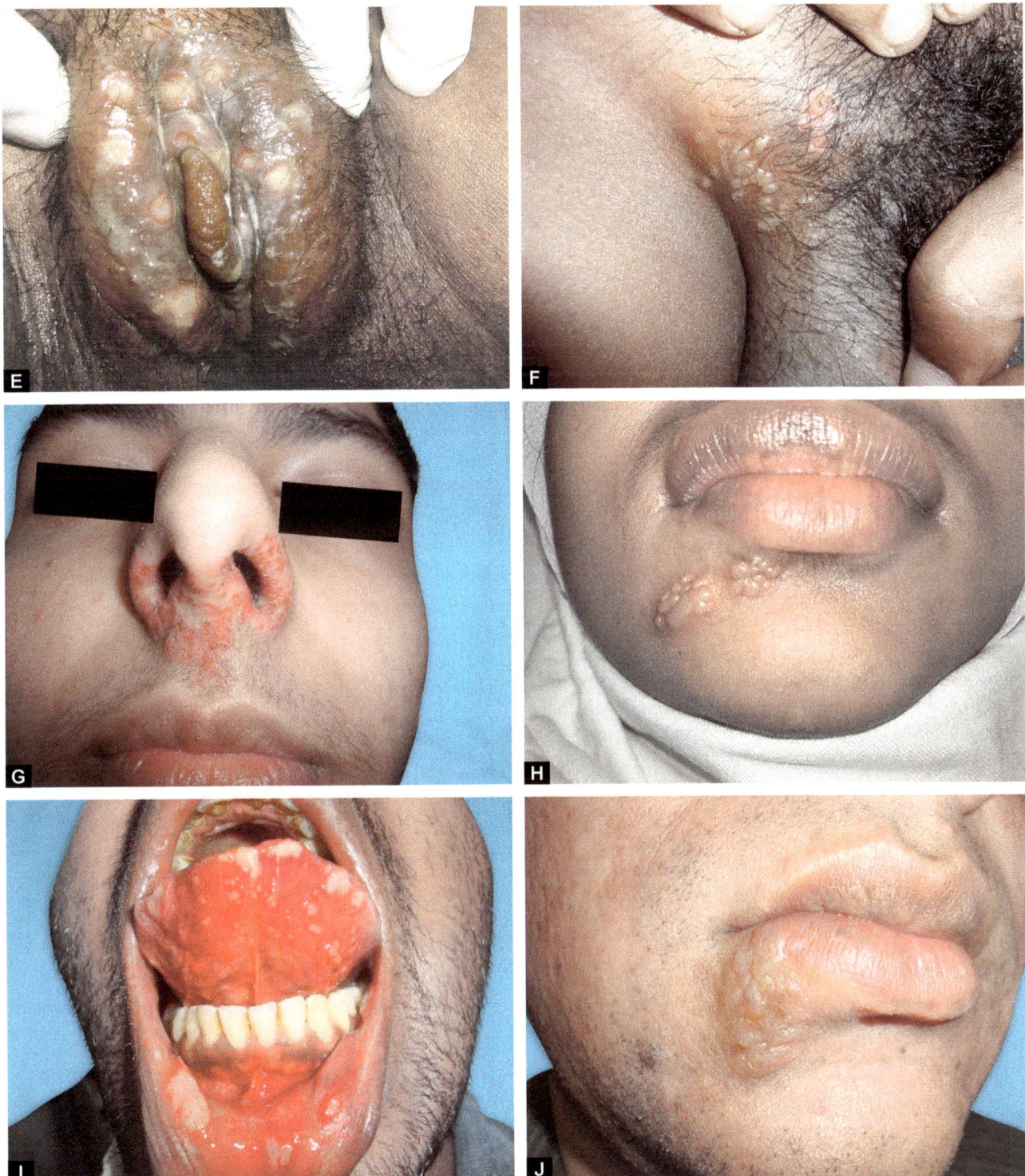

FIGS. 45A TO L: *Continued*

Continued

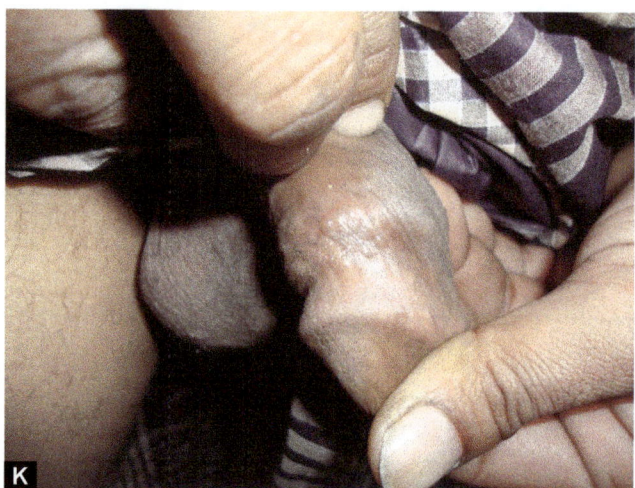
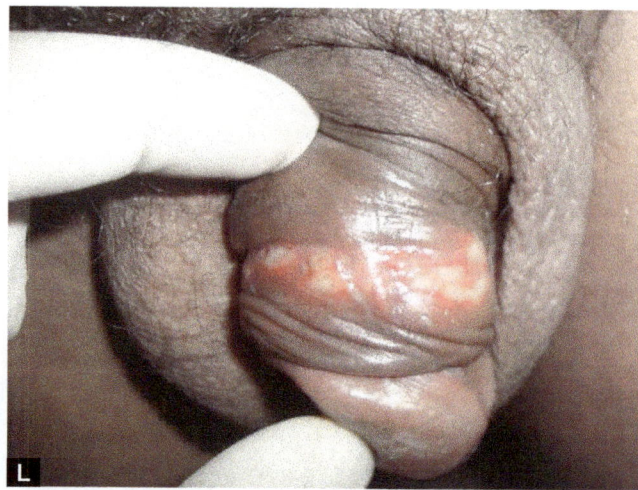

FIGS. 45A TO L: Herpes simplex infections.

Primary Infection

- Onset is usually 3–7 days after exposure.
- Generalized prodrome of tender lymphadenopathy, fever and malaise, localized pain, burning, and tenderness.
- Initial lesion—small round vesicle on an erythematous base followed soon by grouped, often umbilicated vesicles which may become umbilicated or pustular, followed by erosions or ulcerations with hemorrhagic crusts. Lesion resolves over 2–6 weeks.

Reactivation Infection

- Localized prodrome of dysesthesia (e.g., burning/tingling, pain, and pruritus) and tenderness.
- Mucocutaneous lesions similar as in primary but fewer in number, less severe, and shorter duration.

Diagnosis

- Antigen detection by direct fluorescent antibody (DFA)
- Dermatohistopathology
- Culture
- Polymerase chain reaction
- Serology immunoglobulin M (IgM) and immunoglobulin G (IgG) against HSV-1/HSV-2

Treatment

Systemic drug first episode:
- Acyclovir—400 mg three times daily or 200 mg five times daily.
- Valacyclovir—1 g twice daily for 7–10 days.
- Famciclovir—250 mg three times per day for 5–10 days.

TABLE 1: Correlation human papillomavirus (HPV) type with disease.

Skin lesions	Frequent detected HPV type
Common, palmar, plantar, and myrmecial warts	1, 2, 4
Flat warts	3, 10
Epidermodysplasia verruciformis	5, 8
Condyloma accuminate (anogenital warts)	6, 11
High-grade squamous intraepithelial neoplasia (cervical lesion, bowenoid polyposis, and erythroplasia of Queyrat)	16, 18, 31, and 33
Cervical cancer	16, 18
High-grade malignant potential	16, 18, 31, 33, 35, and 39

Recurrences

- No benefit from pulse therapy in severe recurrent disease. Start therapy at the beginning of the prodrome or within 2 days after onset of lesions.

■ Human Papillomaviruses (Table 1)

- Human papillomavirus (HPV) comprises at least 200 genotypes of deoxyribonucleic acid (DNA) viruses that infect skin and mucosa.
- Commonly infection in keratinized skin
- Transmission—transmitted via person-to-person contact or contact with contaminated surfaces or objects.
- More than 30% cases are self-regress within 1–2 years.

CHAPTER 12 Cutaneous Manifestation of Bacterial, Viral, Protozoal, Worm, Fungal Infection, and Other...

Common Warts (Figs. 46A to L)

- It is also known as verruca vulgaris.
- Any site—commonly triggers dorsal hands and/or sites prone to trauma.
- Hyperkeratotic, exophytic, or dome-shaped papules or plaques with punctuate black dot (thrombosed capillaries).

- *Plantar/Palmar warts* **(Figs. 47A to F)**: Thick exo- and endophytic hyperkeratotic papules and plaques, coalescence of lesions can lead to extensive areas of involvement referred to as mosaic warts.
- *Flat warts* **(Figs. 48A and B)**: Commonly on dorsum of hands, arms, and face as well as on the legs (exacerbating by shaving).

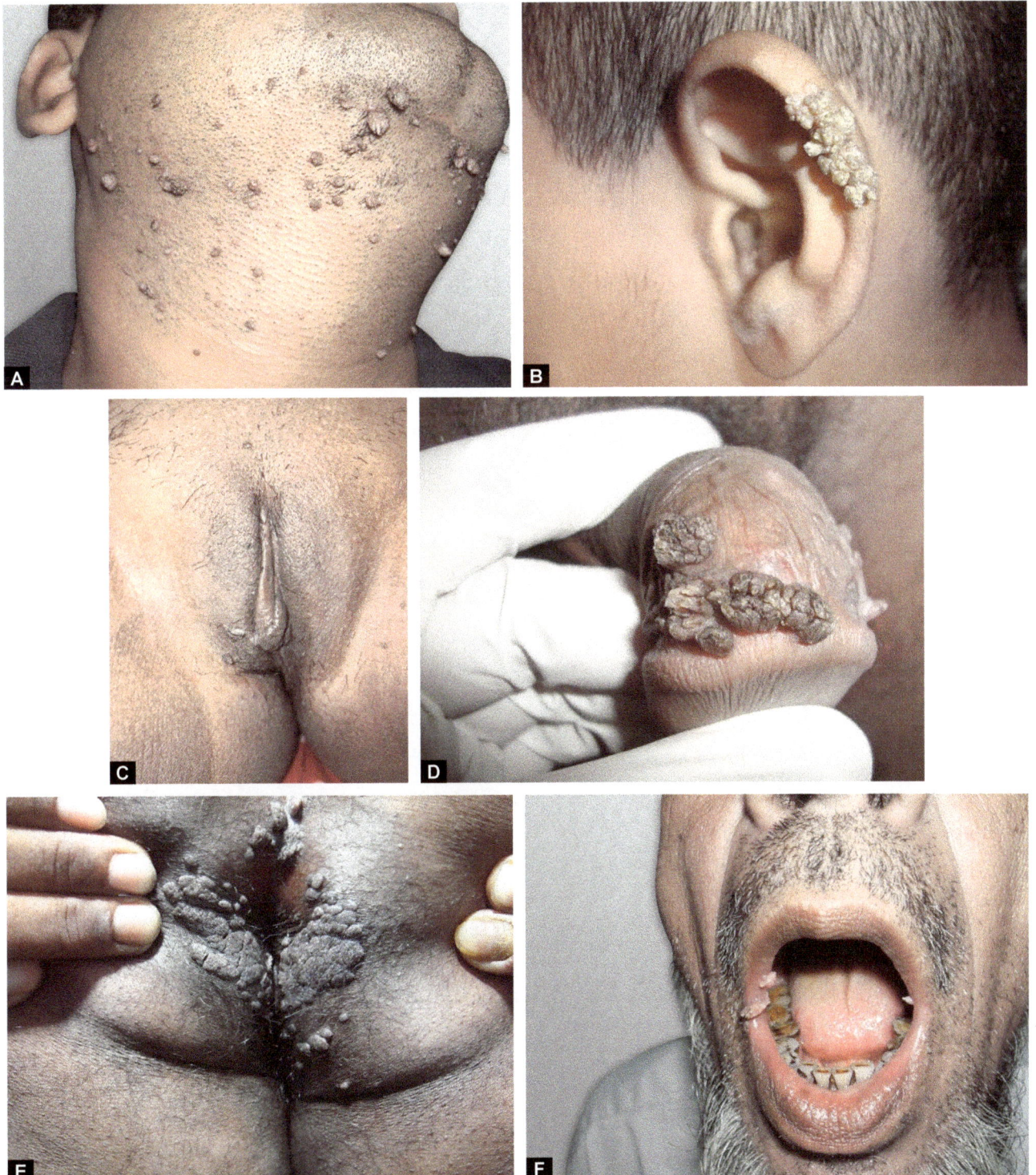

FIGS. 46A TO L: *Continued*

Continued

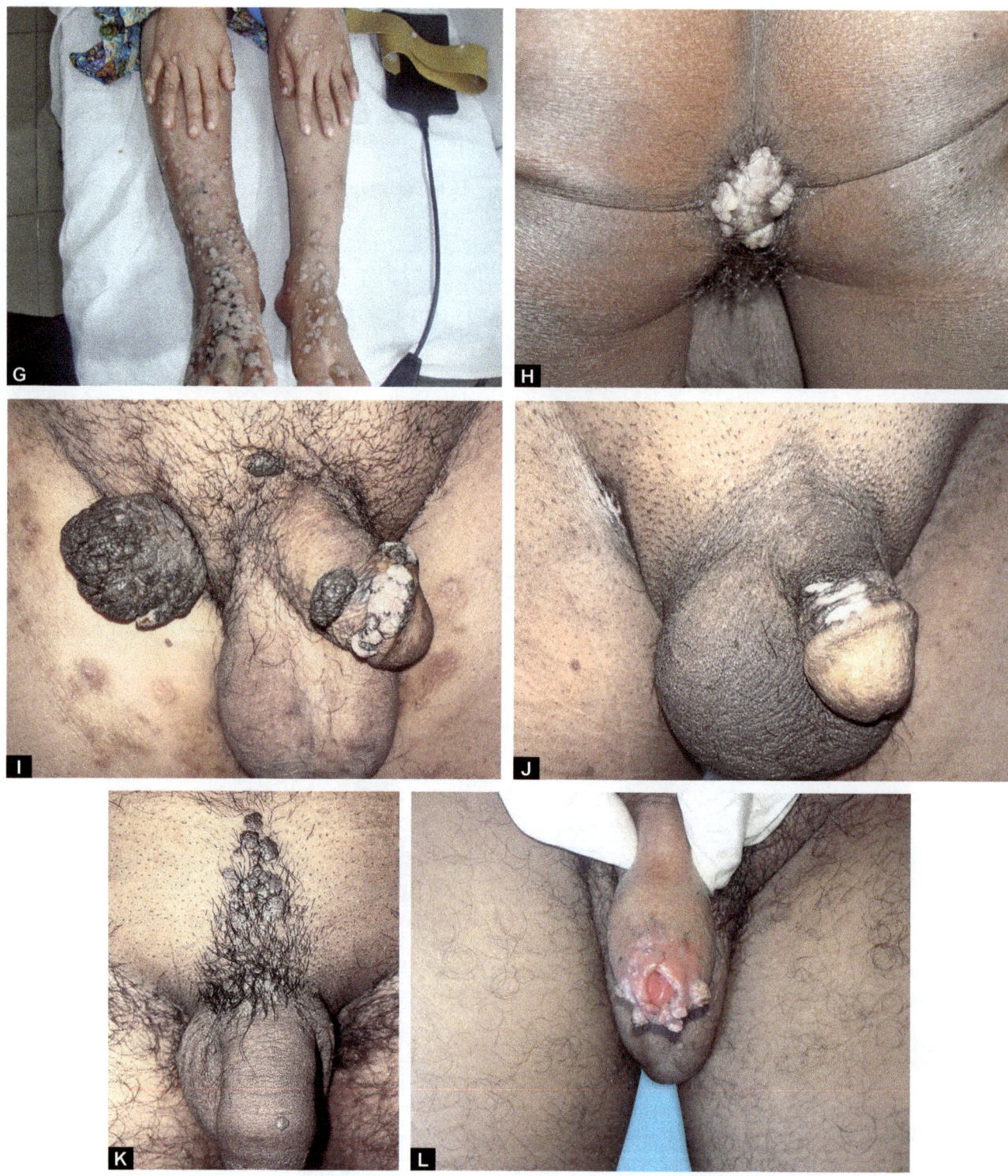

FIGS. 46A TO L: Warts.

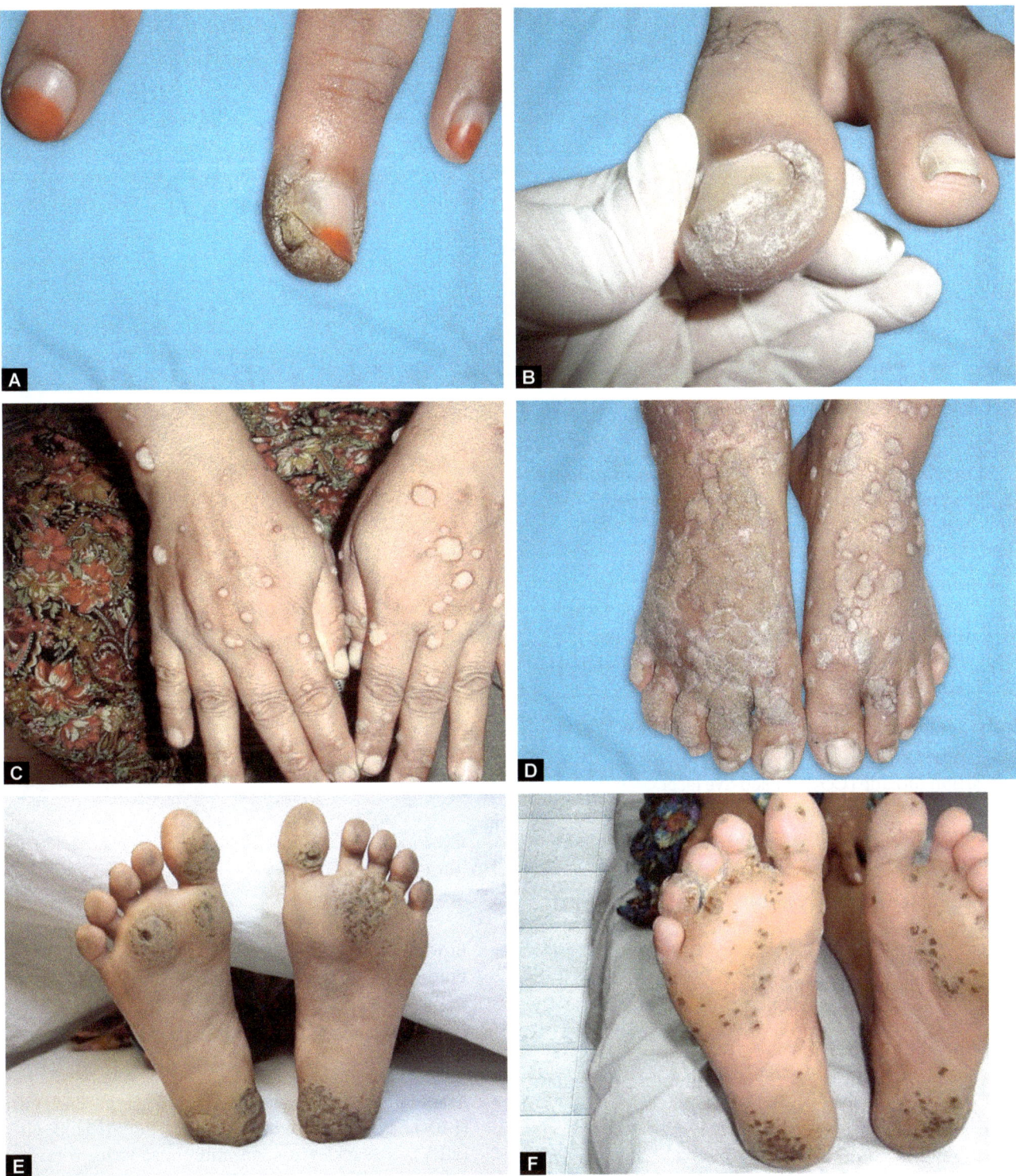

FIGS. 47A TO F: Plantar/palmar warts.

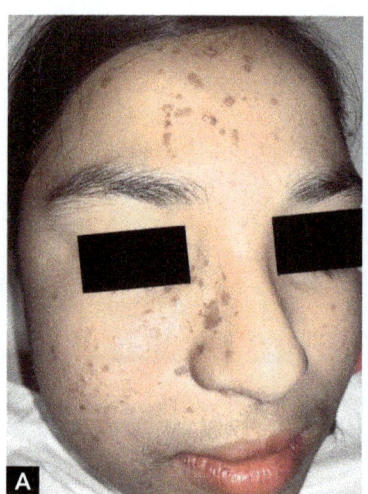
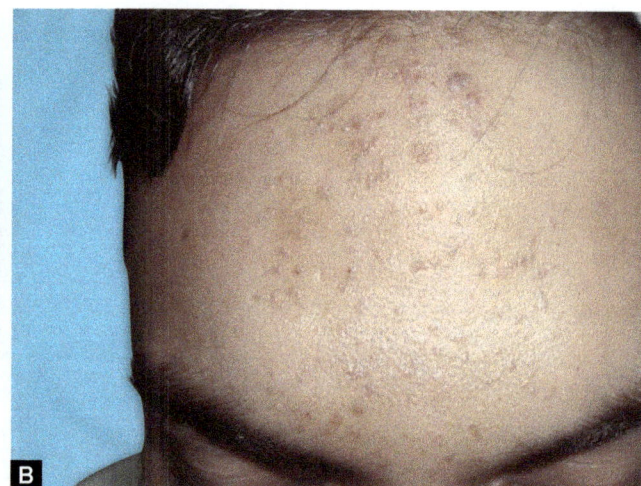

FIGS. 48A AND B: Flat warts.

Skin colored to pink, brown, or hypopigmented papules, surface is smooth, and often flat topped.

Treatment of Warts
- *Dermatologist decides treatment based on:*
  - Number, morphology, and distribution of warts
  - Present immunological status of the patient
  - Motivation and ability to use patient/parent administered therapy

Considerations if Single or Relatively Few Warts
- Cryotherapy
- Carbon dioxide (CO_2)/pulsed dye laser
- Curettage + Electrodesiccation
- Cantharidin + Podophyllotoxin + Salicylic acid (if many warts)

Considerations if Many and/or Recalcitrant Warts
- Cryosurgery
- Intralesional immunotherapy
- Topical immunotherapy

Combinations recommended.

Additional Considerations
- Local hyperthermia (44°C for 30 minutes on the days 1, 2, 3, 17, and 18)
- Intralesional bleomycin
- Intravenous cidofovir (severe disease in immuno-compromised host)
- Topical cidofovir
- Oral cimetidine
- Oral retinoids
- Oral warts
- *Condyloma accuminata*: It involves primarily in the anogenital region.

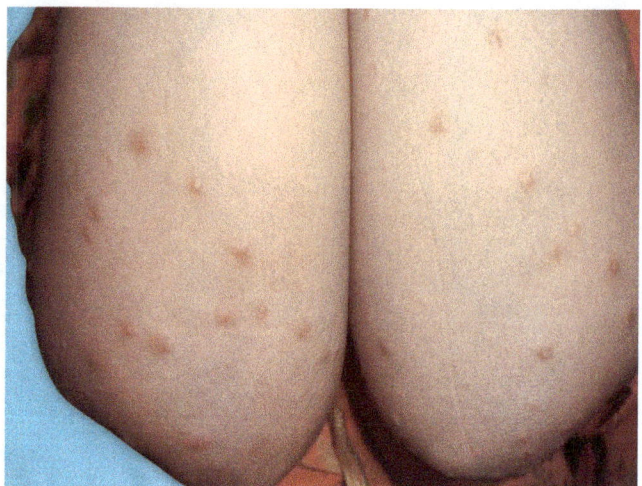

FIG. 49: Gianotti–Crosti syndrome.

- Bowenoid papulosis
- Epidermodysplasia verruciformis

Gianotti–Crosti Syndrome (Papular Acrodermatitis of Childhood) (Fig. 49)
- Associated with viruses such as Epstein–Barr virus (EBV), cytomegalovirus (CMV), hepatitis B virus (HBV), coxsackievirus, parainfluenza virus, rotavirus, poxvirus, HIV, hepatitis A virus (HAV), hepatitis C virus (HCV), parvovirus, and poliovirus.
- Bacteria—*Mycoplasma pneumoniae*, *Borrelia burgdorferi*, and group A *Streptococcus*.
- Vaccines-influenza, diphtheria, tetanus, Bacillus Calmette-Guérin (BCG), *Haemophilus influenzae* type b, and oral polio.

- Most common in the spring and early summer favoring young children.
- Other preceded by a low-grade fever and/or upper respiratory symptoms.
- Rapid onset of monomorphic, skin-colored pink, red, edematous papules, papulovesicles in a symmetric distribution on the extensor surface of extremities, buttocks, and face. Pruritus, purpuric lesions, and extension to the trunk occasionally occur.

Molluscum Contagiosum

- Caused by poxvirus
- Spread by skin-to-skin contact and fomites (towels)
- Favoring young children but also occur via sexual contact in adults; larger and more numerous lesions may be seen in immunocompromised hosts.
- Firm, skin colored to pearly white papules or papulonodules with a waxy surface and central umbilication **(Figs. 50A to D)**.

Dengue (*Flavivirus*)

- Caused by dengue virus carried by *Aedes* mosquitoes.
- Approximately 50% patients develop maculopapular or macular confluent rash over the face, trunk, and flexor surfaces with islands of skin sparing **(Figs. 51A and B)**. The rash usually begins on third day and may persist another 2–3 days. Often petechiae are present.

Chikungunya (Togavirus) (Figs. 52 and 53)

Around 50% cases appear erythematous morbilliform eruption occasionally ulcers (oral, genital, and intertriginous area), vesiculobullous, and post-inflammatory hyperpigmentation (freckles-like lesion but diffuse).

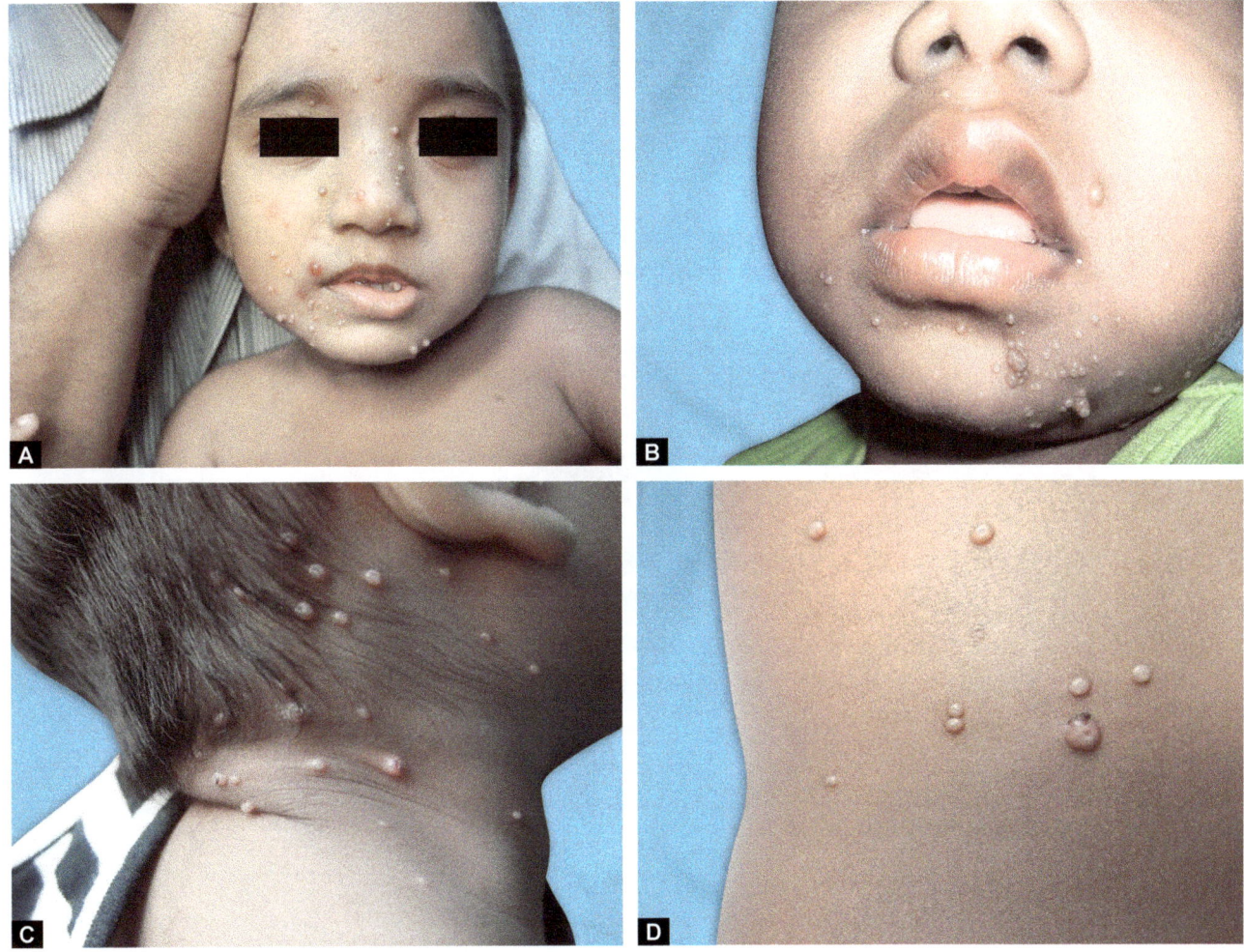

FIGS. 50A TO D: Multiple pearly and umbilicated papules.

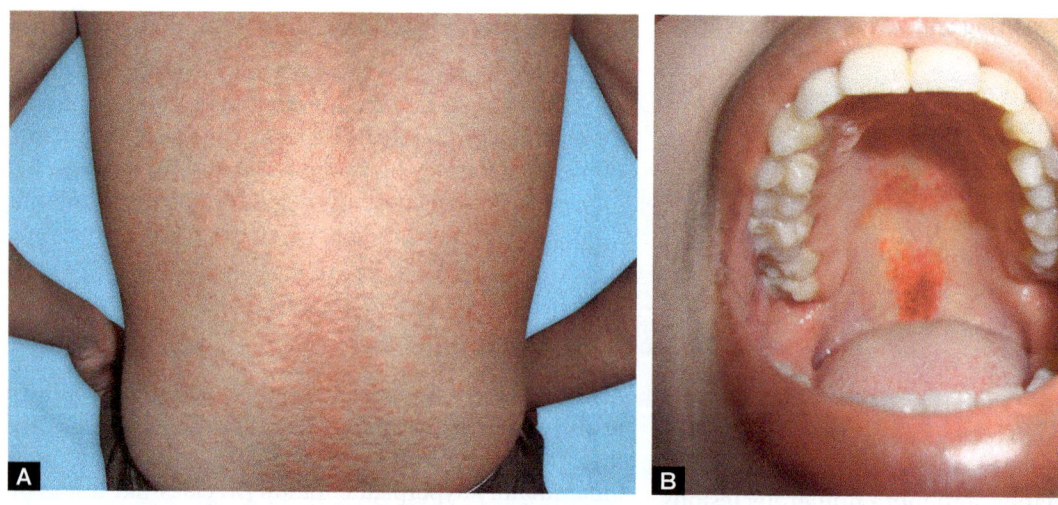

FIGS. 51A AND B: Maculopapular rash and purpuric hemorrhage.

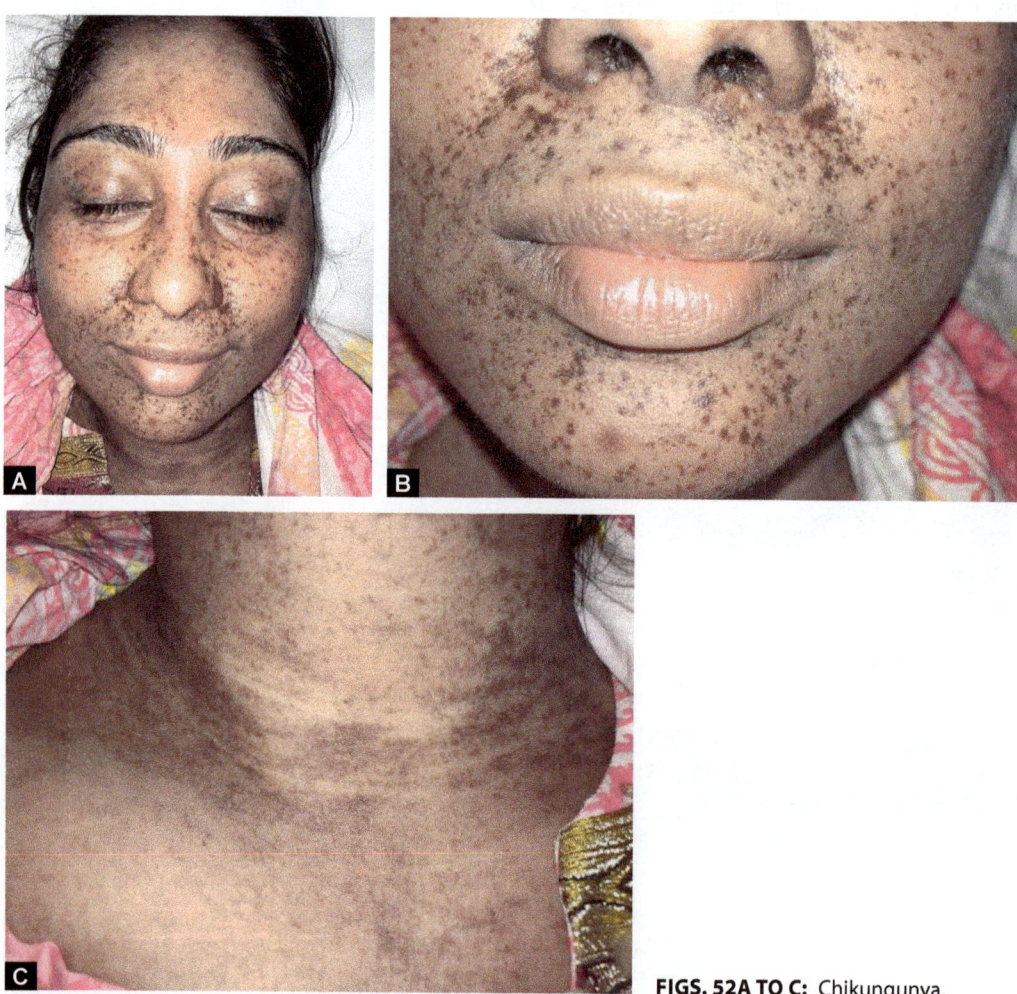

FIGS. 52A TO C: Chikungunya.

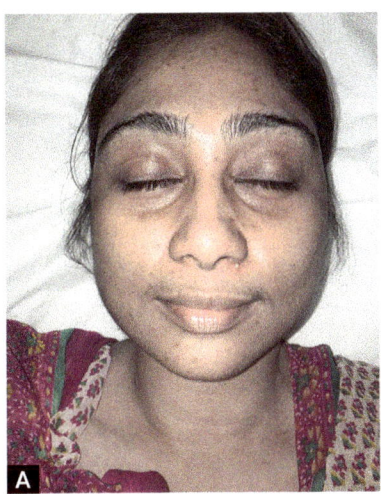
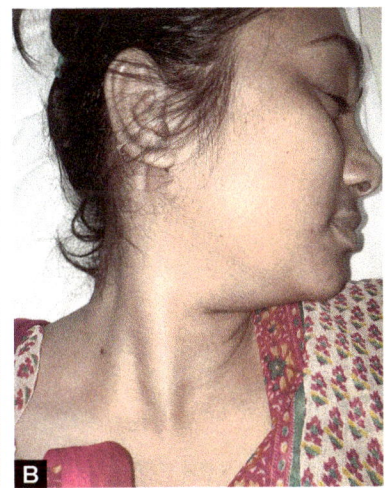

FIGS. 53A AND B: After recovery.

Coronavirus Disease 2019

About 20% of hospitalized coronavirus disease 2019 (COVID-19)-positive patient may present with following skin findings:
- Acute urticaria
- Acral ischemia
- Morbilliform eruption
- Palpable purpura
- Livedo reticularis
- Petechial hemorrhage **(Figs. 54A to F)**

PROTOZOAL INFECTIONS

Leishmaniasis

- Caused by >15 different species of obligate intracellular protozoa *Leishmania*; prominent species are:
  o New World cutaneous leishmaniasis (NWCL)—*Leishmania mexicana, Viannia* subgenus
  o Old World cutaneous leishmaniasis (OWCL)—*Leishmania tropica, Leishmania major,* and *Leishmania aethiopica.*
- Vector—Sandflies, OWCL—*Phlebotomus,* and NWCL—*Lutzomyia.*
- Incubation period is inversely proportional to size of inoculum.
- Three major forms—(1) Cutaneous leishmaniasis, (2) Mucocutaneous leishmaniasis, and (3) Visceral leishmaniasis.
- Noduloulcerative lesions are usually asymptomatic. It may become painful, if secondarily infected.
- New World cutaneous leishmaniasis—after 2–8 weeks of inoculation develop small erythematous papule which becomes ulcerated nodule. It enlarges to 3–12 cm with raised border. Nonulcerating nodules may become verrucous. Lymphangitis and regional lymphadenopathy may present. Lesion with heals with a depressed scar is also present. Ear and nose lesions may persist for years, destroying cartilage **(Figs. 55A and B)**.
- Old World cutaneous leishmaniasis—after 2–4 weeks of inoculation develop small papule which slowly enlarges to 2 cm over a period of several weeks that become violaceous and crusted with an ulcer in its center and raised border. In some cases, nodule develops which becomes hyperkeratotic forming cutaneous horn.

Doctor's Prescription

- Confirmed by intracellular nonflagellated amastigote in a biopsy of skin, mucosa, lymph node, or aspiration from liver, spleen, lymph node, or bone marrow.
- Flagellated promastigote in culture of tissue is present (needs 21 days).

Medical Prescription

Injection of sodium stibogluconate (Pentostam) 15 mg/kg/day intramuscular (IM) for 21 days.

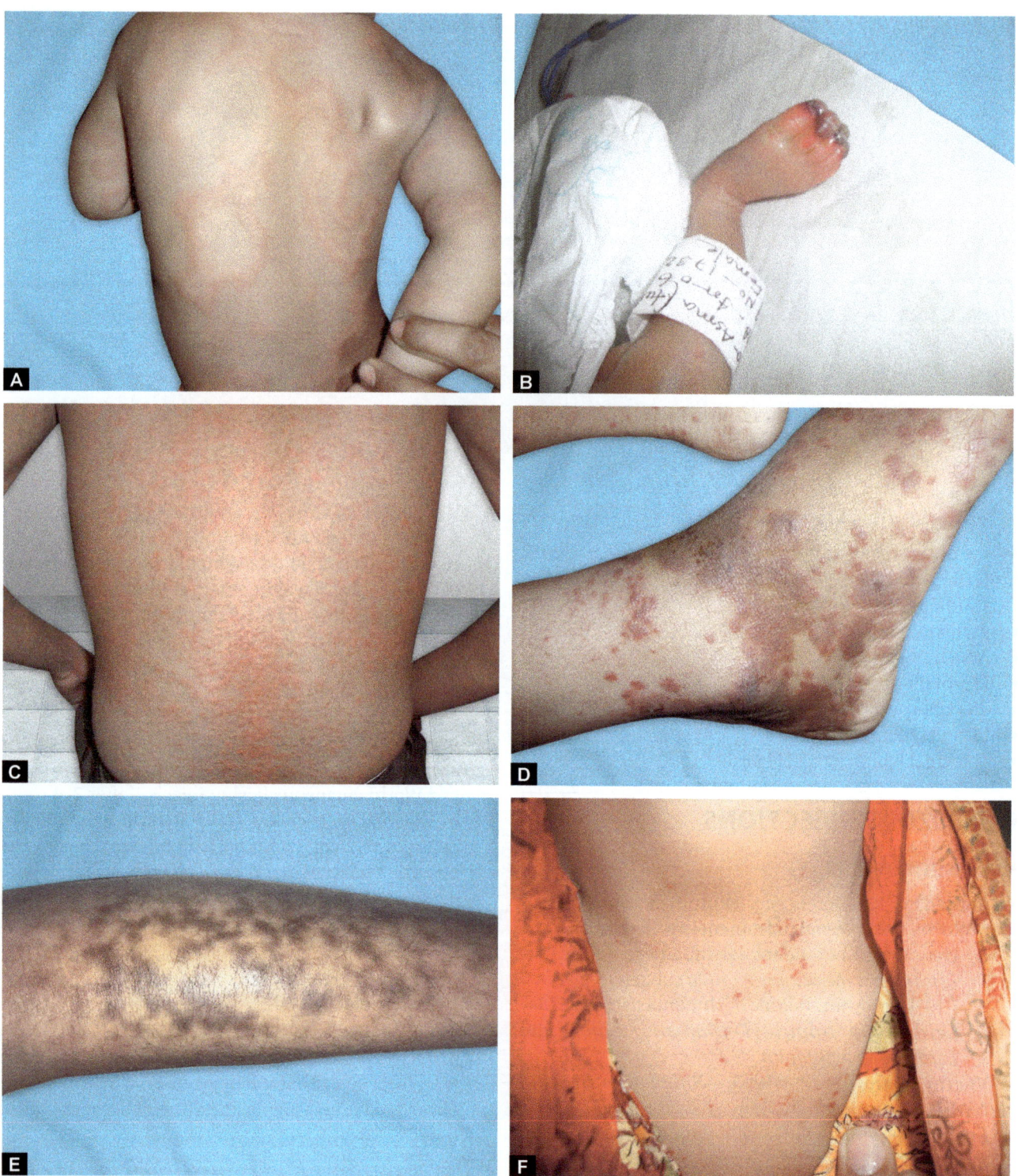

FIGS. 54A TO F: Showing skin lesions in coronavirus disease 2019 (COVID-19), respectively.

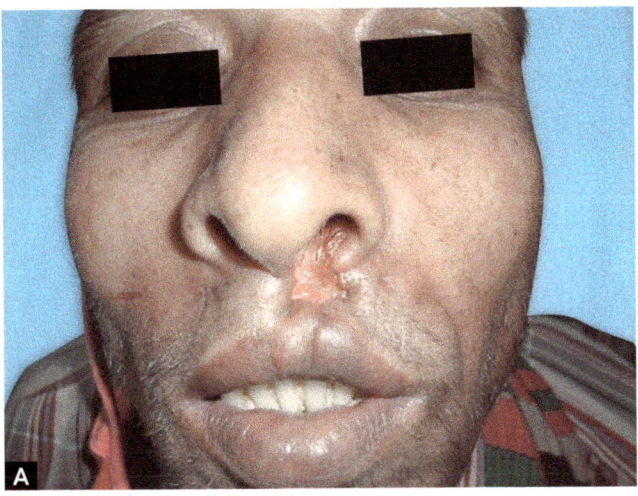
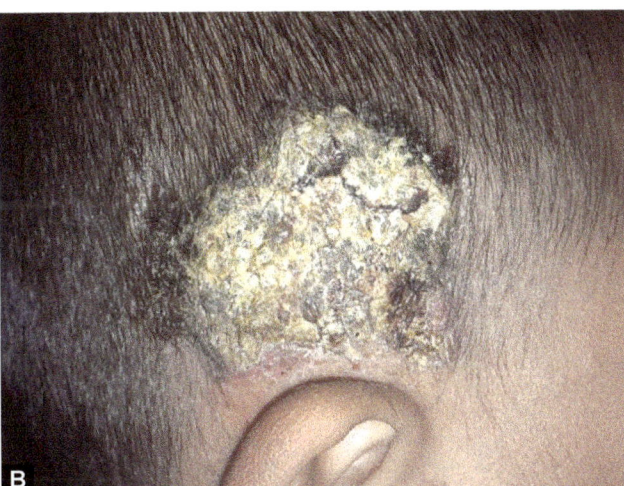

FIGS. 55A AND B: Cutaneous leishmaniasis.

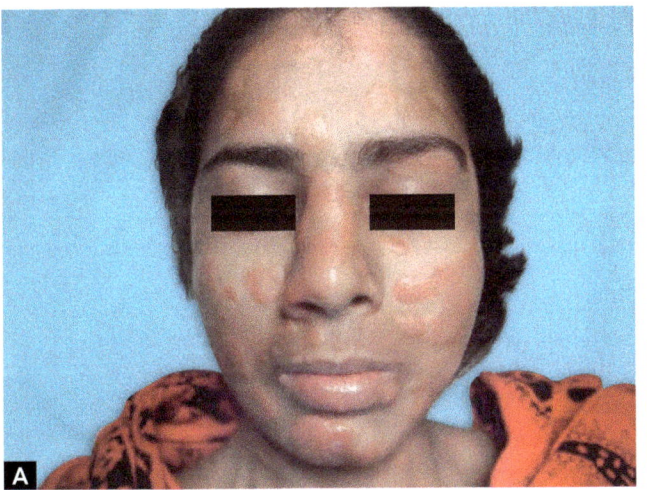
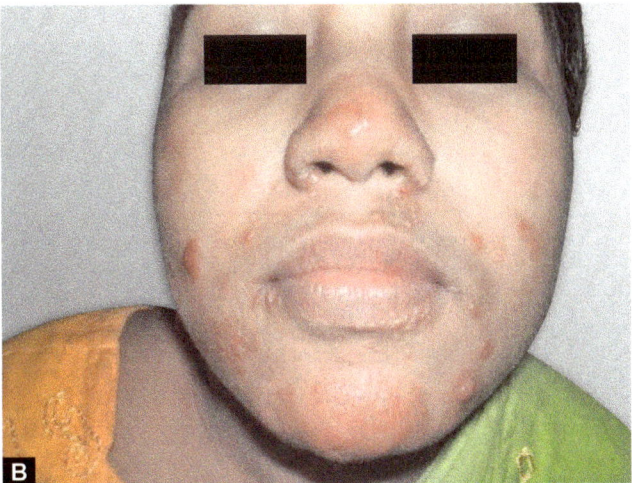

FIGS. 56A AND B: Erythematous papule, plaque, and nodule in post-kala-azar dermal leishmaniasis (PKDL).

Post-kala-azar Dermal Leishmaniasis (Figs. 56A and B)

During and recovery from kala-azar, a special type of dermal disease known as post-kala-azar dermal leishmaniasis develops. It may happen after 10 years of recovery.

Cutaneous Larva Migrans (Figs. 57A and B)

- Secondary to larvae of animal hookworms, e.g., *Ancylostoma braziliense*.
- After penetration into the skin, larvae produce pruritic, inflamed, and serpiginous tracks that are produced by migrating organisms. Migration rate is average 1–2 cm/day. Secondary bacterial infection may occur.

Medical Prescription

Self-limiting disease. It may be given by albendazole or ivermectin or topical thiabendazole.

Filariasis (Figs. 58A to D)

- Infestation by tissue nematodes (*Wuchereria bancrofti* or *Brugia malayi* or *Brugia timori*) of the lymphatic system characterized by lymphedema, with resulting hypertrophy of skin and subcutaneous tissues, resulting in enlarged and deformity of the affected parts, usually the legs, scrotum, penis, or labia majora.
- Vector mosquito (*Culex*, *Anopheles*, and *Aedes* species)
- *Acute form*: Lymphangitis and orchitis.
- *Chronic form*: Lymphedema, elephantiasis (enlarged limb becomes indurated with skin folds and overlying verrucous changes), hydrocele, and chyluria.

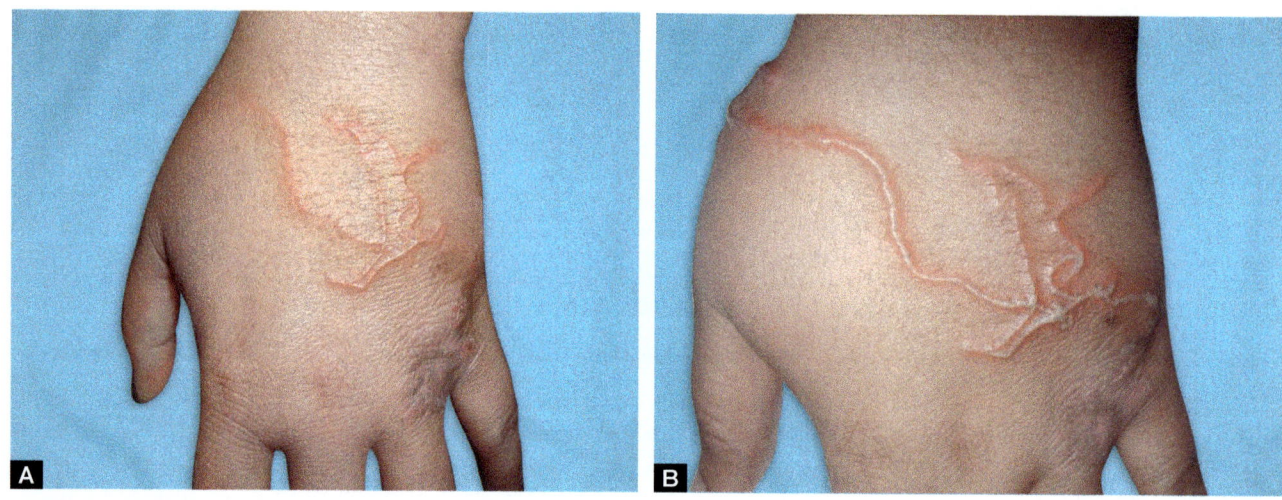

FIGS. 57A AND B: Cutaneous larva migrans.

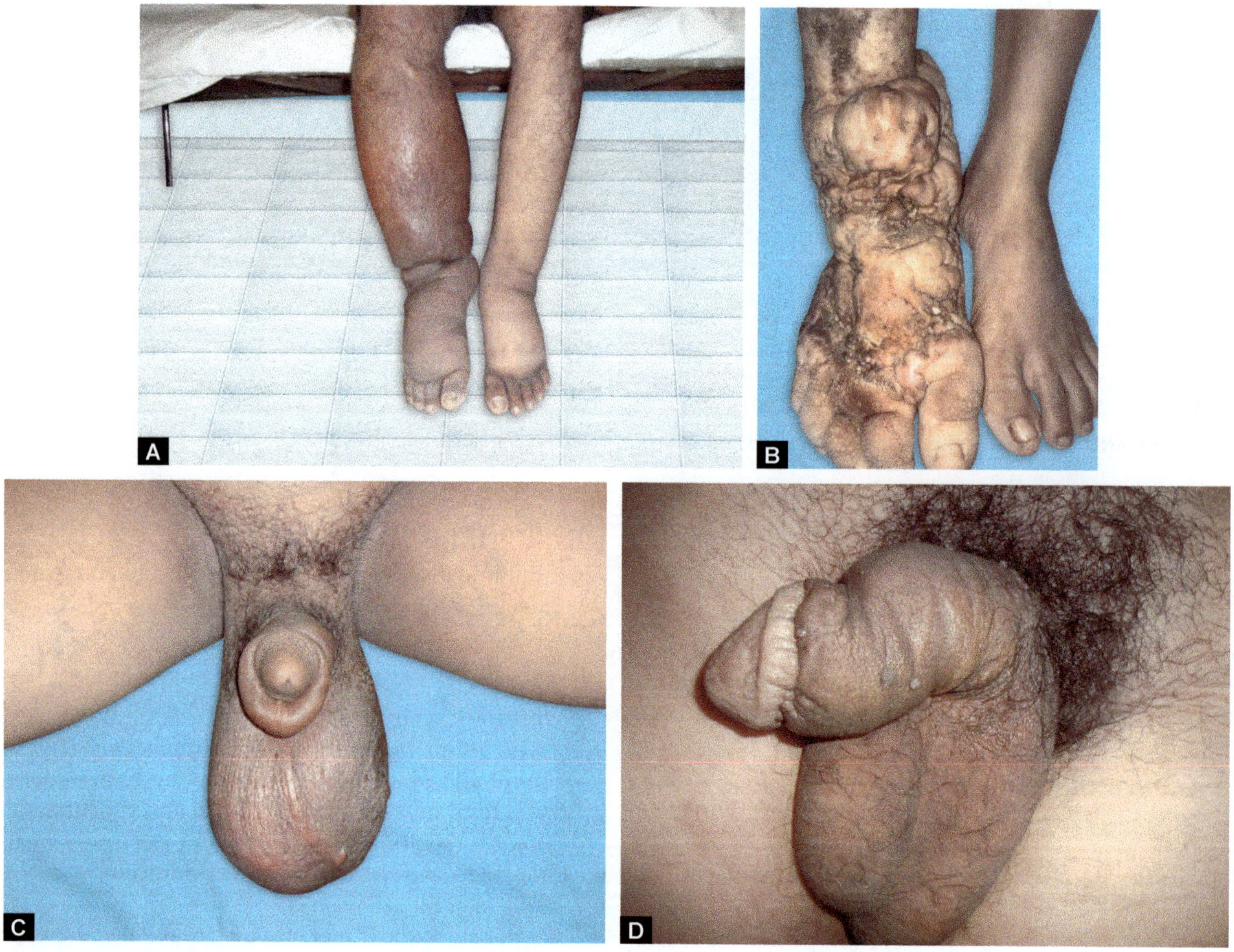

FIGS. 58A TO D: Filariasis.

Doctor's Prescription

- Microfilariae should be sought on fresh cover slip films of blood at midnight sample, urine, or other body fluids and examined with low-power lens.
- Calcified adult worms may be found by X-ray or ultrasonography (USG).
- Serological test.

Medical Prescription

Diethylcarbamazine, in increasing doses over a 14-day period, is the treatment of choice.

■ Scabies (Figs. 59A to V)

- Infestation by *Sarcoptes scabiei hominis*, a mite that lives within the stratum corneum of human skin.
- Transmission is primarily by direct contact with an infected person and occasionally by fomites (e.g., clothing).
- Incubation period may be up to 6 weeks (sensitization begins about 2–4 weeks after onset of infection).
- Asymptomatic (carriers of scabies) infestation is not uncommon.
- Pruritus is severe and often worsens at night or after a hot shower. It begins with sensitization of host. If secondarily infected pain, fever may be present.
- Skin lesions are present in finger webs, flexor surfaces, and genitalia and patient may come with generalized distribution.
- Skin lesions include erythematous papules with scale crust, eczematous change, erosions, excoriations, ulcer, vesicle, nodules, and pathognomonic linear burrow.
- Mite usually lives outside of human = 3 days.

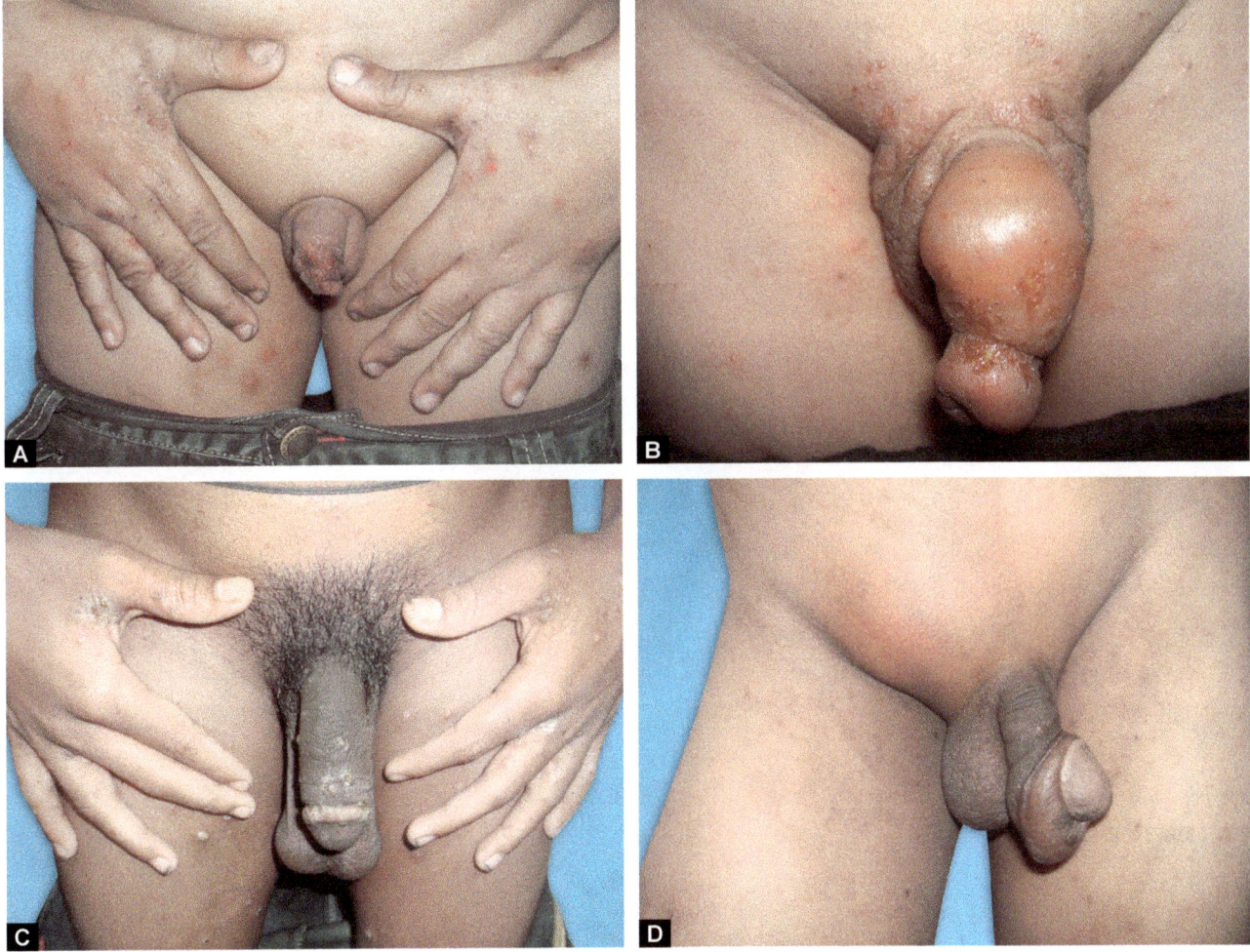

FIGS. 59A TO V: *Continued*

Continued

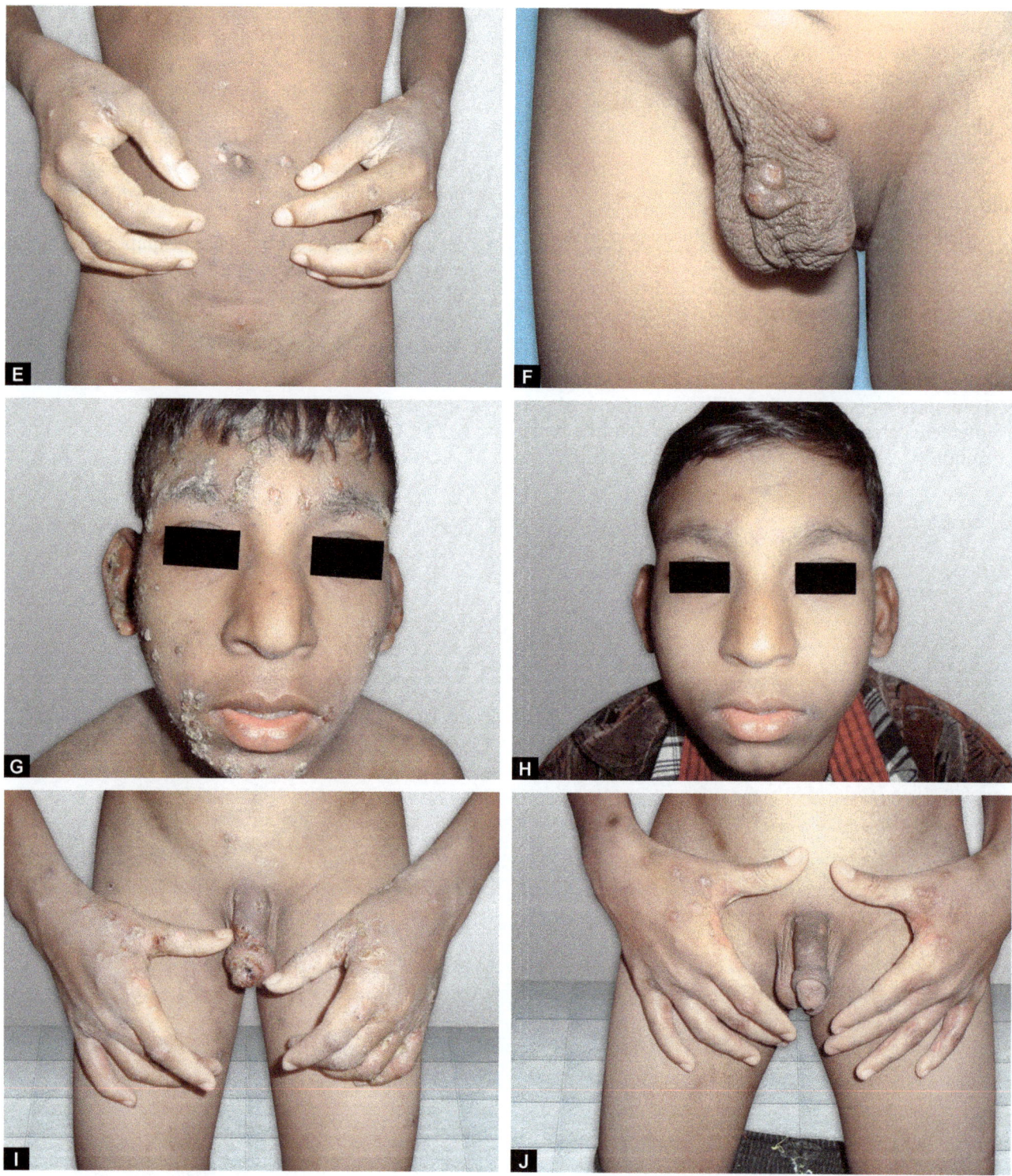

FIGS. 59A TO V: *Continued*

CHAPTER 12 Cutaneous Manifestation of Bacterial, Viral, Protozoal, Worm, Fungal Infection, and Other...

Continued

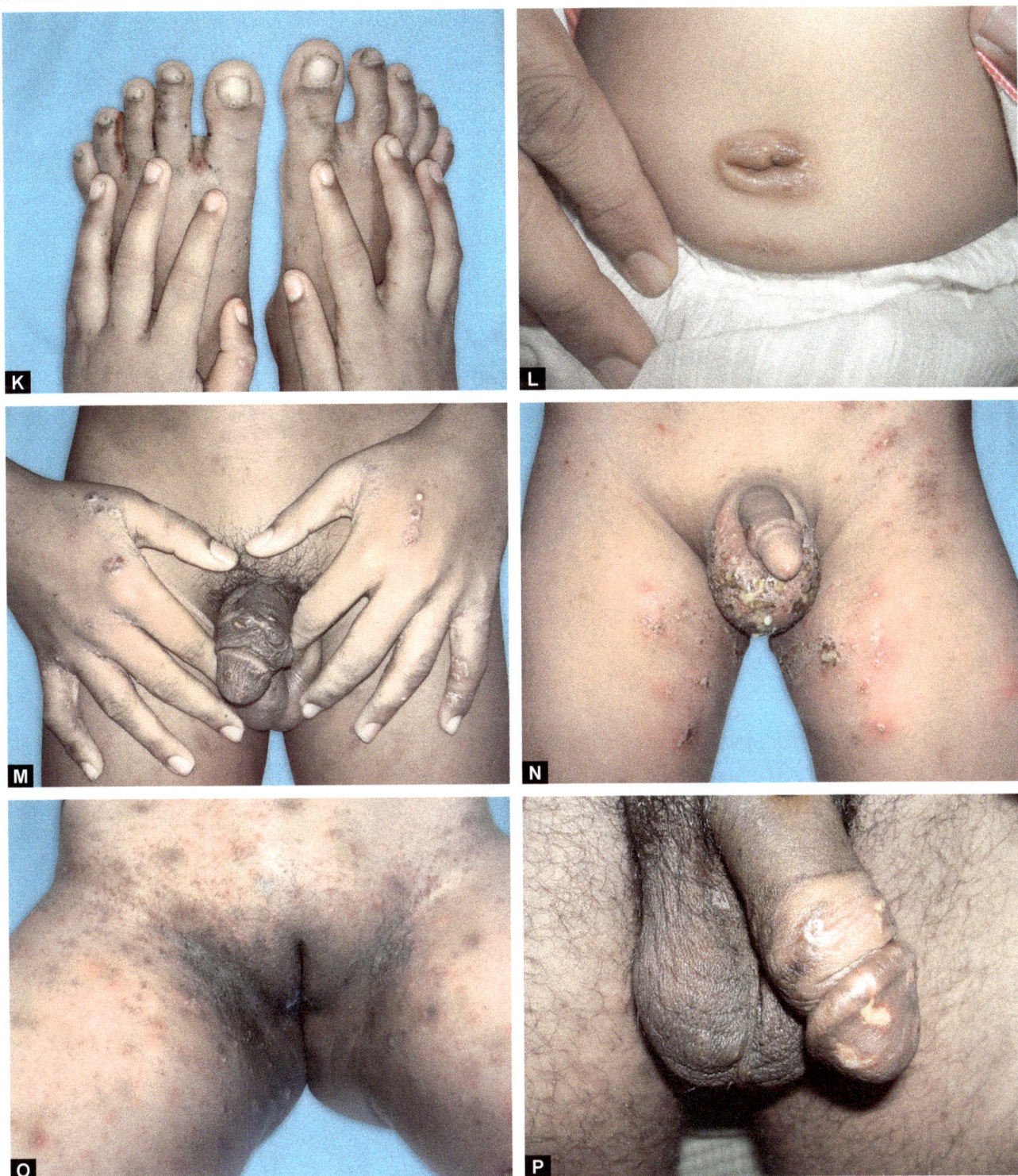

FIGS. 59A TO V: *Continued*

Continued

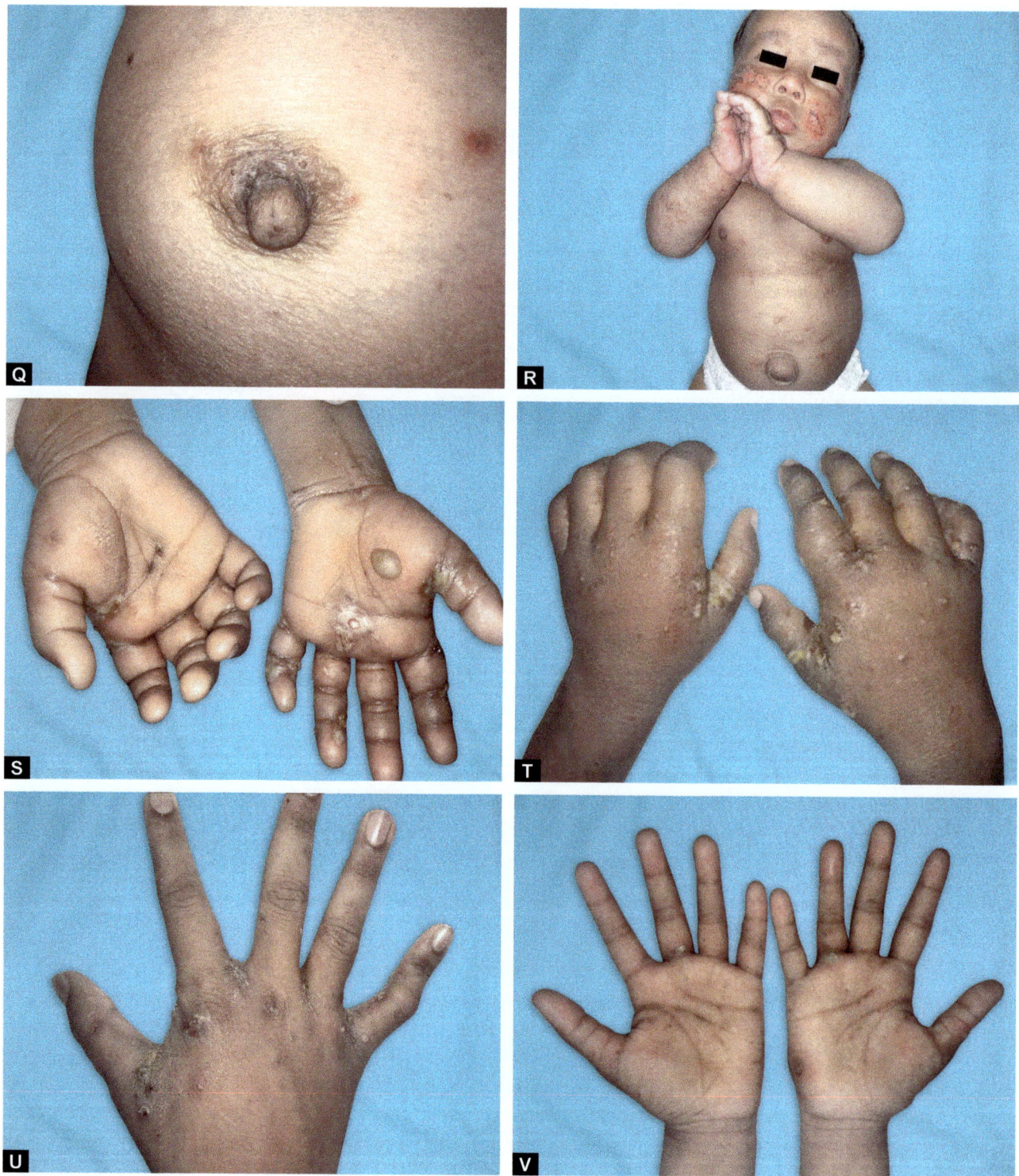

FIGS. 59A TO V: Common presentation of scabies.

Doctor's Prescription

Diagnosis is made by identification of mite or burrow. Using mineral or immersion oil on the skin and after scraping the skin material, examined under microscope to identify mite.

Medical Prescription

- Two overnight applications of topical antiscabetic medication, 1 week apart, to the entire body from the neck to toe; in infants, the elderly or immunocompromised needs to include the face and scalp.
- Permethrin 5% cream is the preferred topical agent.
- Oral ivermectin (200–400 µg/kg given on the days 1 and 8)

Pediculosis Capitis (Head Lice) (Fig. 60)

- A blood sucking six-legged insect, they lay its eggs near the base of hairs on the scalp, and they stay there after egg hatches and migrate outward with growth of hair shaft.
- Transmission is by direct contact with an infected person or fomites (hats, brushes, etc.).
- Pruritus is variable.
- In addition to the presence of lice and eggs, there may be erythema, scaling, excoriation, and crust and secondary bacterial infection is present.

Medical Prescription

Same as scabies, but permethrin is 1% instead of 5%.

Syphilis (Lues)

- Contagious, sexually transmitted disease caused by the spirochete *Treponema pallidum*, transmitted through skin and mucous membrane resulted in systemic infection with manifestations in nearly every organ system.
- After 10–90 days of inoculation (average 3 weeks), primary syphilis (chancre) develops with one or more ulcers, usually anogenital regions (**Figs. 61A and B**). The ulcers are painless and on palpation, the base is firm; regional lymphadenopathy may be present.
- Up to 3–10 weeks after appearance of chancre, secondary syphilis develops with some constitutional symptoms. Maculopapular rash, condylomata lata, generalized lymphadenopathy, and mucosal patches are four common features of secondary syphilis (**Figs. 62A and B**).
- After 1–2 years of secondary syphilis, disease enters into latent phase.
- After 2–20 years of latency, one-third of untreated patient develops tertiary syphilis with formation of gummas at different sites in different systems of body and two-thirds of patient becomes disease free in time.

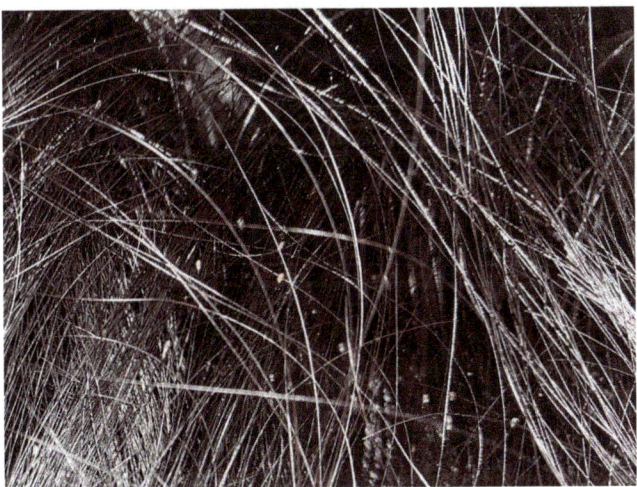

FIG. 60: Head lice.

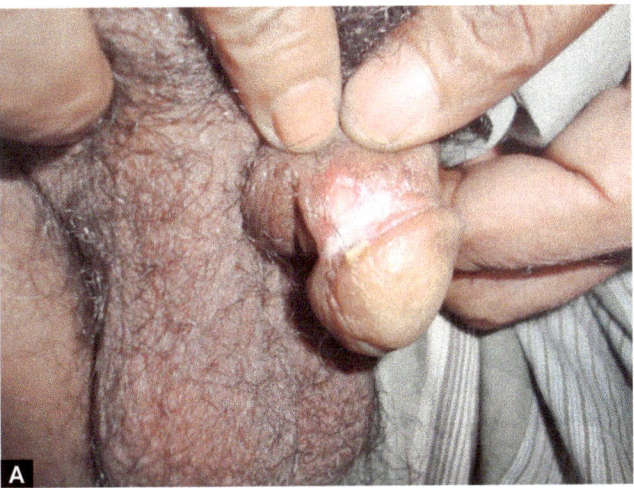
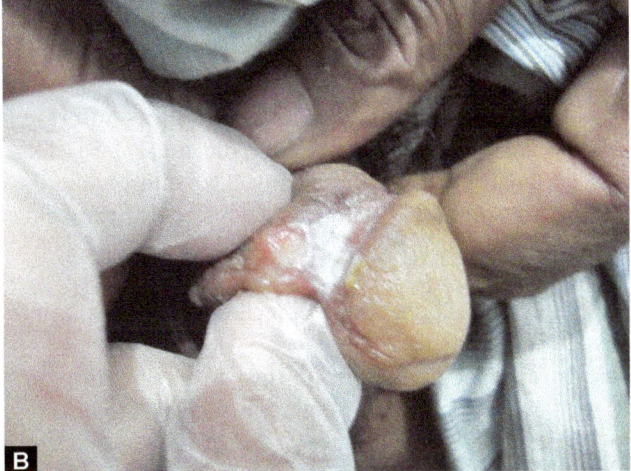

FIGS. 61A AND B: Chancre, hard consistency.

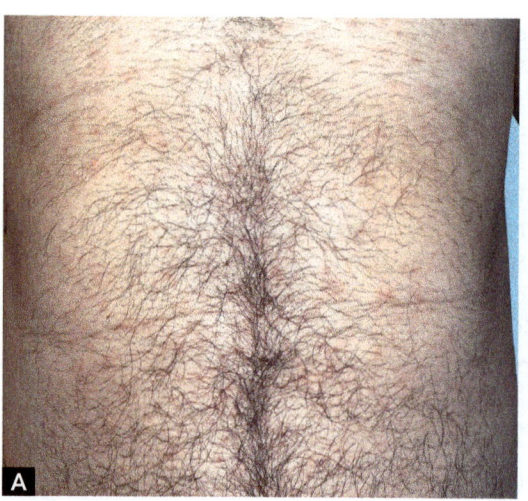
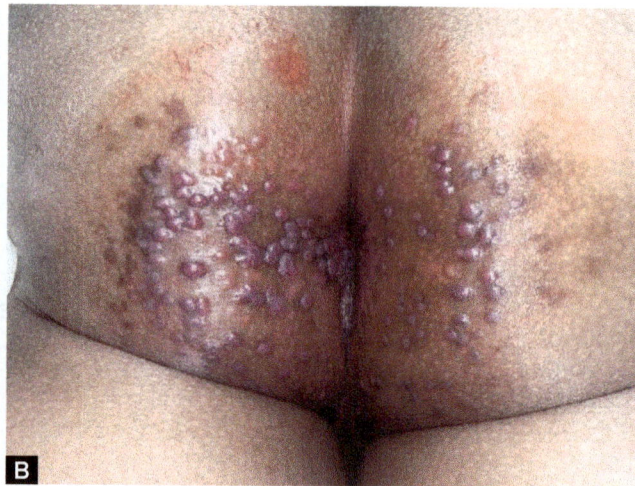

FIGS. 62A AND B: Maculopapular rash and condylomata lata in secondary syphilis.

Doctor's Prescription

- Dark-field microscopy—positive in primary syphilis and papular lesions of secondary syphilis such as condylomata lata.
- Direct fluorescent antibody-*T. pallidum* (DFA-TP) test—used to detect TP in exudates of lesions from lymph node aspiration or tissue.

Serological Tests

- Venereal disease research laboratory (VDRL)—positive around 80% in primary syphilis and 99% in secondary syphilis.
- Anti-TP antibodies—microhemagglutination assay (MHA-TP) and fluorescent treponemal antibody absorption (FTA-ABS) around 90% positive in primary syphilis and 99% in secondary syphilis.

Medical Prescription

- *Recommended treatment for early syphilis (primary, secondary, and early latent)*:
  - Injection of benzathine penicillin 2.4 million units in single dose.
  - Alternative regimens for penicillin—allergic patients having doxycycline 100 mg PO BD for 14 days or tetracycline 500 mg PO qid for 14 days or ceftriaxone 1 g IV daily for 14 days or azithromycin 2 g single dose.
- *In pregnancy*:
  - Injection of benzathine penicillin 2.4 million units in single dose.
  - In case of penicillin allergy, desensitization to penicillin or alternate regimens such as ceftriaxone 1 g IV daily for 14 days or azithromycin 500 mg daily for 10 days.

FUNGAL INFECTIONS OF SKIN, HAIR, NAIL, AND MUCOUS MEMBRANE

Superficial Fungal Infections

It is caused by fungi that are capable of colonizing and superficially invade in skin, hair, nail, and mucous membrane.
- Dermatophytes
- *Malassezia* species
- *Candida* species

Deep Fungal Infections

It occurs after percutaneous inoculation.
- Maduromycosis
- Sporotrichosis

Systemic Fungal Infections

Primary lung infection is disseminated hematogenously to multiple organs.

Fungi Causing Infections

- *Dermatophytes*: Infect keratinized epithelium, hair follicles, and nail apparatus.
- *Candida* species: Requires a worm humid environment.
- *Malassezia* species: Requires a humid micro-environment and lipids for growth.

Dermatophytosis

Dermatophytes are unique group of fungus capable of infecting keratinized cutaneous structures including serum, hair, and nails.

CHAPTER 12 Cutaneous Manifestation of Bacterial, Viral, Protozoal, Worm, Fungal Infection, and Other...

Tinea Corporis (Figs. 63 and 64)

- Synonym—ringworm.
- Dermatophyte infection of the trunk, legs, arms, and/or neck excluding the feet, hands, groin, scalp, and face.

Key Points

- Small-to-large scaling, sharply marginated plaques with or without pustules or vesicles, usually sharp margins.
- Peripheral enlargement and central clearing are classic presentation.
- Psoriasiform plaques
- Verrucous plaques

Laboratory Examination

Approach is same for other dermatophyte infections.
- Direct microscopy with potassium hydroxide (KOH) preparation—dermatophytes are recognized as septated, tube-like structures (hyphae or mycelia).

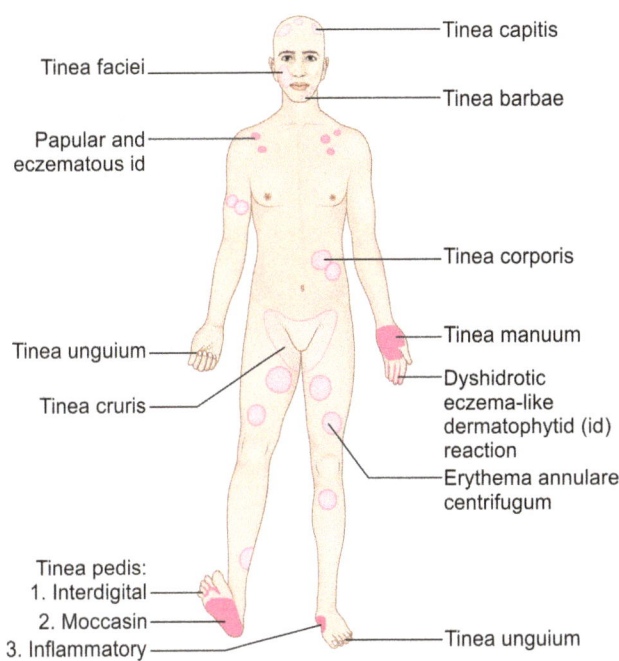

FIG. 63: Name of dermatophyte infections according to their sites.

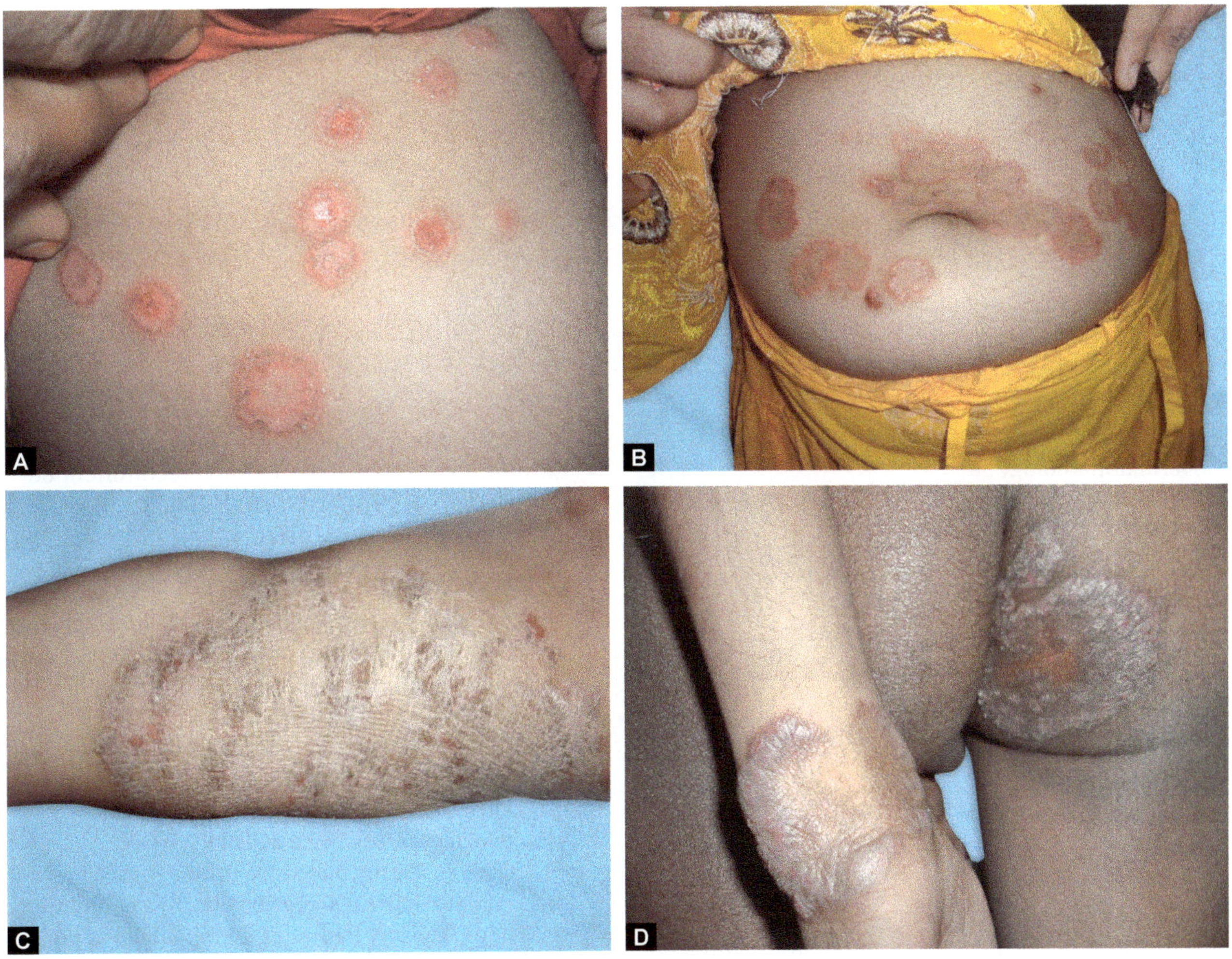

FIGS. 64A TO H: *Continued*

Continued

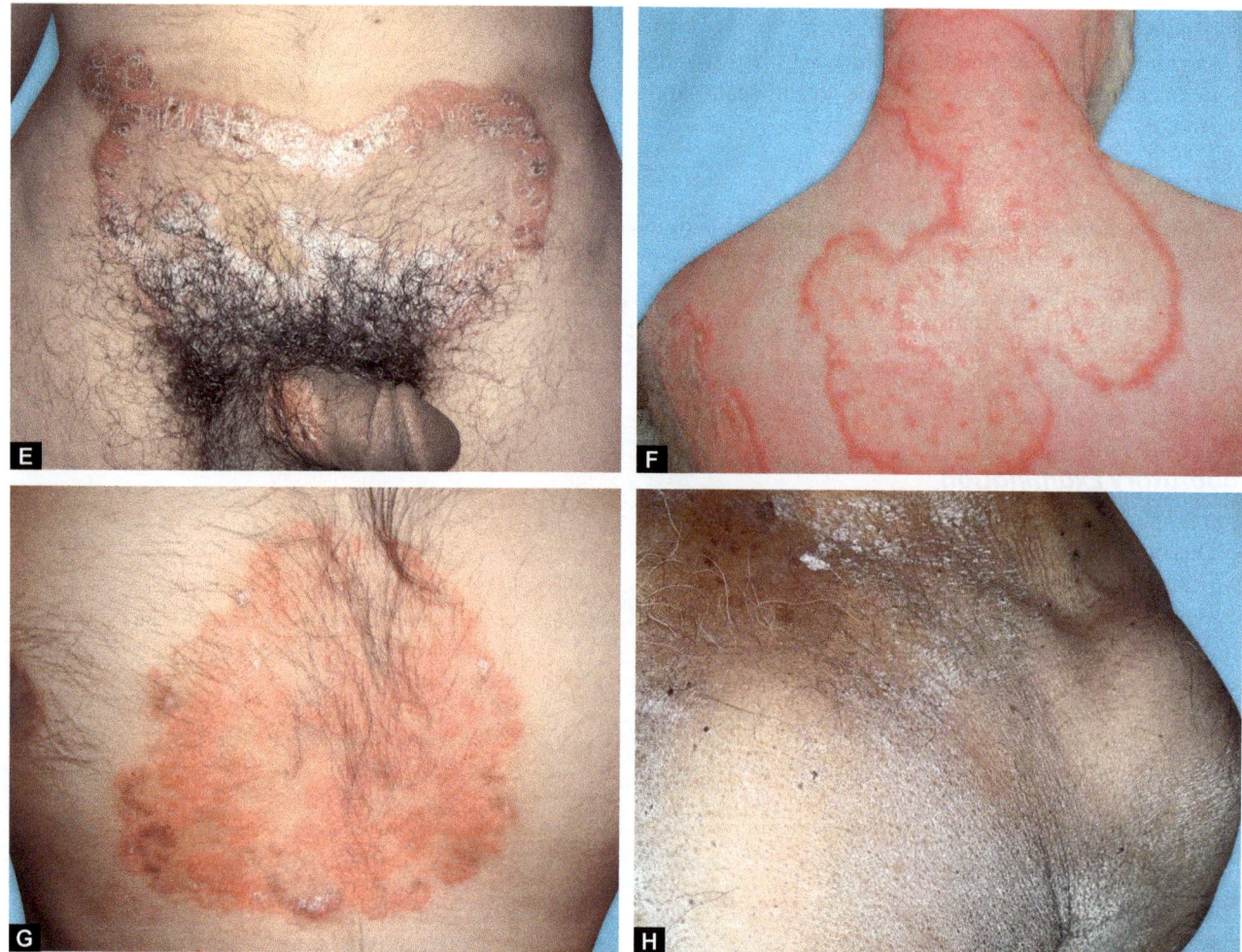

FIGS. 64A TO H: Tinea corporis.

- Wood's lamp
- Fungal culture
- Dermatopathology

Treatment

General Measures

Avoid and correction of triggering factors.
- Correction of hyperhidrosis (DM, anxiety, humid environment, hyperthyroidism, obesity, etc.).
- Avoid tight-fitting clothes.
- Prophylactic measures in immunosuppressive conditions.

Specific Measures

Topical treatment is usually sufficient in limited disease conditions.
- Miconazole, clotrimazole, terbinafine, tolnaftate, naftifine, ciclopirox, ketoconazole, econazole, oxiconazole, butenafine, or sulconazole until 1–2 weeks after clearance.
- Minimum duration of therapy recommended is 4 weeks.
- Treat until there is no scaling.

Systemic Antifungal Drugs

- Needed for poor response in topical antifungal drug or in extensive diseases such as tinea capitis, tinea unguium, and tinea pedis.
- *Terbinafine 250 mg tablet*:
  - Most effective oral antidermatophyte.
  - Low efficacy against other fungal infections.
  - One tablet daily for 1–2 weeks duration.
- Itraconazole 200 mg twice daily for 1 week.
- Fluconazole 150 mg once a week for 4 weeks.
- Griseofulvin 500–1,000 mg/day. Dosage of children is 10–20 mg/kg/day. Period of therapy depends on the response of the lesions.

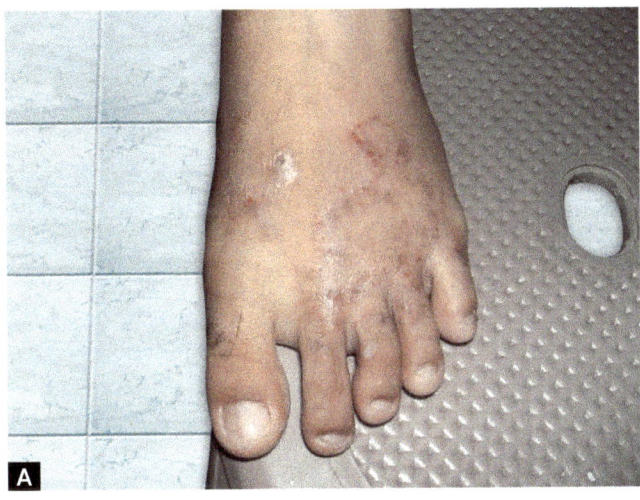
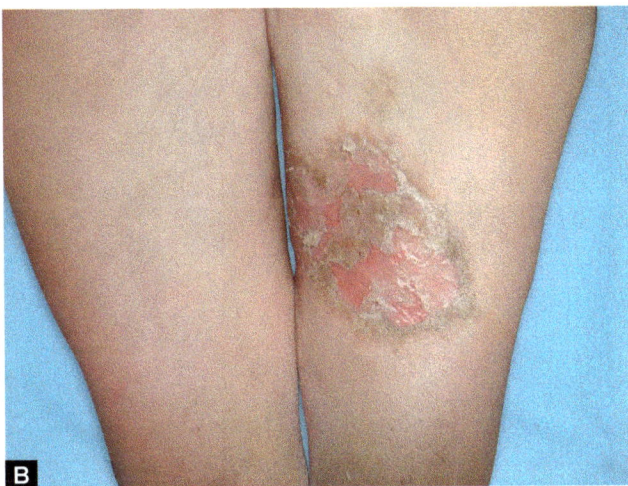

FIGS. 65A AND B: Typical presentation.

Tinea Pedis (Figs. 66 and 67)

Synonym: Athlete's foot fungus.

Key Points

- Scaly, pruritic, and erythematous eruption on the plantar and dorsal surfaces of the feet with maceration, peeling, and fissuring.
- Hypersensitivity reaction to the fungus (dermatophytid or "id" reaction) may be present on the hands and feet with pruritus, vesicles, and papules.
- Usually asymptomatic, mild pruritus, and pain with bacterial superinfection.

Types

- *Interdigital type* (**Figs. 66C and 68A**):
  - Dry scaling, maceration, peeling, and fissure of toe web
  - Most common between the fourth and fifth toes.
  - Hyperhidrosis is common.
  - Infection may spread to adjacent of feet.
  - May be associated with tinea unguium.
- *Moccasin type* [**Figs. 65A and B, 66A and B (after treatment) 66D, 67A and B, 68B**]:
  - Well-demarcated erythema with minute papules on margin, fine white scaling, and hyperkeratosis is confined to the heels, soles, and lateral border of feet.
  - Bilateral involvement is more common.
- *Inflammatory/bullous type*:
  - Vesicles or bullae are filled with clear fluid.
  - Pus usually indicates secondary bacterial infection.
  - May be associated with "id" reaction.
  - *Site*: Sole, web spaces, and instep.

Treatment

- General and topical management like tinea corporis; however, topical treatment should be continued for 2–4 weeks.
- Systemic antifungal drug indicated for extensive infection, for failures of topical treatment, or for those with tinea unguium and moccasin-type tinea.
  - *Terbinafine*: 250 mg daily for 14 days.
  - *Itraconazole*: 200 mg twice daily for 7 days or 200 mg daily for 14 days.
  - *Fluconazole*: 150–200 mg daily for 4–6 weeks.

Tinea Manuum (Figs. 69A to D)

Synonym: Tinea hand.

Key Points

- Often unilateral, most commonly on the dominant hand.
- Well-demarcated scaling patches and hyperkeratosis.
- Scaling is confined to palmer creases and fissure on palm hand. Borders are well-demarcated and central clearing may present.

Management

- General and topical measures—same as tinea corporis.
- *Systemic*:
  - Because of thickness of palmar stratum corneum and especially if associated with tinea unguium of figure nails, tinea manuum is impossible to cure with topical agents.

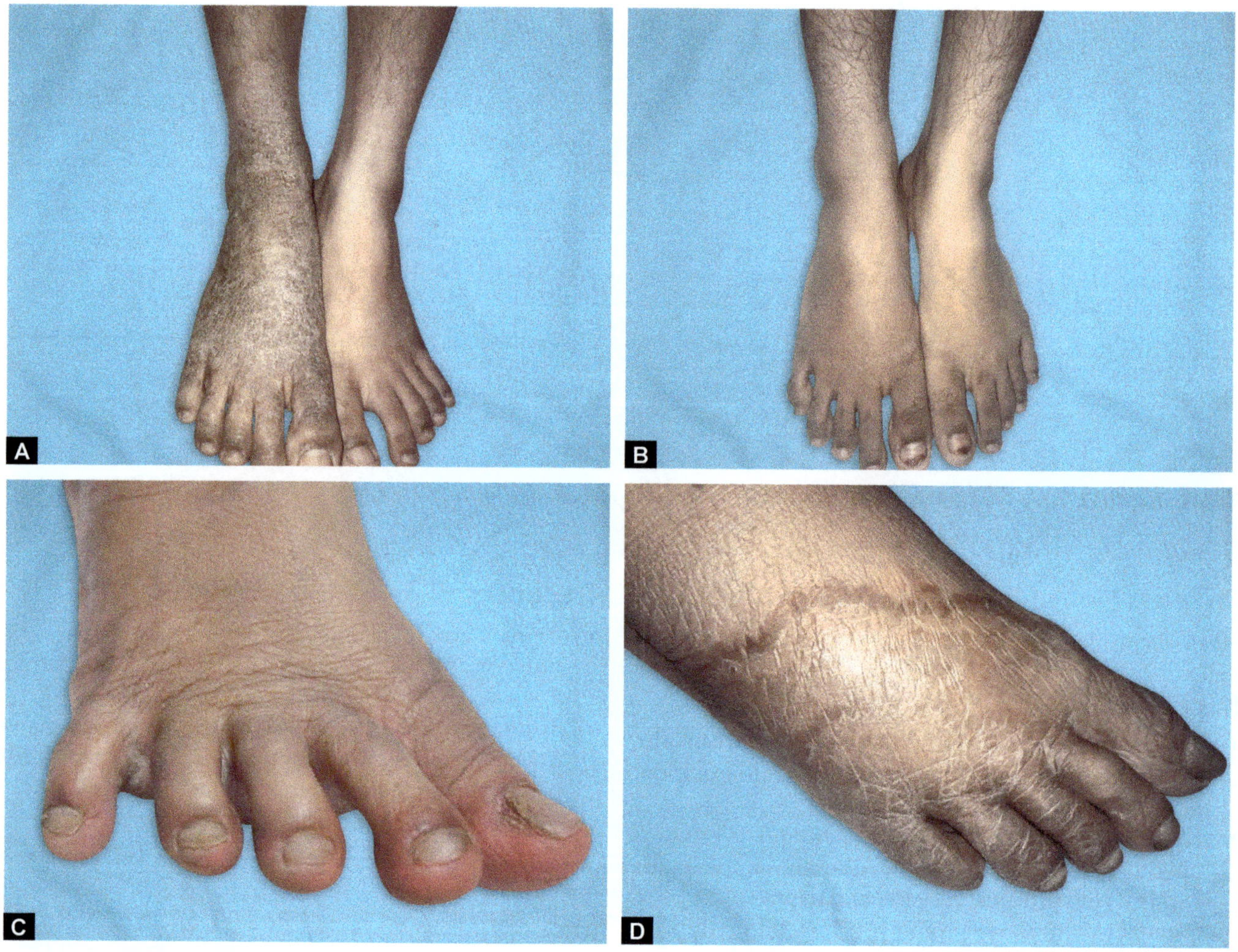

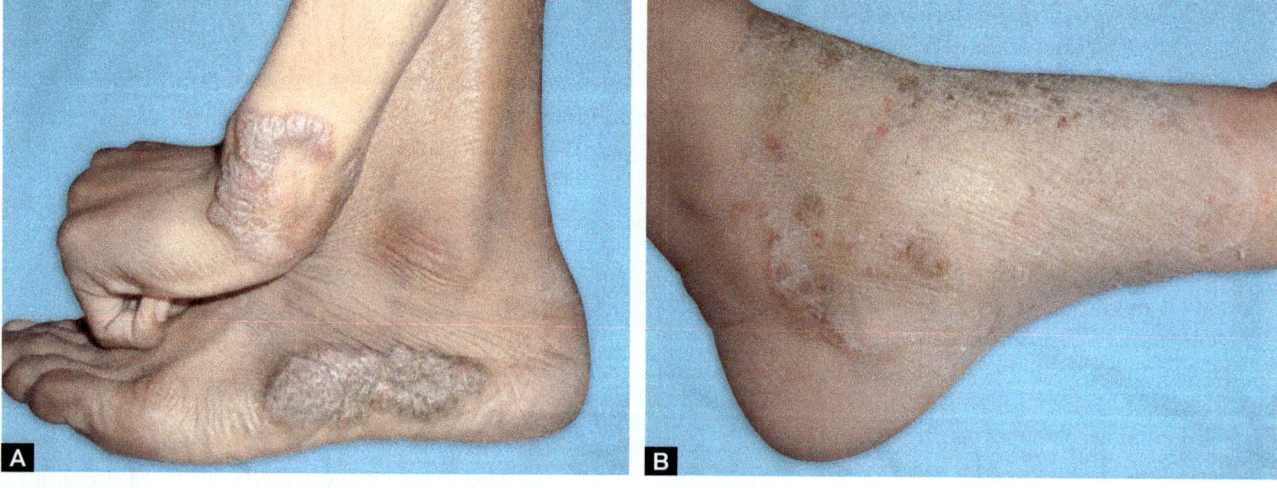

FIGS. 66A TO D: Before and after treatment.

FIGS. 67A AND B: Tinea pedis.

CHAPTER 12 Cutaneous Manifestation of Bacterial, Viral, Protozoal, Worm, Fungal Infection, and Other...

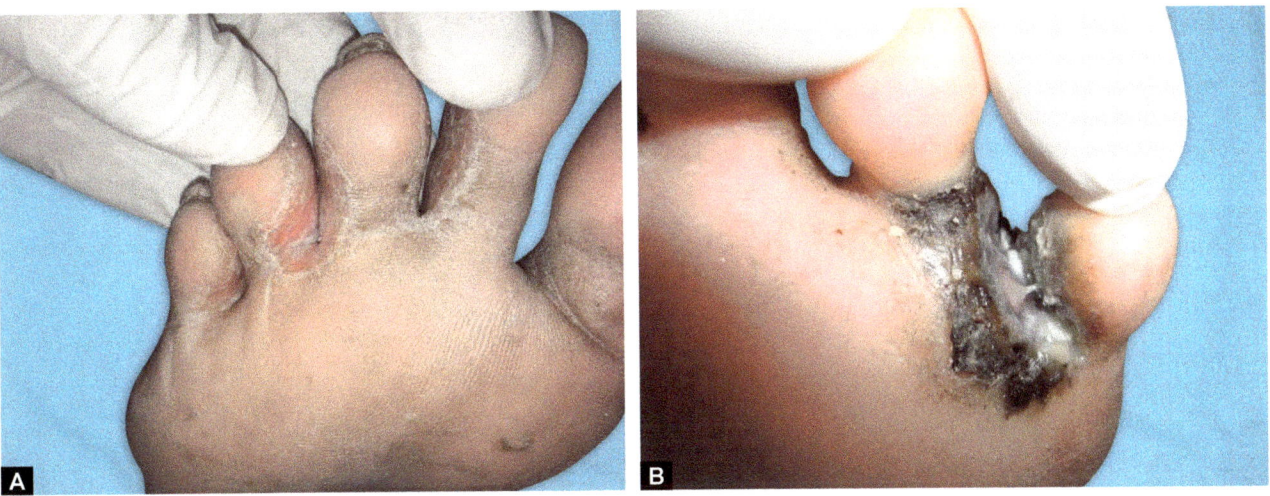

FIGS. 68A AND B: Untreated chronic infection develops squamous cell carcinoma (SCC).

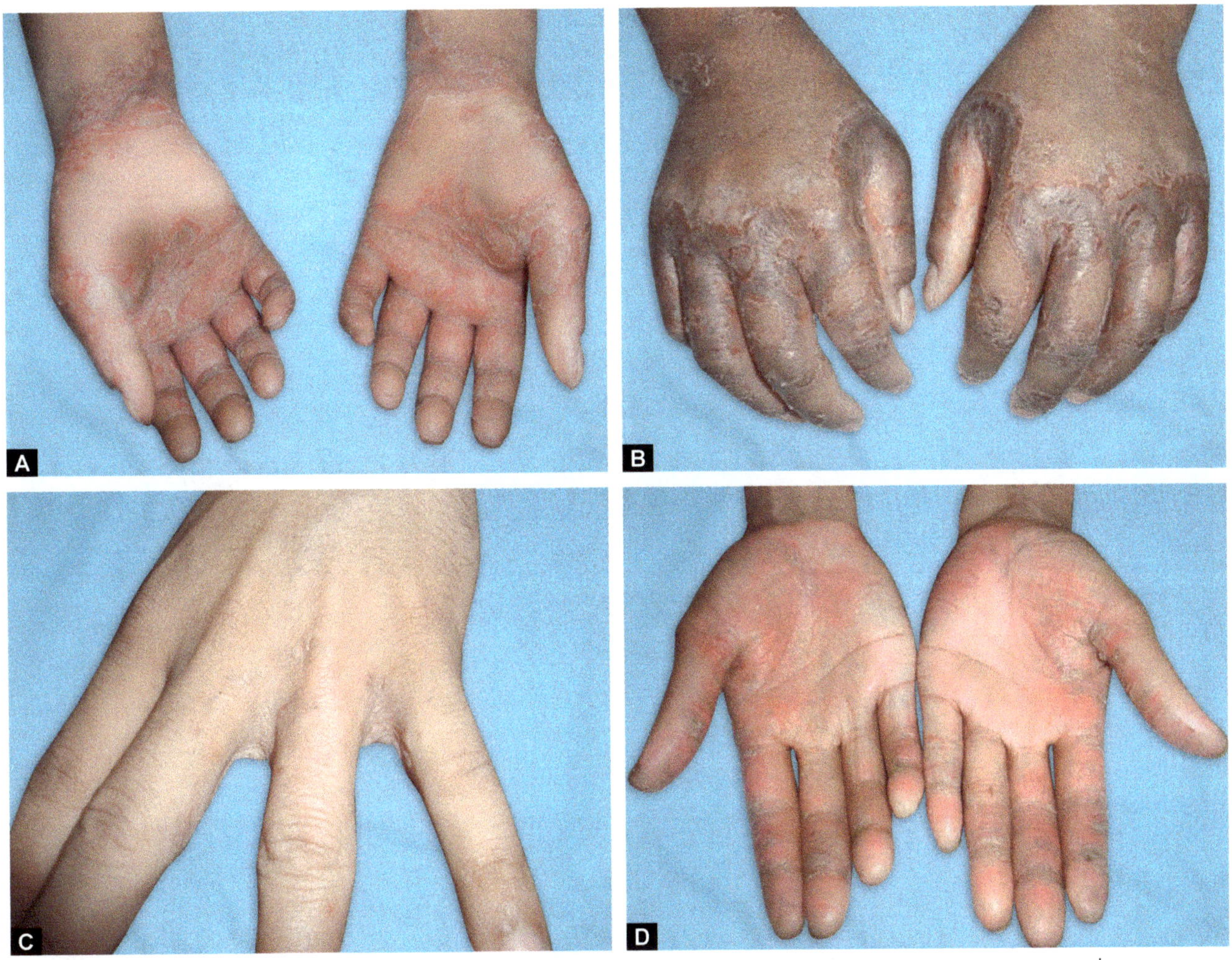

FIGS. 69A TO D: Tinea manuum.

- Oral agents eradicate dermatophytoses of hands and feet:
  - *Terbinafine*: 250 mg daily for 14 days.
  - *Itraconazole*: 200 mg daily for 7 days.
  - *Fluconazole*: 150–200 mg daily for 2–4 weeks.

Tinea Cruris (Figs. 70A to J)

- *Synonym*: "Jock itch."
- Subacute or chronic dermatophytoses of the groin, pubic regions, and thighs.

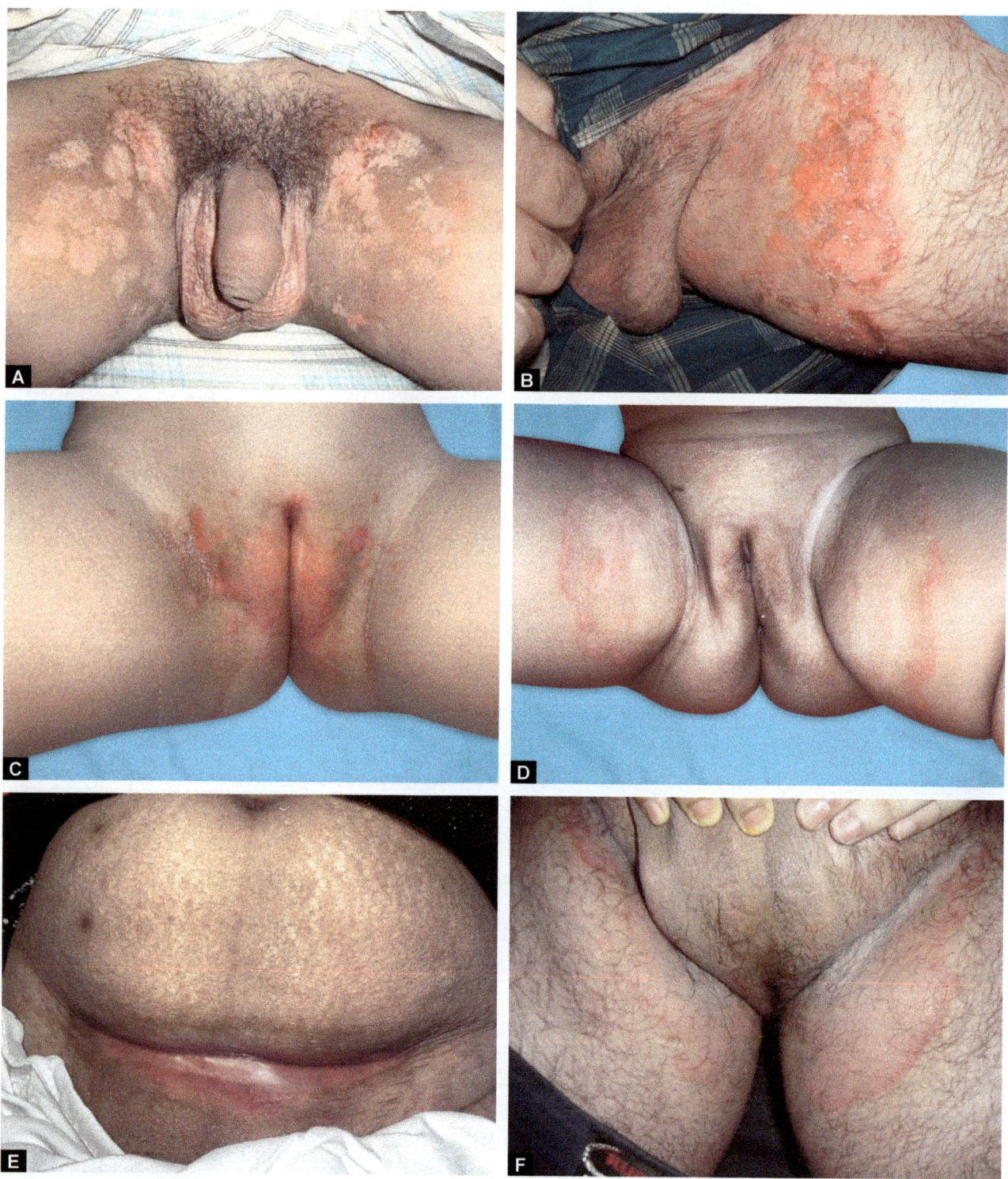

FIGS. 70A TO J: *Continued*

Continued

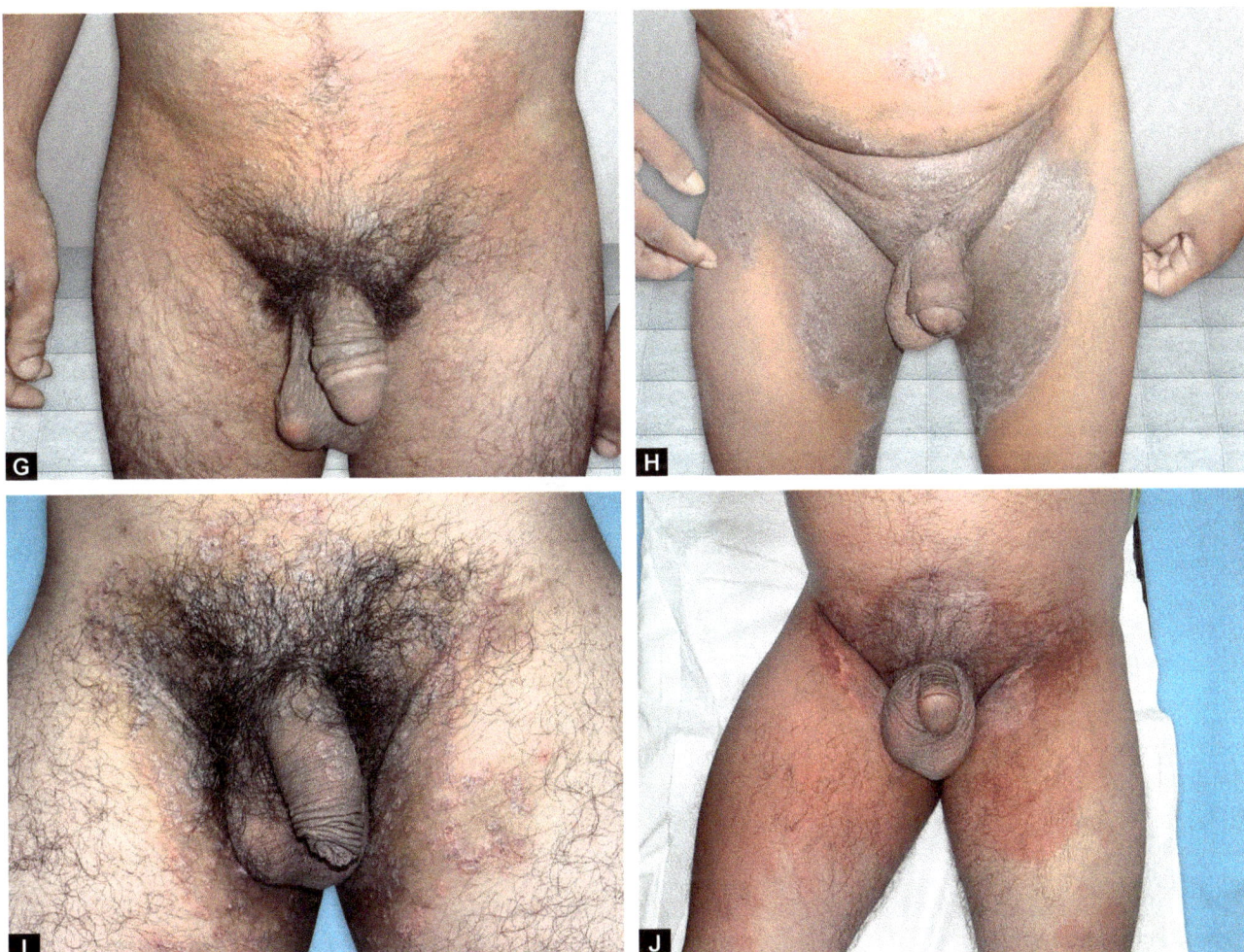

FIGS. 70A TO J: Tinea cruris.

Key Points
- Usually associated with tinea pedis and tinea unguium of toenails.
- Large, scaling, and well-demarcated dull red/tan/brown plaque.
- Central cleary.
- Papules and pustules may be present of mycosis and dermatophytic folliculitis.
- Treated cases—lack of scale and postinflammatory hyperpigmentation in dark-stained person.

Laboratory Examination
Same as tinea corporis.

Management
- *General measures*:
  - Avoid warm, humid environment and tight-fitting clothes.
  - Control obesity and topical glucocorticoid therapy.
- *Topical and systemic treatment*: Same as tinea corporis.

Tinea Facialis (Figs. 71A to F)
- *Synonym*: Tinea faciei.
- Dermatophytosis of the glabrous facial skin.

Key Points
- Well-circumscribed macule to plaque of variable size, elevated border, and clearing.
- Scaling is often minimal but can be pronounced.

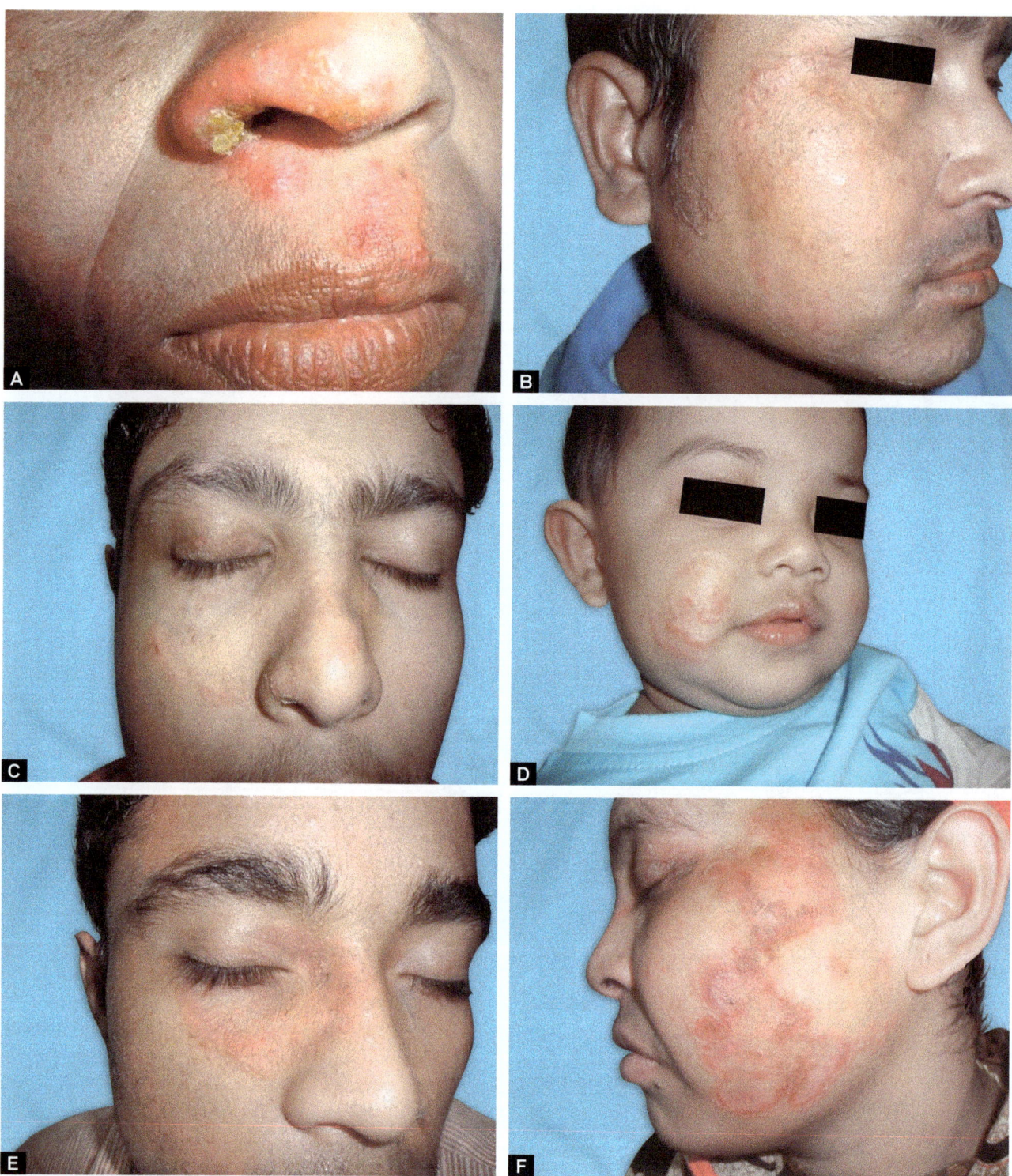

FIGS. 71A TO F: Tinea faciei.

CHAPTER 12 Cutaneous Manifestation of Bacterial, Viral, Protozoal, Worm, Fungal Infection, and Other...

- Pink to erythematous.
- Any area of face, but usually not symmetric.

Management
Same as tinea corporis.

Tinea Capitis (Figs. 72A to H)
Synonym: Scalp ringworm.

Key Points
- Incidence is higher in black children.
- Asymptomatic scaling
- Widespread scaling with minimal loss.
- "Black dot" tinea—discrete areas of hair loss with shafts of brown hairs reassembly "dots".
- "Gray patch"—partial alopecia, inflammation minimal, but massive scaling is usually found.
- Kerion—painful, inflamed, and crusted mass with purulent discharge, often associated with fever and regional lymphadenopathy.
- *Favus*: Inflammatory and scarring characterized by yellow cup-shaped crust (scutula) around a hair.

Management
- *Griseofulvin*:
  - *Microsized*: 20 mg/kg/day; maximum 1 g/day for 6 weeks to 1–2 months.
  - *Ultramicrosize griseofulvin*: 10 mg/kg/day; maximum 750 mg/kg/day.
- Terbinafine—250 mg/day.
- Itraconazole—200 mg/day for 4–8 weeks.
- Fluconazole—100 mg, 150 mg, and 200 mg for children 6–8 mg/kg/day for 3–4 weeks.
- Ketoconazole—200 mg/day for 4–6 weeks.

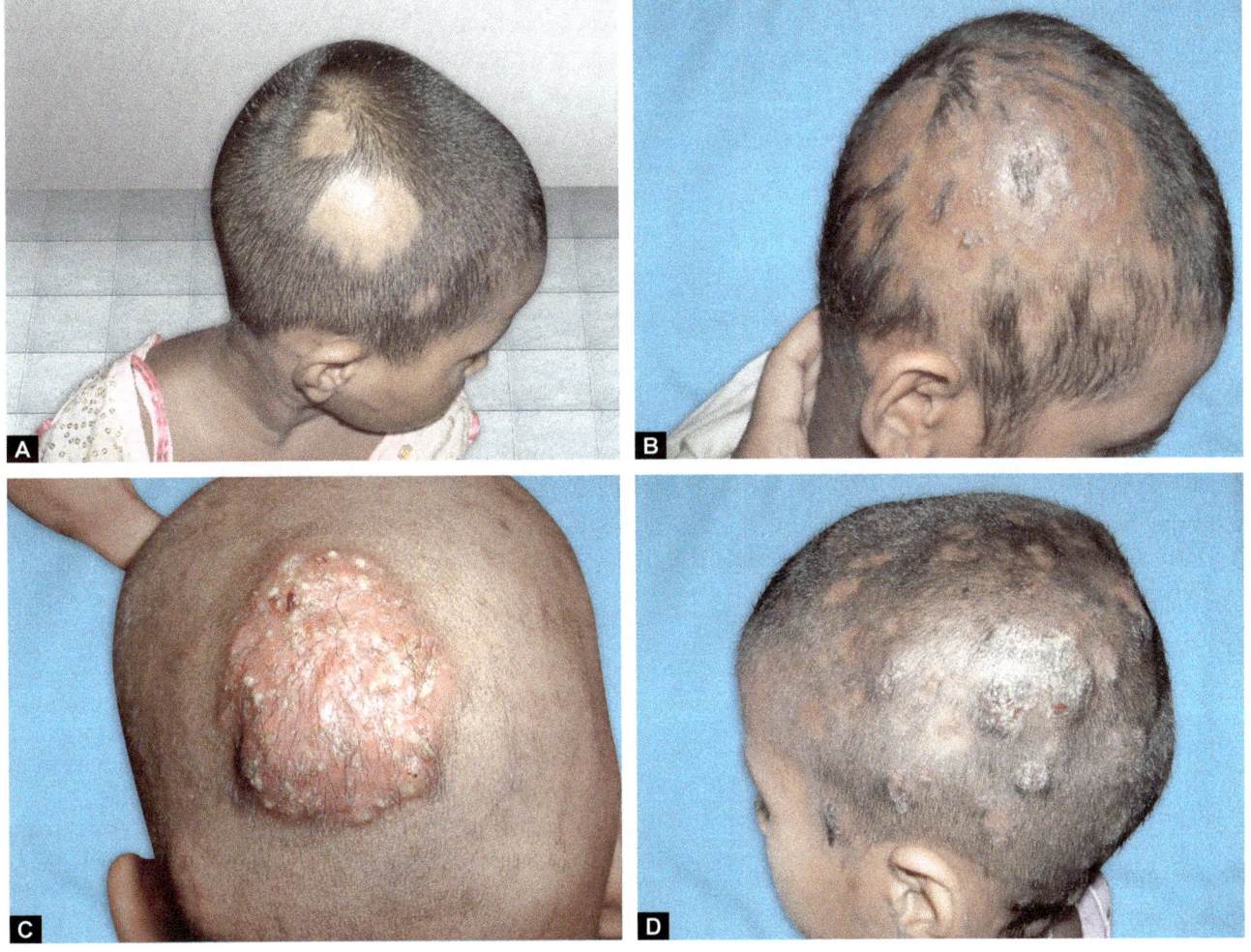

FIGS. 72A TO H: *Continued*

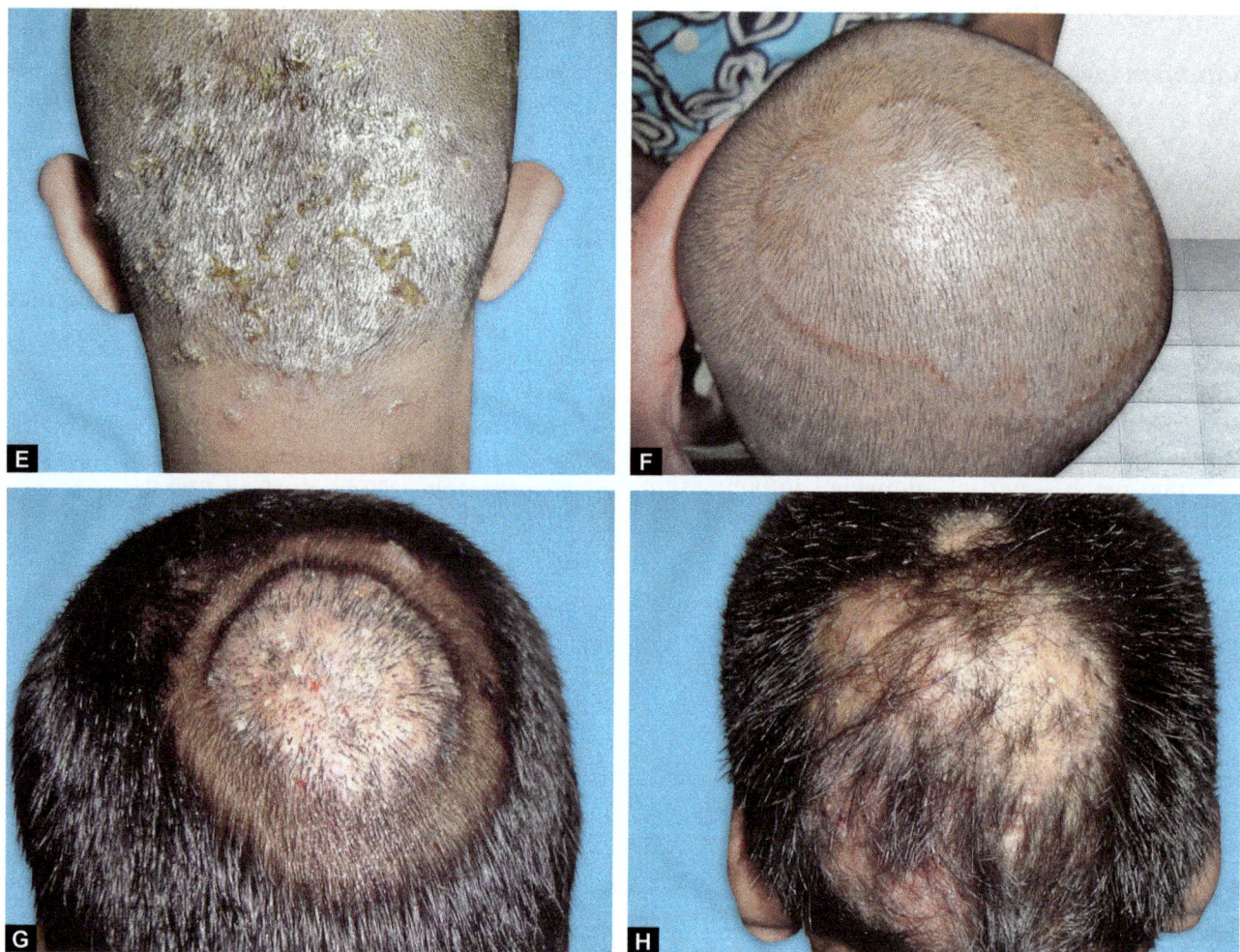

FIGS. 72A TO H: Tinea capitis.

■ Tinea Barbae (Figs. 73A to D)
- *Synonym*: Ringworm of the beard.
- Dermatophytic trichomycosis involving the beard and moustache area.

Key Points
- It is more common in farmers.
- Pustular folliculitis
- Involved hairs are loose and easily removed.
- Papules may coalesce to inflammatory plaques topped by pustules.

Management
Same as tinea capitis.

■ Candidiasis
Most commonly caused by the yeast *Candida albicans* and less often by other *Candida* species.

Cutaneous Candidiasis
Key Points
- *Intertrigo*—sharply demarcated, polycyclic erythematous, eroded patches with small pustular lesion at the periphery. Distributed usually submammary folds, axillae, groins, perineal, and intergluteal cleft.
  - Differential diagnosis—bacterial intertrigo, psoriasis, erythrasma, and dermatophytosis.

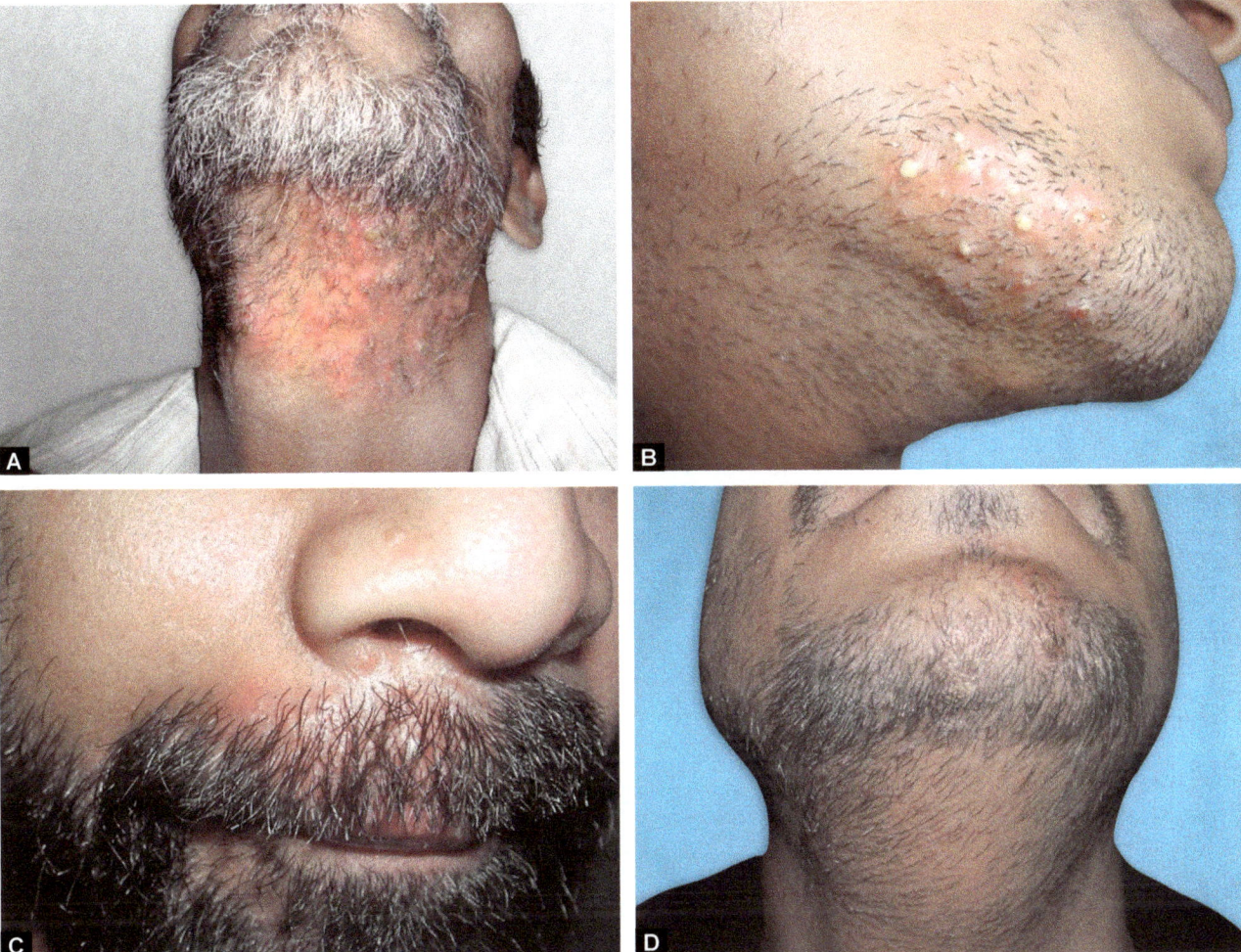

FIGS. 73A TO D: Tinea barbae.

- *Interdigital*—most common among obese elderly. Superficial erosion or fissure, surrounded by thickened white skin usually between third and fourth fingers and fourth and fifth toes.
  - Differential diagnosis—same as intertrigo.
- *Diaper dermatitis*—brightly erythematous (beefy red) confluent patches with a sharply demarcated serpiginous border and satellite pustules, small healing of scales, and edema and oozing are present in perigenital, perianal, inner aspect of thighs and buttocks **(Figs. 74A to F)**.
  - Differential diagnosis—atopic dermatitis, psoriasis, and irritant dermatitis.
- *Follicular candidiasis*—discrete pustule in ostia of hair follicle.
  - Differential diagnosis—bacterial folliculitis.

Oropharyngeal Candidiasis (Figs. 75A to D)

Synonym: Oral thrush.

Key Points
- Occurs in minor variations of host factors such as antibiotic therapy, glucocorticoid therapy, age (very young and very old), and significant immunocompromised condition.
- Pseudomembranous candidiasis—white-to-creamy plaques on any mucous surface variable in size 1–2 mm to extensive and widespread. Removal with dry gauze leaves an erythematous mucosal surface.
  - Differential diagnosis—oral hairy leukoplakia, geographic tongue, and lichen planus.
- Erythematous (atropic) candidiasis—smooth, red, and atrophic patches over hard or soft palate buccal mucosa on the dorsal surface of tongue.
  - Differential diagnosis—lichen planus.

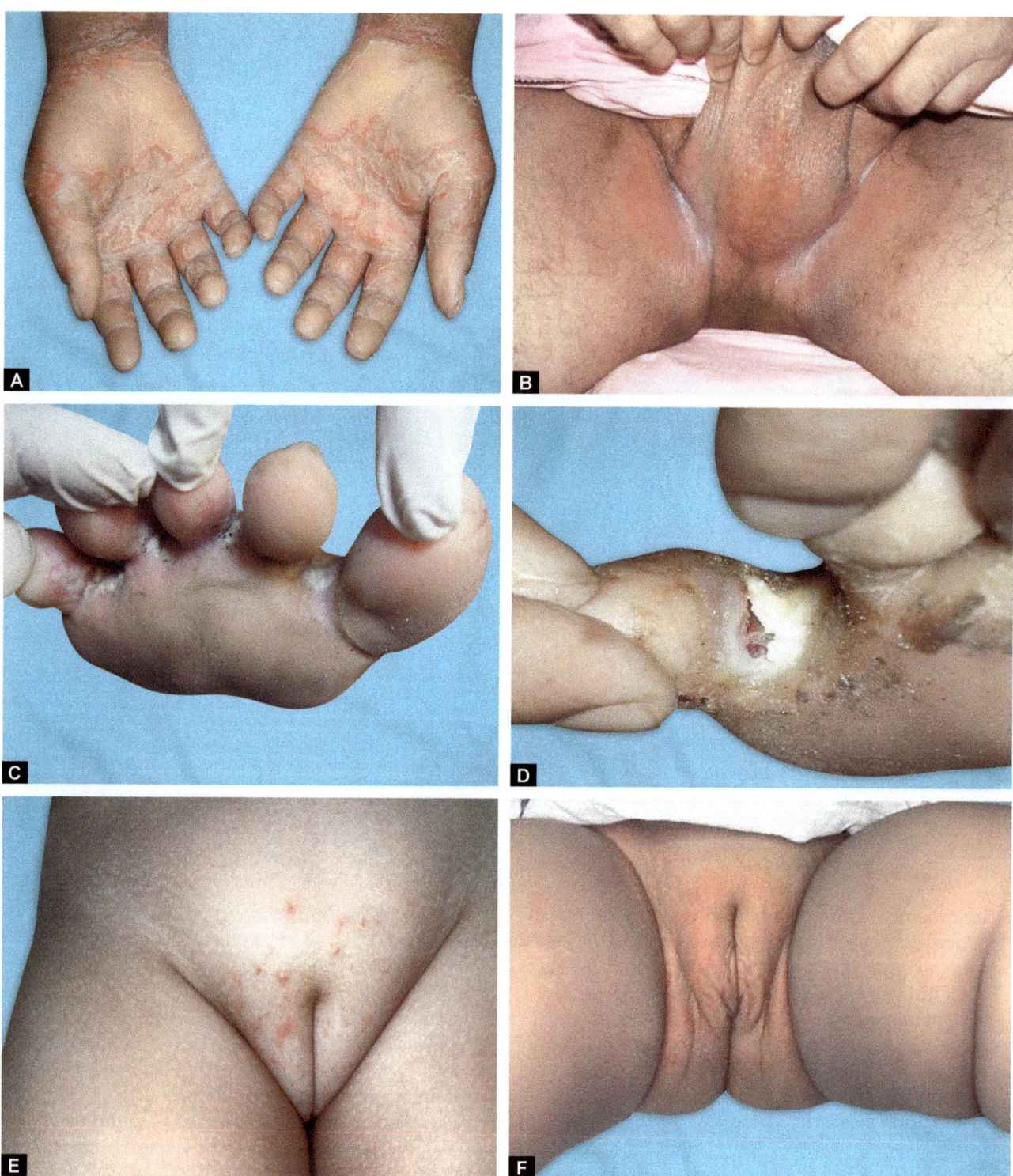

FIGS. 74A TO F: Candidiasis in different sites and last one is diaper dermatitis.

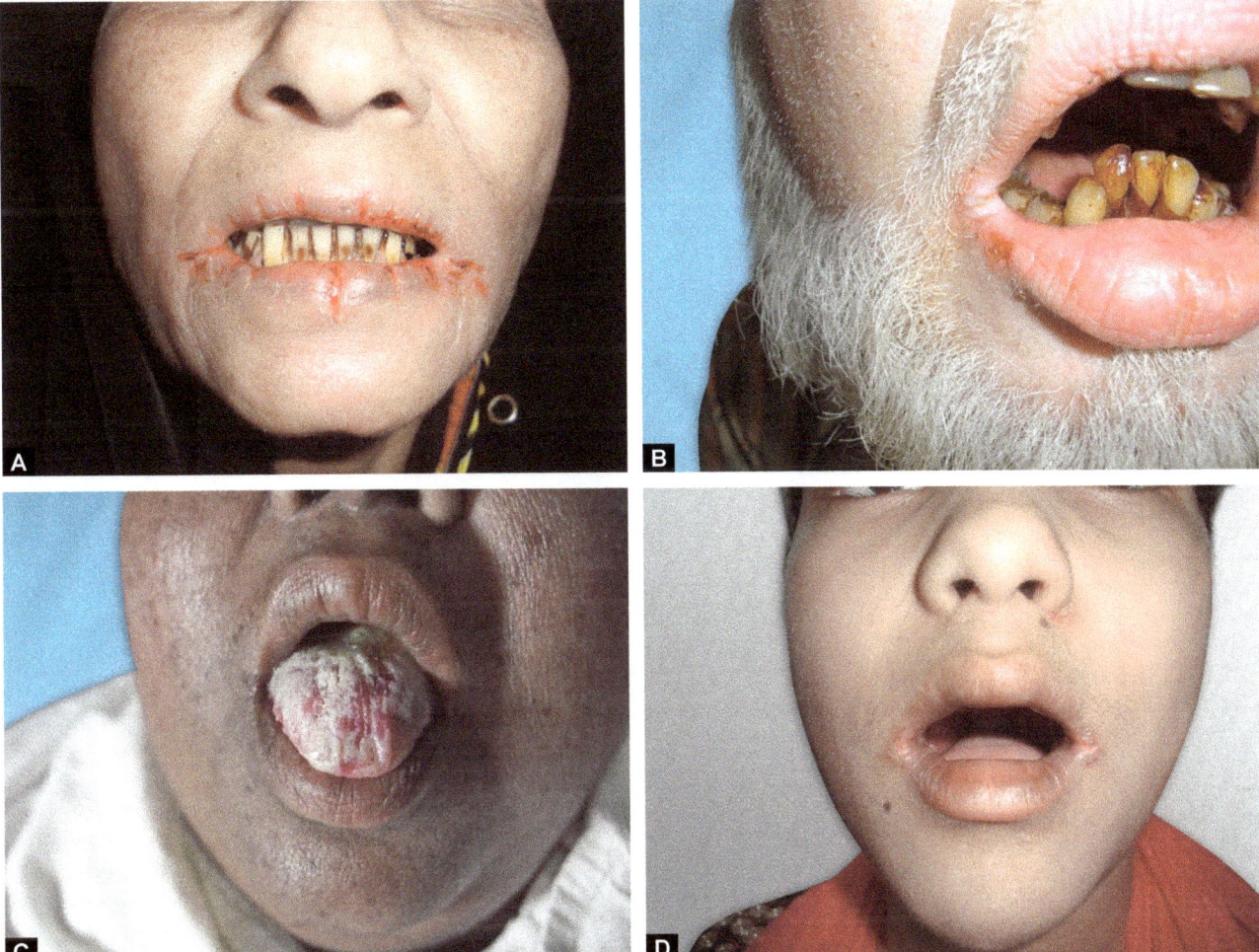

FIGS. 75A TO D: Oropharyngeal candidiasis.

- *Candida leukoplakia* (hyperplastic candidiasis)—white plaques cannot be wiped off with dry gauze pad. Usual sites are buccal mucosa, tongue, and hard palate.
- Angular cheilitis—intertrigo at the corner of lips and erythema and erosion are present.

Genital Candidiasis (Figs. 76A to D)

Synonym: Yeast infection.

Key Points

- *Vulvitis/vulvovaginitis*—vaginitis with white discharge, vaginal erythema and edema, and white plaques are present that can be wiped off on vagina and/or cervical mucosa.
- *Balanoposthitis, balanitis*—papules, pustules, and erosions are present on glans and preputial sac. Maculopapular lesions with diffuse erythema, edema, ulceration, and fissuring are often present.

Management

Keep the areas dry and topical and systemic measures are done accordingly.

- *Topical treatment*: Nystatin cream or oral suspension, imidazole creams.
- *Oral antifungal*: Nystatin tablet, clotrimazole tablet, fluconazole 100 mg/day, itraconazole 200 mg/day, and ketoconazole 200 mg/day for 1-2 weeks.

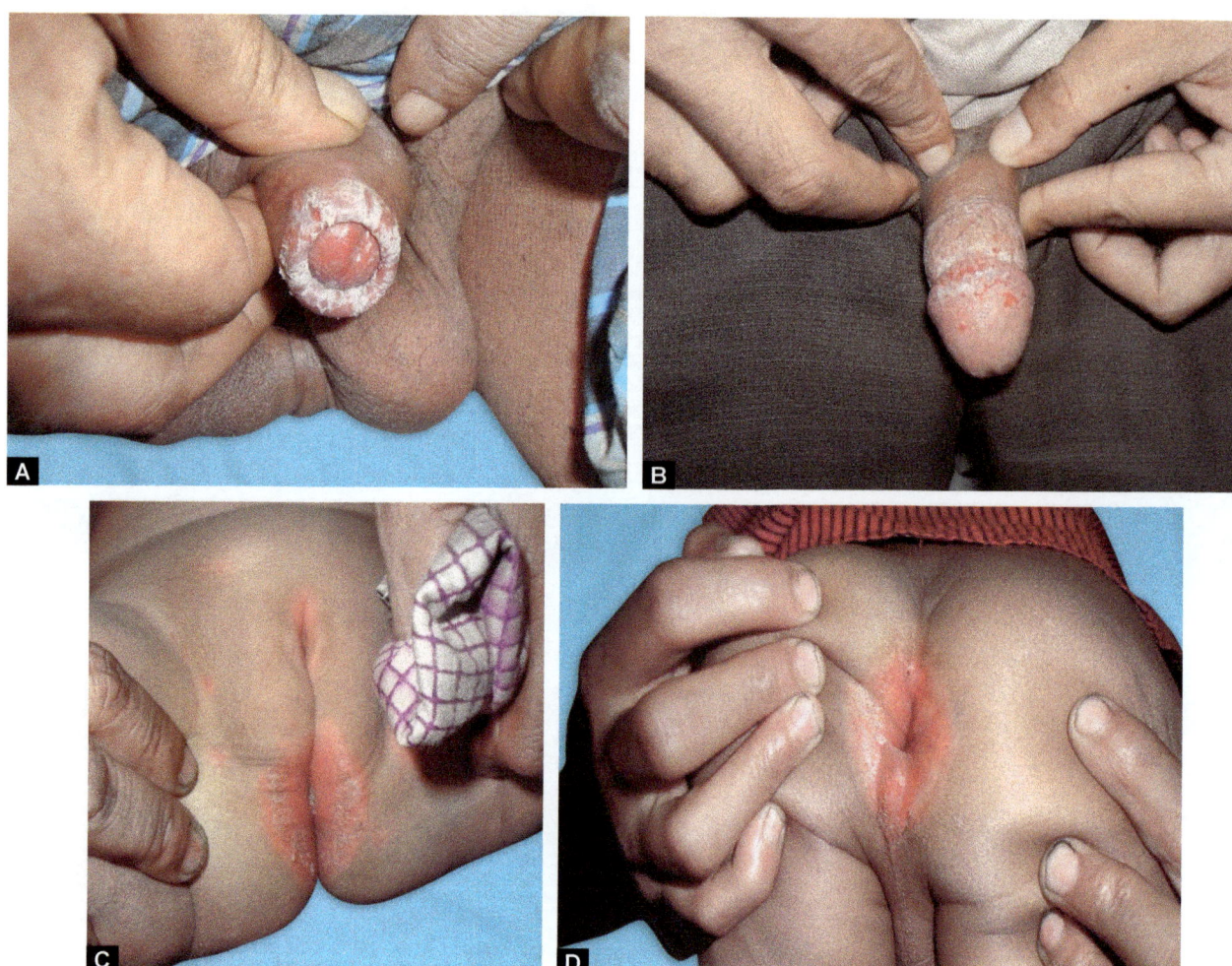

FIGS. 76A TO D: Genital candidiasis.

Pityriasis Versicolor (Figs. 77A to D)

Synonym: Tinea versicolor.

Key Points

- *Malassezia furfur* is a lipophilic yeast that normally resides in the keratin of skin and hair follicle of individuals at puberty and beyond.
- Warm season, tropical climate, hyperhidrosis, aerobic exercise, glucocorticoid therapy, and immunocompromised conditions are the common predisposing factors.
- In untanned skin, lesions are light brown.
- On tanned skin, lesions are hypopigmented.
- Discrete or oval macules and patches with slight, fine scale distributed over back, upper chest, shoulders, neck, proximal extremities, and face (in case of children).

Management

Main aim of treatment is removal of precipitating factors.
- *Topical agents*: Application over affected areas one to twice daily for 7 days recommended.
  - Selenium sulfide (2.5%) lotion or shampoo
  - Ketoconazole shampoo
  - Azole creams (ketoconazole, econazole, miconazole, and clotrimazole)
  - Terbinafine 1% solution
- *Systemic agents*:
  - Ketoconazole 400 mg stat (takes 1 hour before exercise)
  - Fluconazole 400 mg stat
  - Itraconazole 400 mg stat

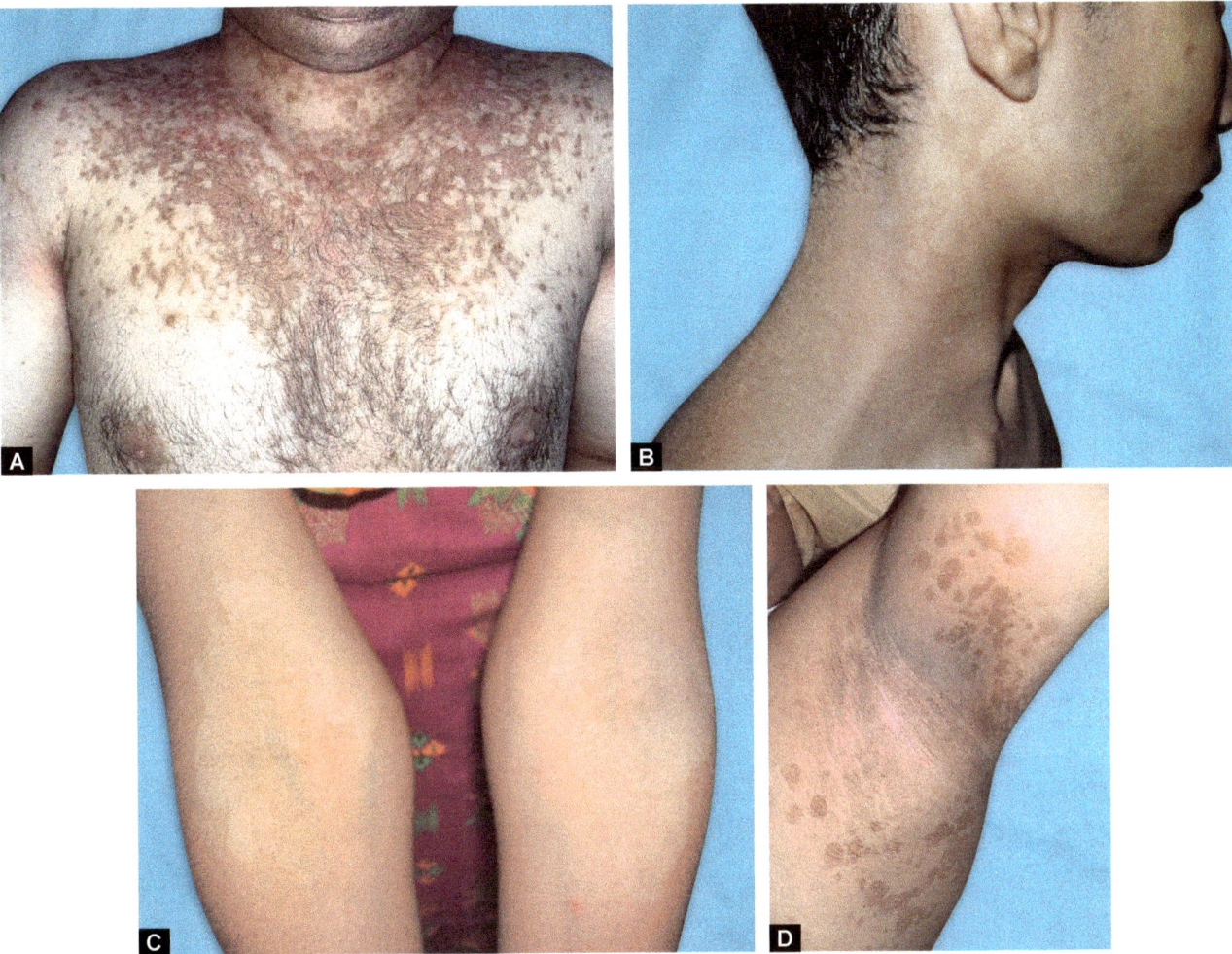

FIGS. 77A TO D: Pityriasis versicolor.

Mycetoma

- Also known as Madura foot or maduromycosis (**Figs. 78A to D**). Chronic, granulomatous, subcutaneous, and inflammatory diseases of skin, subcutaneous tissue, fascia, or bone caused by filamentous bacteria (actinomycosis) or true fungi (eumycetoma).
- A triad of progression present in both forms—subcutaneous swelling, sinus tracts, and discharge grains.
- Organism enters through the web area of toe by traumatic puncture. Chest, hands, arms, jaw, and buttocks are the other sites where mycetoma may occur.

Doctor's Prescription

- Diagnosed by triad of signs, tumefaction, sinuses, and granules
- Biopsy for histopathological examination
- X-ray and MRI of affected part

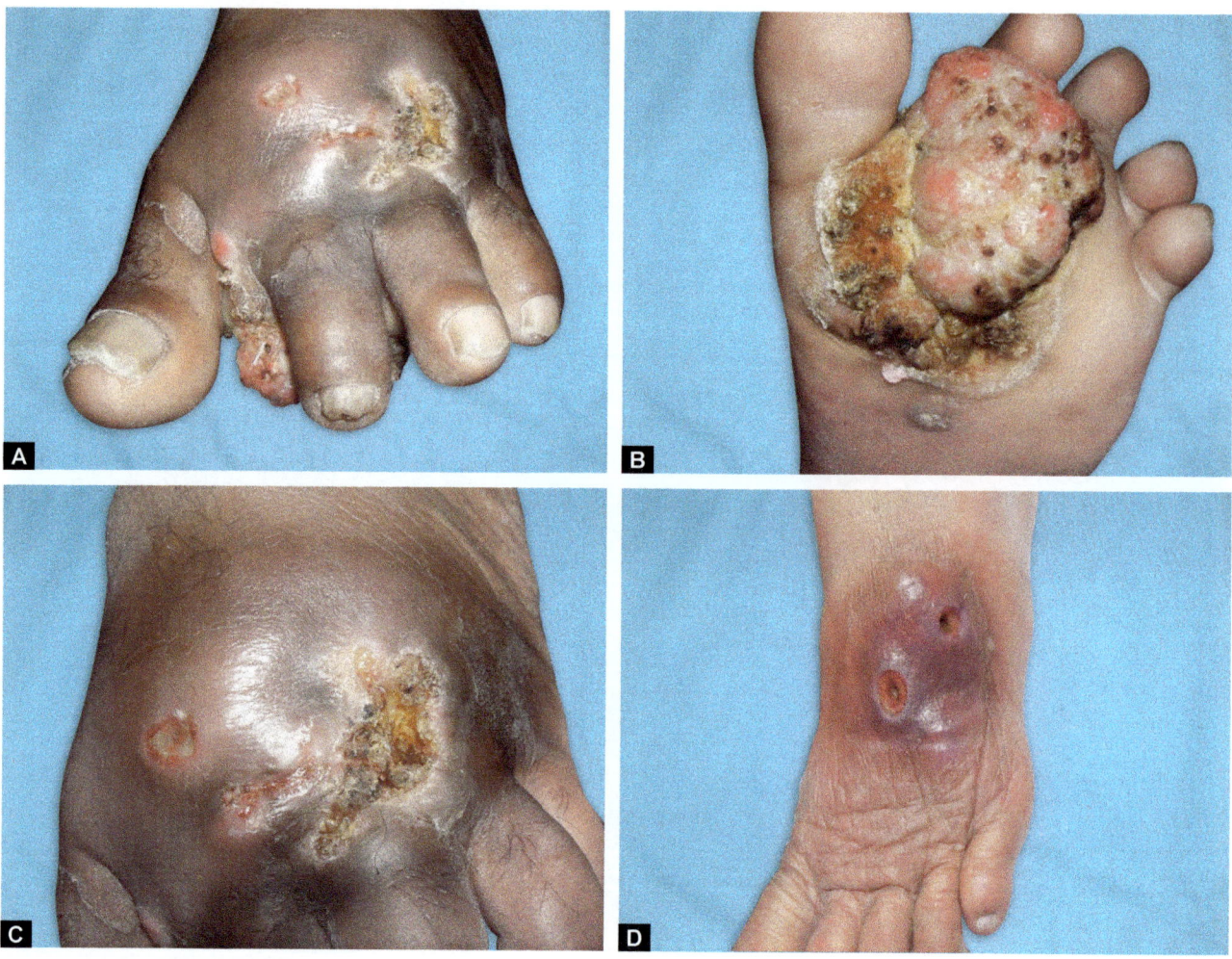

FIGS. 78A TO D: Maduromycosis.

CHAPTER 13
Bullous Diseases (Genetic, Autoimmune and Acquired)

EPIDERMOLYSIS BULLOSA

Epidermolysis bullosa (EB) is a group of genetic disorders characterized by mechanical fragility of the skin that leads to blister formation with minor trauma or friction.

Inherited EB is traditionally divided into three major categories:
1. Epidermolysis bullosa simplex (EBS)
2. Junctional epidermolysis bullosa (JEB)
3. Dystrophic epidermolysis bullosa (DEB)

Clinical Findings

The severity and distribution of blistering vary depending on:
- *Epidermolysis bullosa subtypes*:
    - Epidermolysis bullosa simplex—primarily affects palms/soles, worsens in early childhood **(Figs. 1 and 2)**

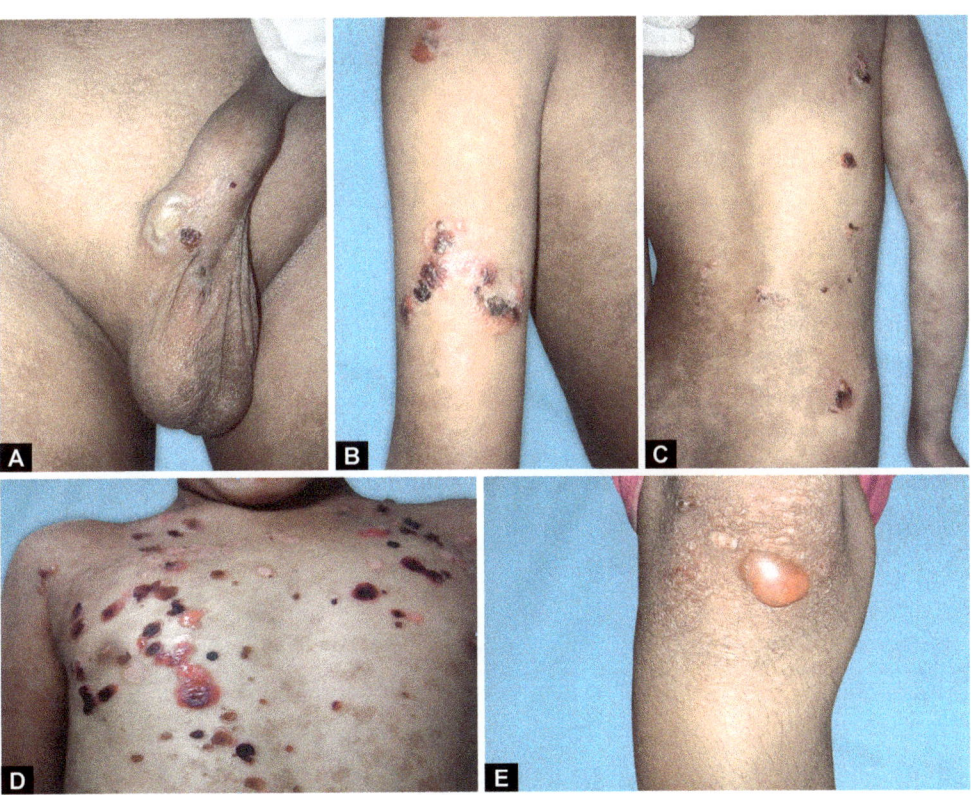

FIGS. 1A TO E: Epidermolysis bullosa simplex (EBS) generalized.

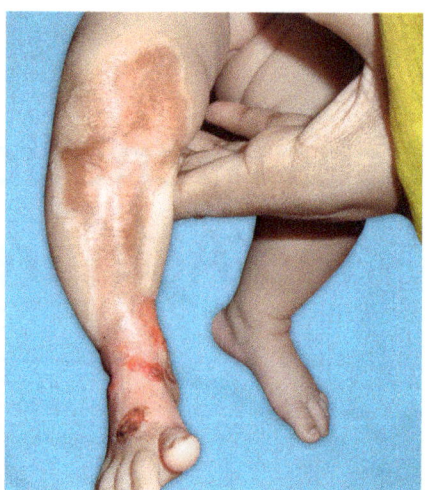

FIG. 2: Epidermolysis bullosa simplex (EBS) localized.

- Junctional epidermolysis bullosa—exuberant granulation tissue, often death during infancy **(Figs. 3A to C)**
- Dystrophic epidermolysis bullosa—prominent scarring, milia, nail dystrophy, pseudosyndactyly of hands/feet, microstomia, excessive dental caries, corneal ulcer/scarring, esophageal or urethral stricture, constipation, anemia, cardiomegaly, renal failure, and 50% risk of cutaneous squamous cell carcinoma (SCC) before 30 years **(Figs. 4A to C)**.
• Patient age—improvement over time, especially for EBS.
• Environmental factors—sweating and friction.

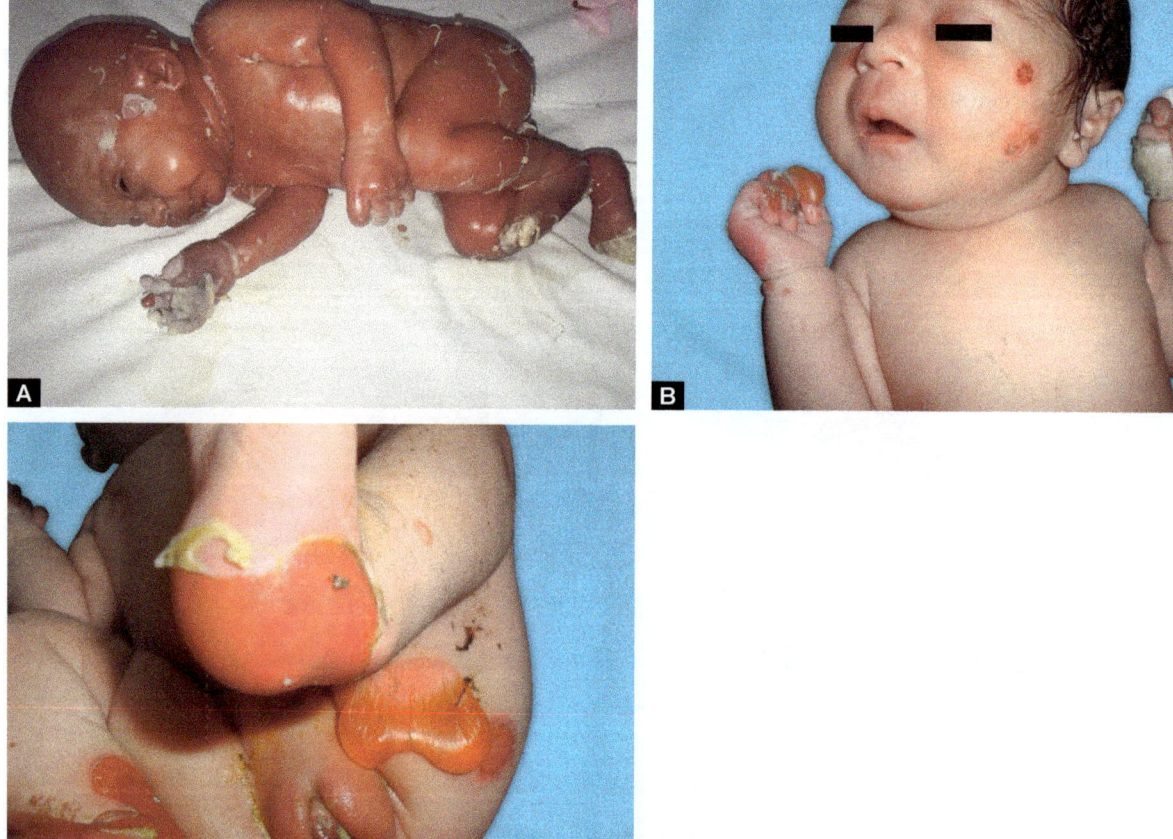

FIGS. 3A TO C: Junctional epidermolysis bullosa (JEB).

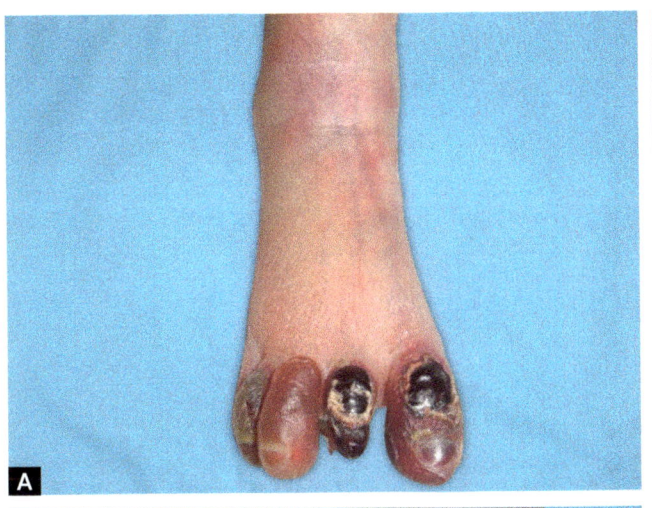
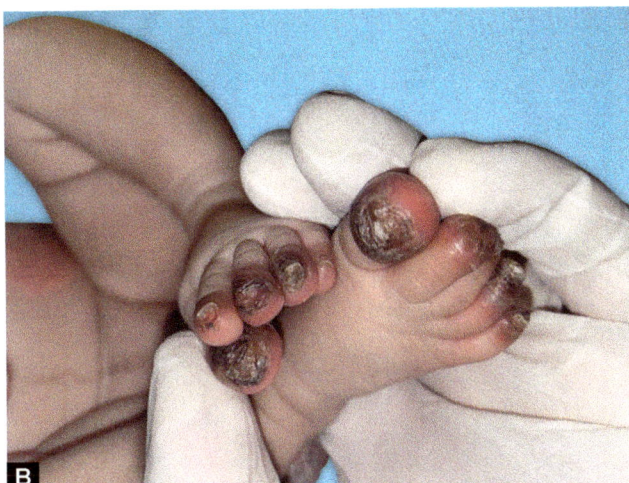
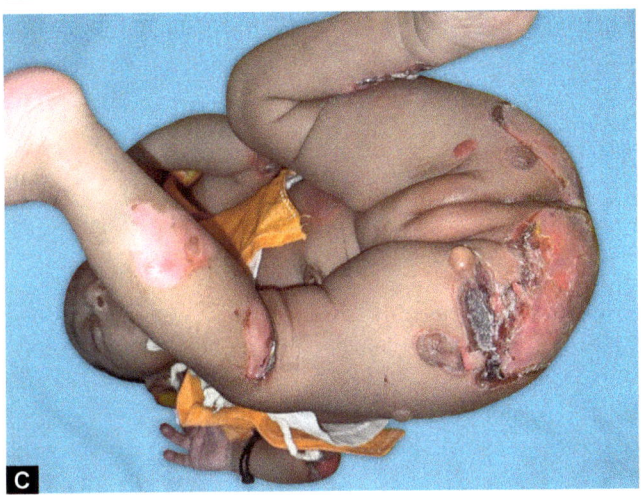

FIGS. 4A TO C: Dystrophic epidermolysis bullosa (DEB).

Medical Prescription

- Avoidance of mechanical trauma
- Prevention of infection
- Petrolatum-impregnated gauze and soft silicon dressing should apply.
- Lancing and draining blisters can relieve pressure and promote healing. Local and systemic antibiotic may be needed.

PEMPHIGUS

Acute or chronic autoimmune bullous disease of skin and mucous membrane based on acantholysis.

Two major types: (1) Pemphigus vulgaris (PV) and (2) Pemphigus foliaceus (PF).

Pemphigus Vulgaris (Figs. 5A to M)

An autoimmune disease where loss of cell-to-cell adhesion in the epidermis (desmoglein-1) and mucous membrane (desmoglein-3) occurs due to circulating antibody of the immunoglobulin G (IgG) class, which binds to desmoglein-1 or -3 or both. Desmosomes hold epidermal cell together.

Mucosal erosions (60% of cases) are thin-walled, relatively flaccid, and easily ruptured bullae that appear on apparently normal skin and mucous membrane or on erythematous base. The fluid in the bulla is clear at first, but may become hemorrhagic or seropurulent. The bullae rupture to form erosions. The denuded areas soon become partially or totally covered with crusts that have little or no tendency to heal. After successful treatment, when the lesions heal, it leaves hyperpigmented patches but no scarring.

164 | CHAPTER 13 Bullous Diseases (Genetic, Autoimmune and Acquired)

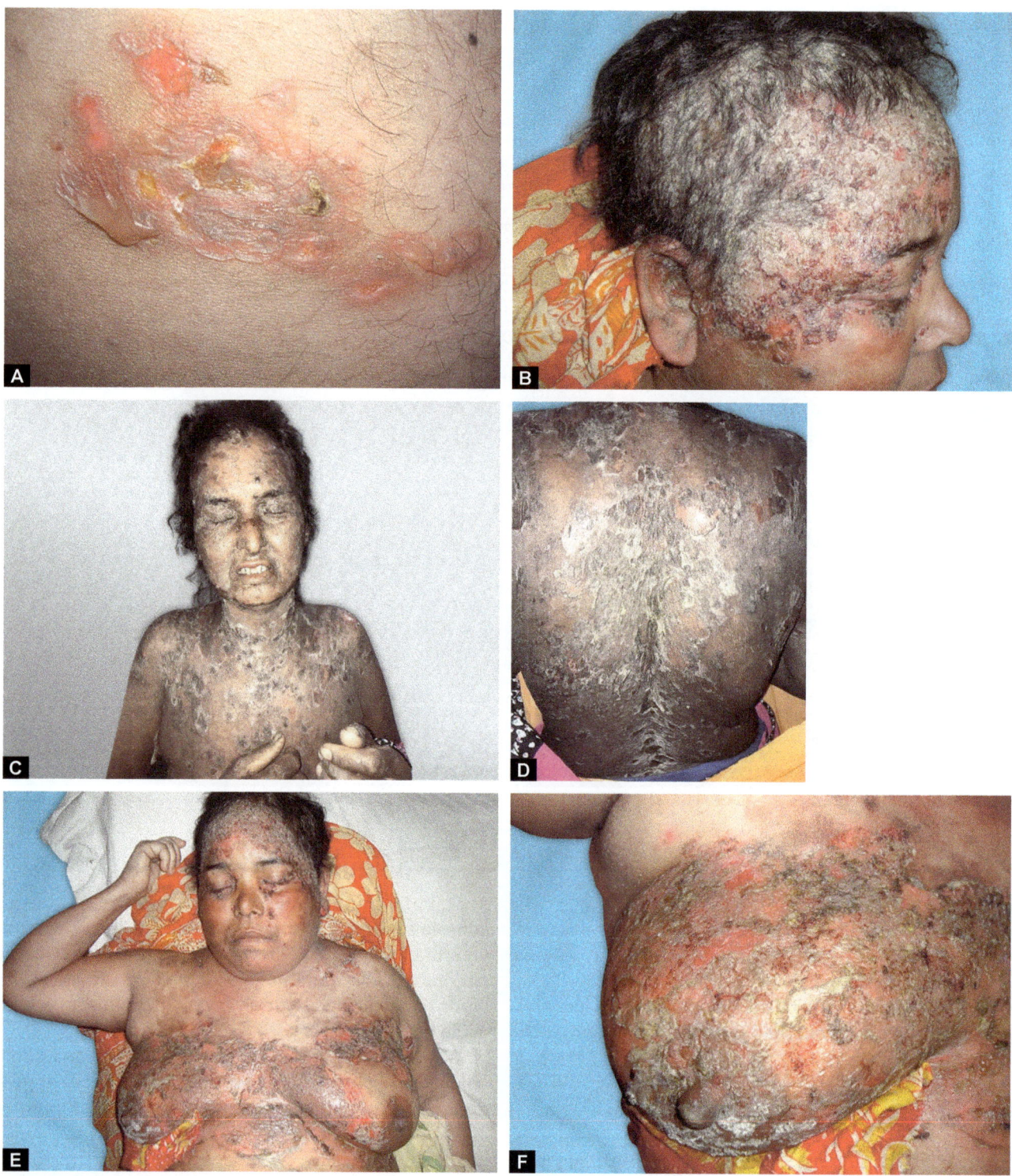

FIGS. 5A TO M: *Continued*

Continued

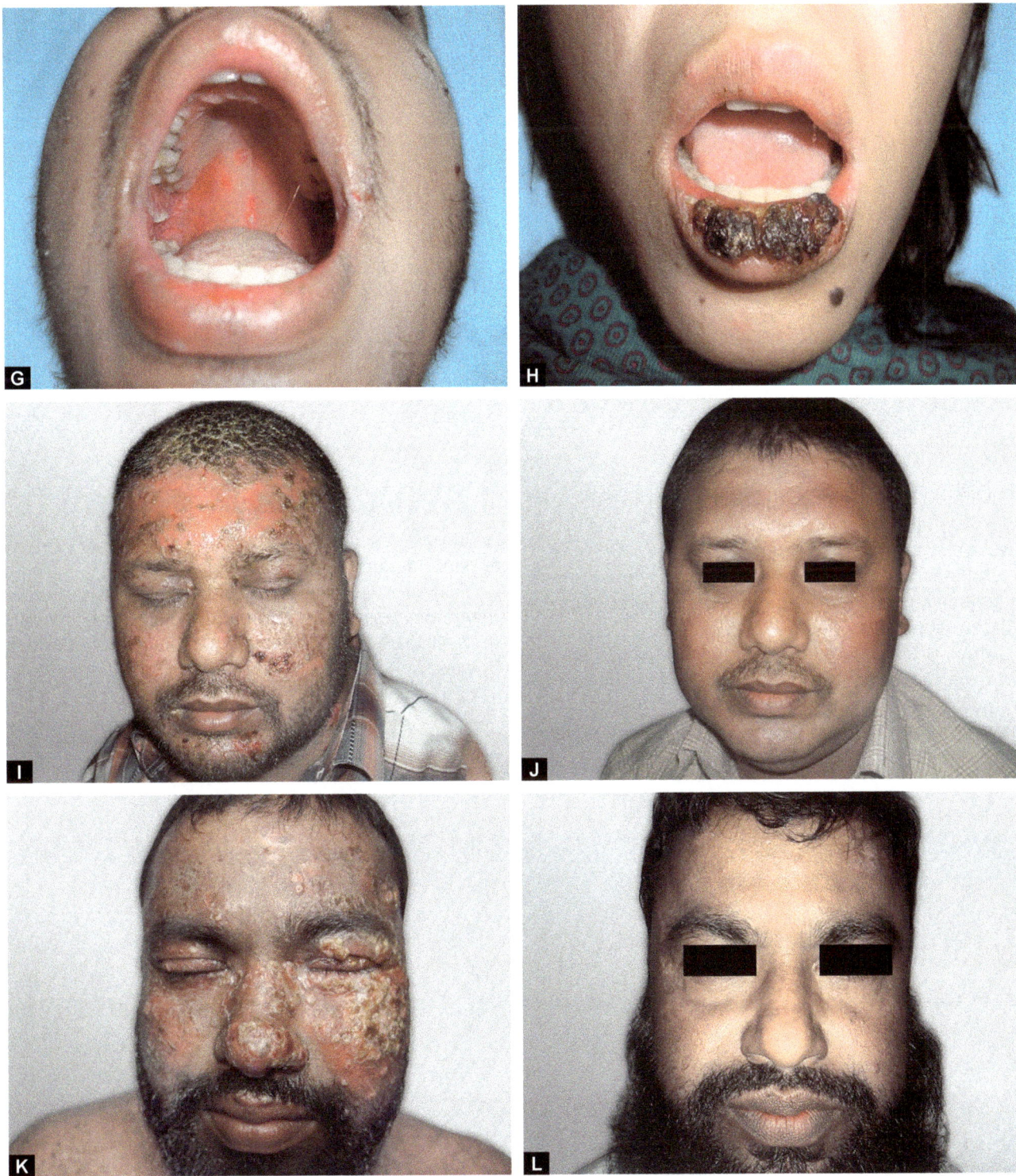

FIGS. 5A TO M: *Continued*

Continued

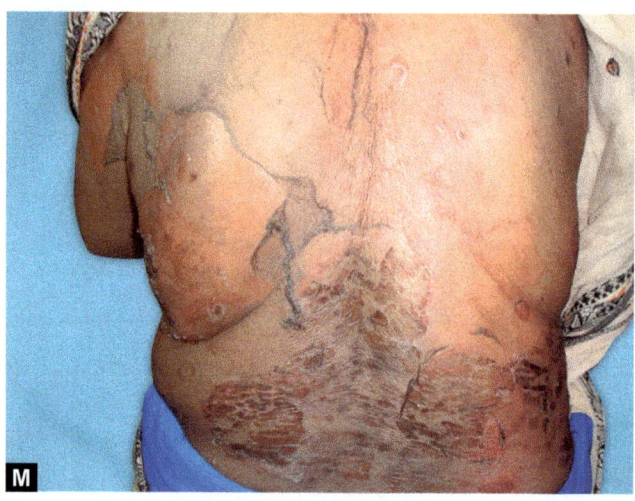

FIGS. 5A TO M: Pemphigus vulgaris.

Nikolsky sign is present (intact epidermis shearing away from underlying dermis leaving moist surface after slight pressure, twisting, or rubbing).

Bulla-spread phenomenon is elicited by pressure on intact bulla, gently forcing the fluid to spread under the adjacent skin.

Mucous lesions usually painful and erosions extend onto the lips and form heavy, fissured crusts on the vermilion. Hoarseness of voice and difficulty in swallowing may develop after involvement of throat. Esophageal mucosa may be involved.

Pemphigus Foliaceus (Figs. 6A to D)

In PF, only desmoglein-1 affected so lesions only confined to skin. No mucous membrane involvement.

Scaly crusted lesions on an erythematous base, initially in seborrheic areas. More superficial and fragile nature of the vesicles leads to erosion with scale crust rather than bullae.

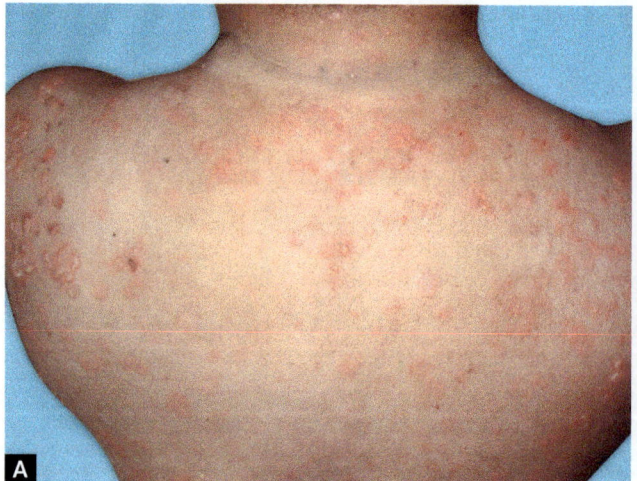
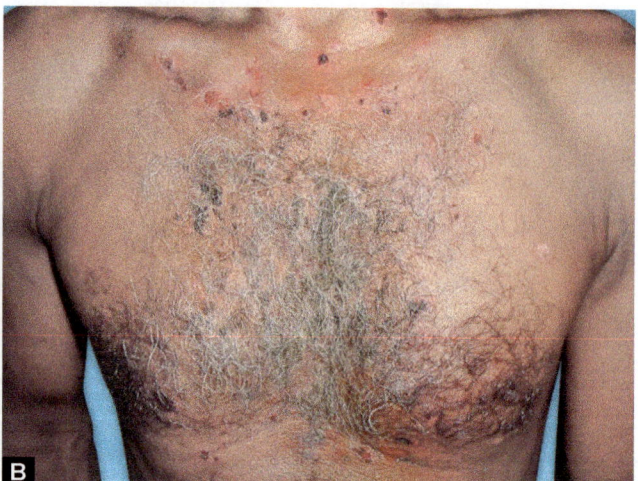

FIGS. 6A TO D: *Continued*

Continued

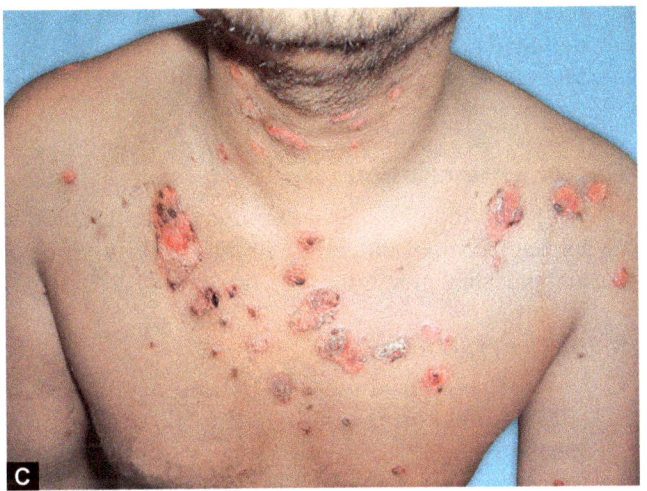
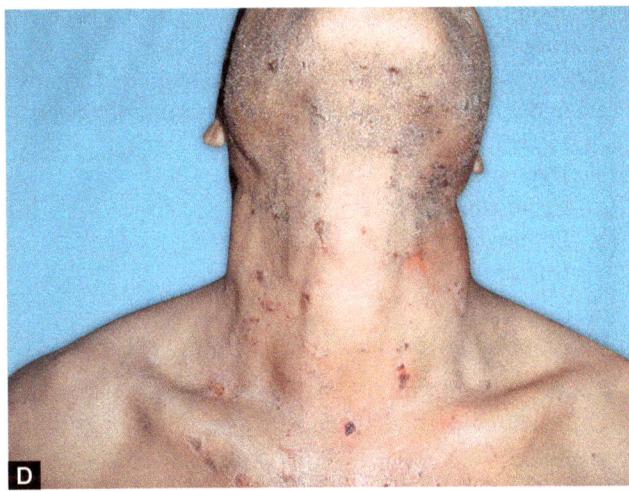

FIGS. 6A TO D: Pemphigus foliaceus.

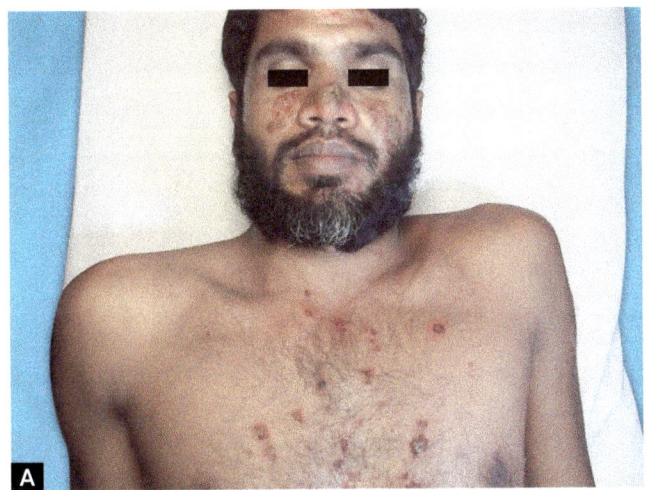
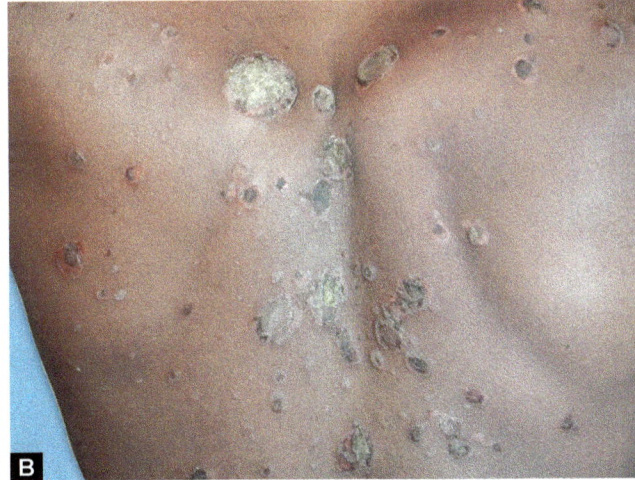

FIGS. 7A AND B: Pemphigus erythematosus.

Pemphigus Erythematosus (Figs. 7A and B)

Localized form of PF is largely confined to seborrheic area. Erythematous, crusted, and erosive lesions are present in butterfly area of face, forehead, presternal, and intrascapular region.

It may be positive antinuclear antibody (ANA) titer.

Doctor's Prescription

- Biopsy for histopathological examination and direct immunofluorescence (DIF).
- *Pemphigus vulgaris*: Suprabasal acantholysis is present. IgG and C3 deposition in lesional and perilesional skin.
- *Pemphigus foliaceus*: Acantholysis in granular layer.

Medical Prescription

- *Glucocorticoid*—2-3 mg/kg of prednisolone until cessation of new blister and disappearance of the Nikolsky sign.
- Concomitant immunosuppressive therapy is given as glucocorticoid-sparing therapy.
- *Azathioprine*—2-3 mg/kg body weight until complete clearance of lesions then tapered.
- *Methotrexate*—25-35 mg/week. Dose adjustments are made as with azathioprine.
- *Cyclophosphamide*—100-200 mg daily, with reduction to maintenance doses 50-100 mg/day.
- *Mycophenolate mofetil*—1 g twice daily.
- *Plasmapheresis*—in conjunction with glucocorticoid and immunosuppressive agents.

- *High dose of intravenous immunoglobulin (IVIG)*—2 g/kg body weight every 3-4 weeks have glucocorticoid-sparing effects.
- *Rituximab*—in refractory cases, intravenous therapy given once a week for 4 weeks shows dramatic effects.
- *In milder cases*:
  - Dapsone
  - Cyclosporine
  - Etanercept
  - Infliximab

Bullous Pemphigoid (Figs. 8A to D)

- Bullous autoimmune disease is characterized by large, tense, subepidermal bullae with a predilection for the groins, axillae, trunk, thighs, and flexor surfaces of forearms.
- Age of onset—60-80 years.
- Most common bullous autoimmune disease.
- Here circulating autoantibodies bind two components of hemidesmosomes that provide adhesion between the epidermis and the dermis.
- Pruritic fixed urticarial plaque and 10 bullae are seen on examination. Later, bullae rupture and large denuded area are seen.
- Mucous membrane involvement sometimes but less severe.

Doctor's Prescription

Biopsy for histopathological examination and DIF bulla in dermoepidermal junction with IgG deposition along dermoepidermal junction.

Medical Prescription

- Systemic prednisolone—50-100 mg/day until clear either alone or in combination of azathioprine 150 mg/day.
- Intravenous immunoglobulin
- Rituximab
- Dapsone
- Methotrexate

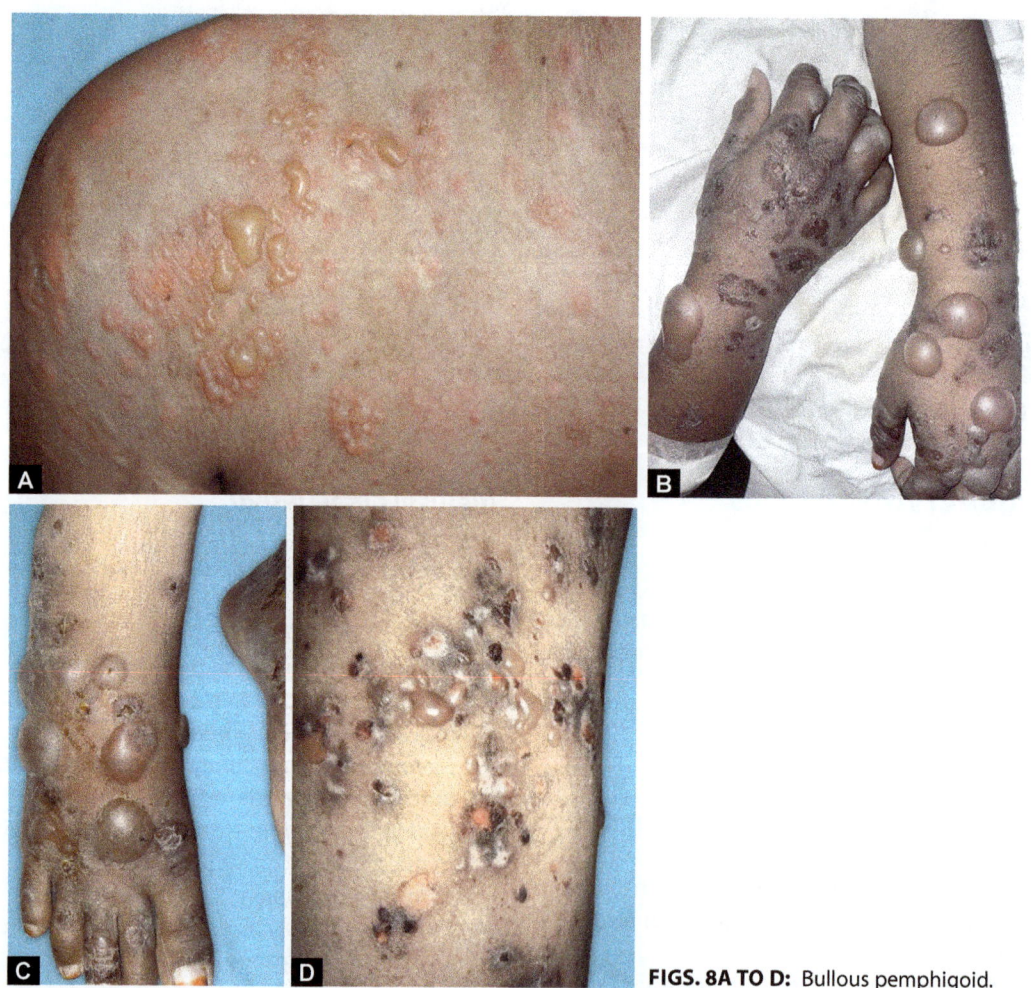

FIGS. 8A TO D: Bullous pemphigoid.

Dermatitis Herpetiformis (Figs. 9A to F)

Autoimmune bullous disease that is a cutaneous manifestation of celiac disease in which >90% of patients have histological evidence of gluten-sensitive enteropathy and almost 20% of patients with dermatitis herpetiformis (DH) have symptomatic celiac disease.

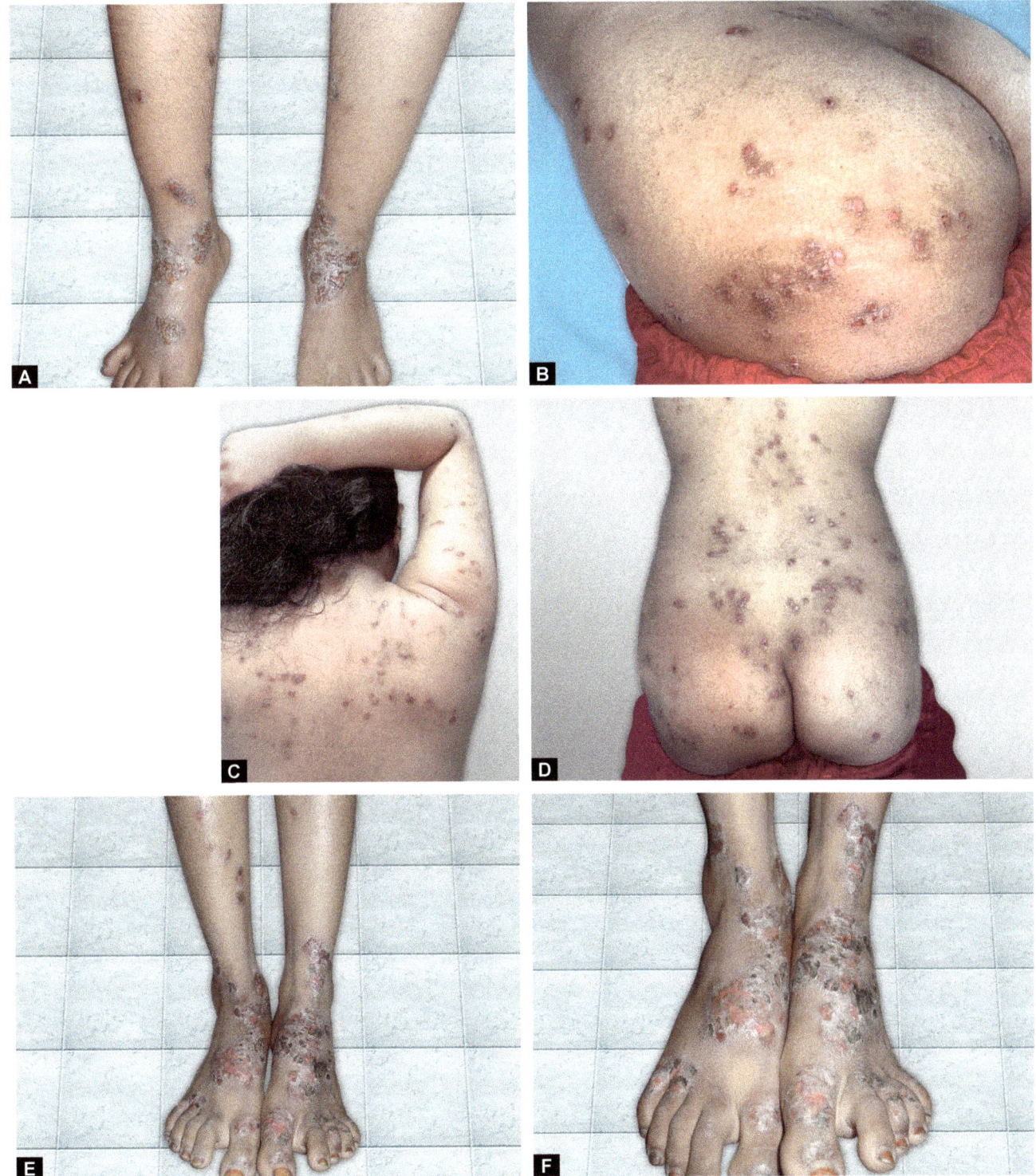

FIGS. 9A TO F: Dermatitis herpetiformis.

Primary lesions consist of pruritic vesicles, papules, and urticarial plaque that are arranged in groups; however, due to scratching, only excoriated papules and hemorrhagic crusts may be present. Lesions are usually symmetric in distribution.

Sites of involvement usually are the elbows, extensor forearms, knees, posterior neck, presacral, and buttock.

Doctor's Prescription

- Biopsy is taken from early erythematous papule. Subepidermal vesicle and microabscesses at the tips of dermal papillae are seen.
- Direct immunofluorescence—perilesional skin is taken (best from buttock) and seen as granular deposition of immunoglobulin A (IgA) in the tip of papillae.

Medical Prescription

- Gluten-free diet
- Dapsone—initially 25–50 mg/day after screening for glucose-6-phosphate dehydrogenase (G6PD) deficiency, average dose 100 mg/day
- Sulfapyridine—improvement of pruritus within a few days.

CHAPTER 14
Rheumatologic Dermatology

LUPUS ERYTHEMATOSUS

A multisystem autoimmune disorder that prominently affects the skin.
- *Broadly divided into*:
  - Small vessel vasculitis
  - Polyarteritis nodosa-like lesion
- *Vasculopathy*:
  - Raynaud phenomenon (RP)
  - Livedo reticularis
- *SLE*: Systemic lupus erythematosus.
- *CLE*: Cutaneous lupus erythematosus.
- *DILE*: Drug-induced lupus erythematosus.

Cutaneous lupus erythematosus is further classified into specific and nonspecific skin lesions.

Three major forms of specific skin lesion are:
1. *CCLE: Chronic cutaneous lupus erythematosus*:
   i. Localized discoid lupus erythematosus (DLE), generalized DLE
   ii. Hypertrophic/verrucous DLE
   iii. Lupus profunda
   iv. Mucosal DLE
   v. Lupus tumidus (urticarial plaque of LE)
   vi. Chilblain LE (chilblain lupus)
   vii. Lichenoid DLE (LE-LP overlap)
2. *SCLE: Subacute cutaneous lupus erythematosus*:
   i. Annular SCLE
   ii. Papulosquamous SCLE
3. *ACLE: Acute cutaneous lupus erythematosus—malar rash, butterfly rash*:
   i. Generalized ACLE

■ Nonspecific Cutaneous Findings of Lupus Erythematosus

- *Vasculitis*:
  - Urticarial vasculitis
  - Nailfold telangiectasias and erythema
  - Palmar erythema
  - Livedoid vasculopathy
- *Cutaneous signs of antiphospholipid antibody syndrome*:
  - Widespread and persistent livedo reticularis
  - Multiple subungual splinter hemorrhage
  - Digital gangrene and cutaneous necrosis
  - Degos-like lesion
  - Atrophic blanche
  - Anetoderma

■ Discoid Lupus Erythematosus (Figs. 1A to I)

It is the most common skin manifestation of LE. Lesions begin as dull red macule or indurated plaques that develop an adherent scale, then evolve with atrophy, scarring, and pigmentary changes. Overall 5-10% of patients of DLE will develop SLE.

Three clinical variants are:
1. *Localized DLE*: Most commonly involves the head and neck regions. Have ≤5% risk of development of SLE.
2. *Generalized DLE*: Total of 20% patient can progress to SLE.
3. *Hypertrophic DLE*: Usual sites are extensor arms, upper trunk, and thick scale overlying or at periphery of DLE lesions.

CHAPTER 14 Rheumatologic Dermatology

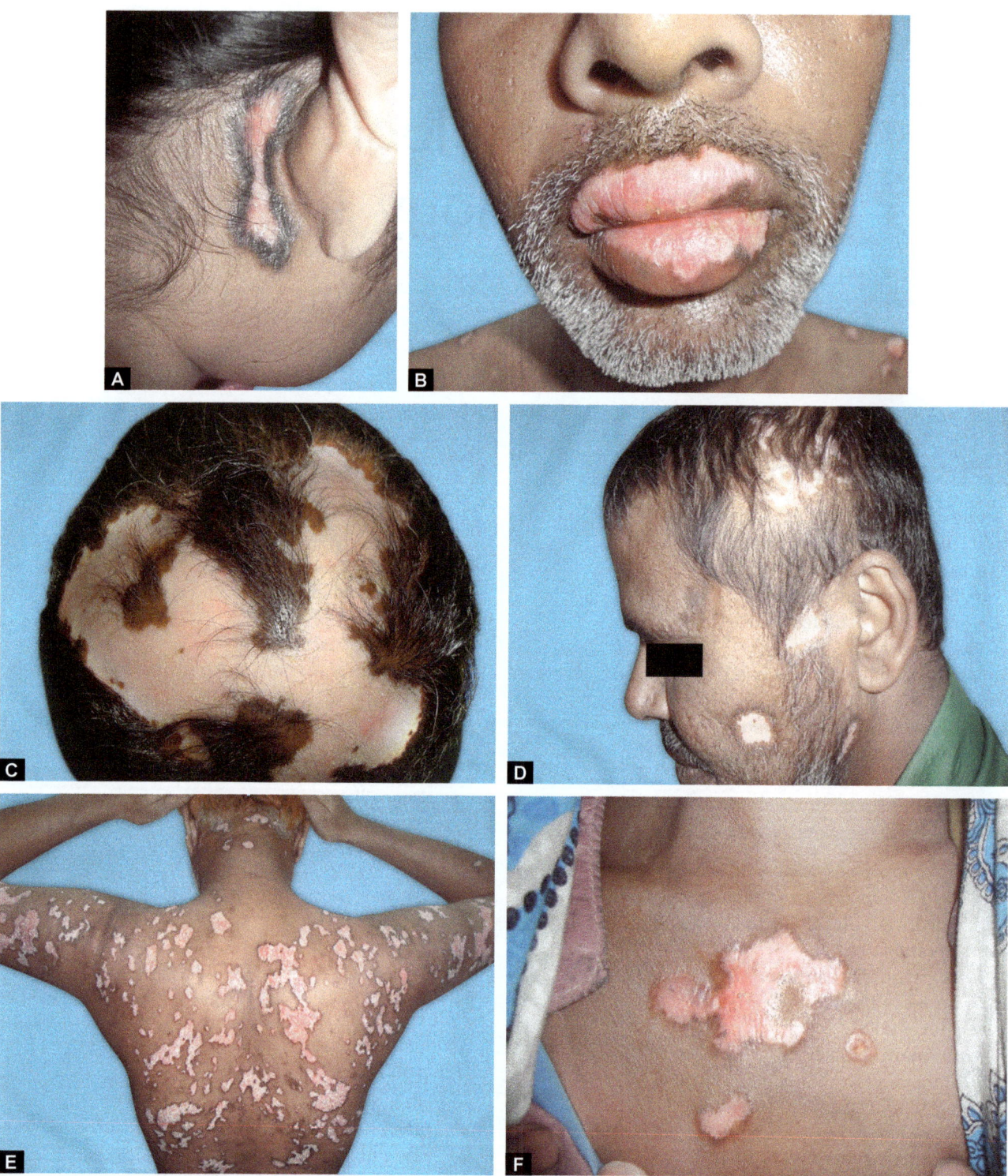

FIGS. 1A TO I: *Continued*

Continued

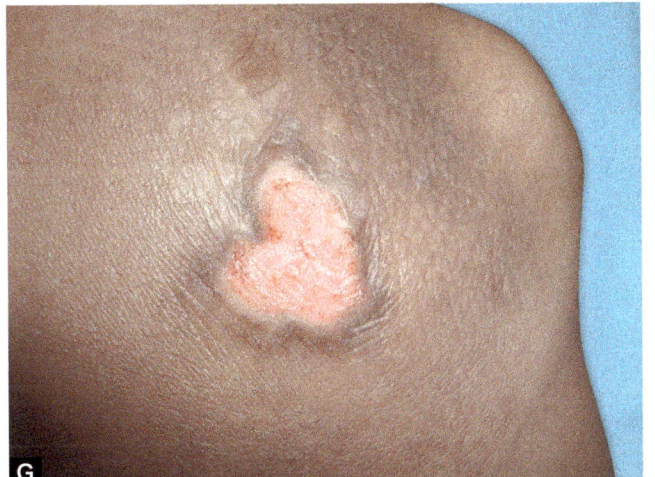
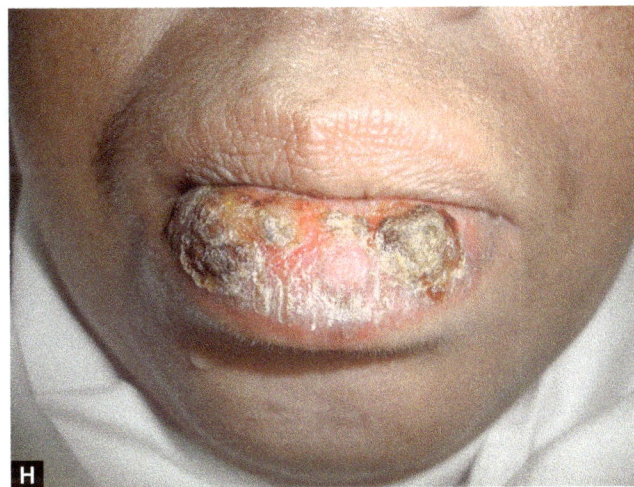
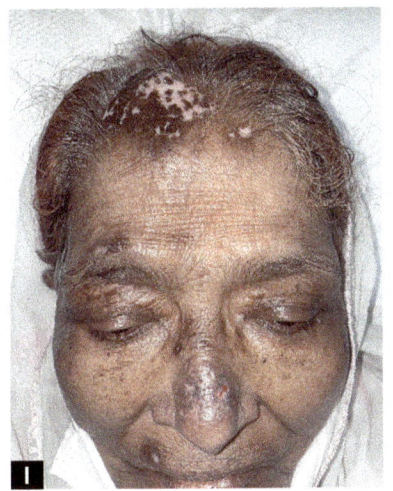

FIGS. 1A TO I: Discoid lupus erythematosus (DLE).

Systemic Lupus Erythematosus (Figs. 2A to O)

Multisystem autoimmune disease is based on polyclonal B-cell immunity, which involves connective tissue and blood vessels.

Male to female ratio is 1:9.

The clinical manifestations include:
- Fever (90%), fatigue (100%), weight loss, and malaise
- Skin lesions (85%)—ACLE, SCLE, and CCLE
- Mucous membrane—ulcer arising from pruritic necrotic lesion on hard palate, buccal mucosa, and gum.
- Hair—diffuse alopecia or discoid lesions associated with patchy alopecia.
- Arthritis (80%).
- NS—peripheral neuropathy (14%), renal (50%), cardiac—pericarditis (20%), pulmonary disease—pneumonitis (20%), and lymphadenopathy (50%).

Doctor's Prescription
- Blood—complete blood count (CBC), anemia—normocytic, normochromic, or hemolytic, and raised erythrocyte sedimentation rate (ESR).
- *Serology*:
  - Antinuclear antibody (ANA)—>95%.
  - Anti-double-stranded deoxyribonucleic acid (dsDNA) 70–80%—skin and kidney involvement.
  - Anti-Sm—kidney involvement.
  - Anti-ribosomal ribonucleoprotein (rRNP)

Medical Prescription
- *General measures*:
  - Sun protection
  - Avoid photosensitizing medication
  - Stop smoking
  - Oral vitamin D3
- *Local*:
  - Topical and intralesional corticosteroid (CS)

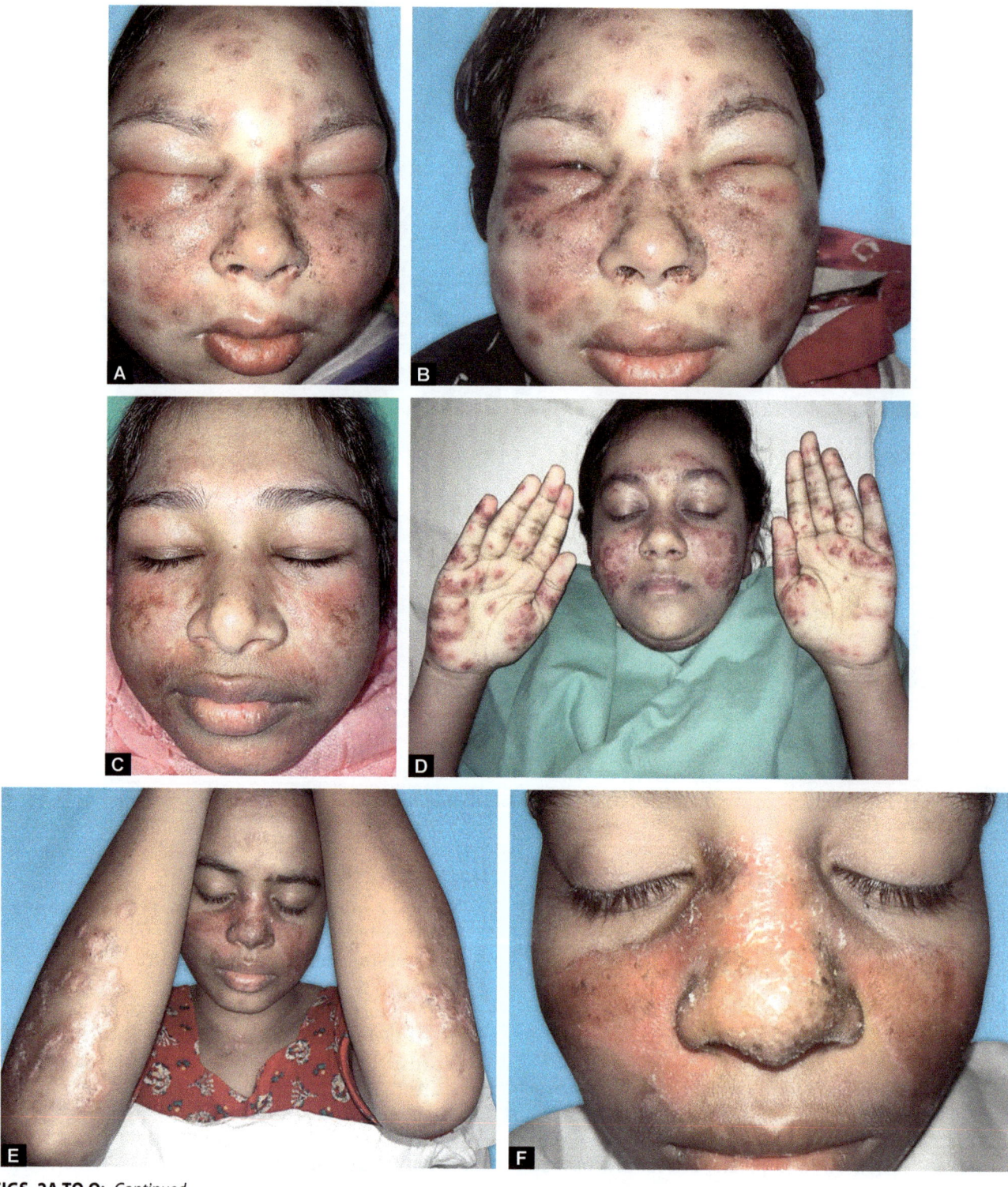

FIGS. 2A TO O: *Continued*

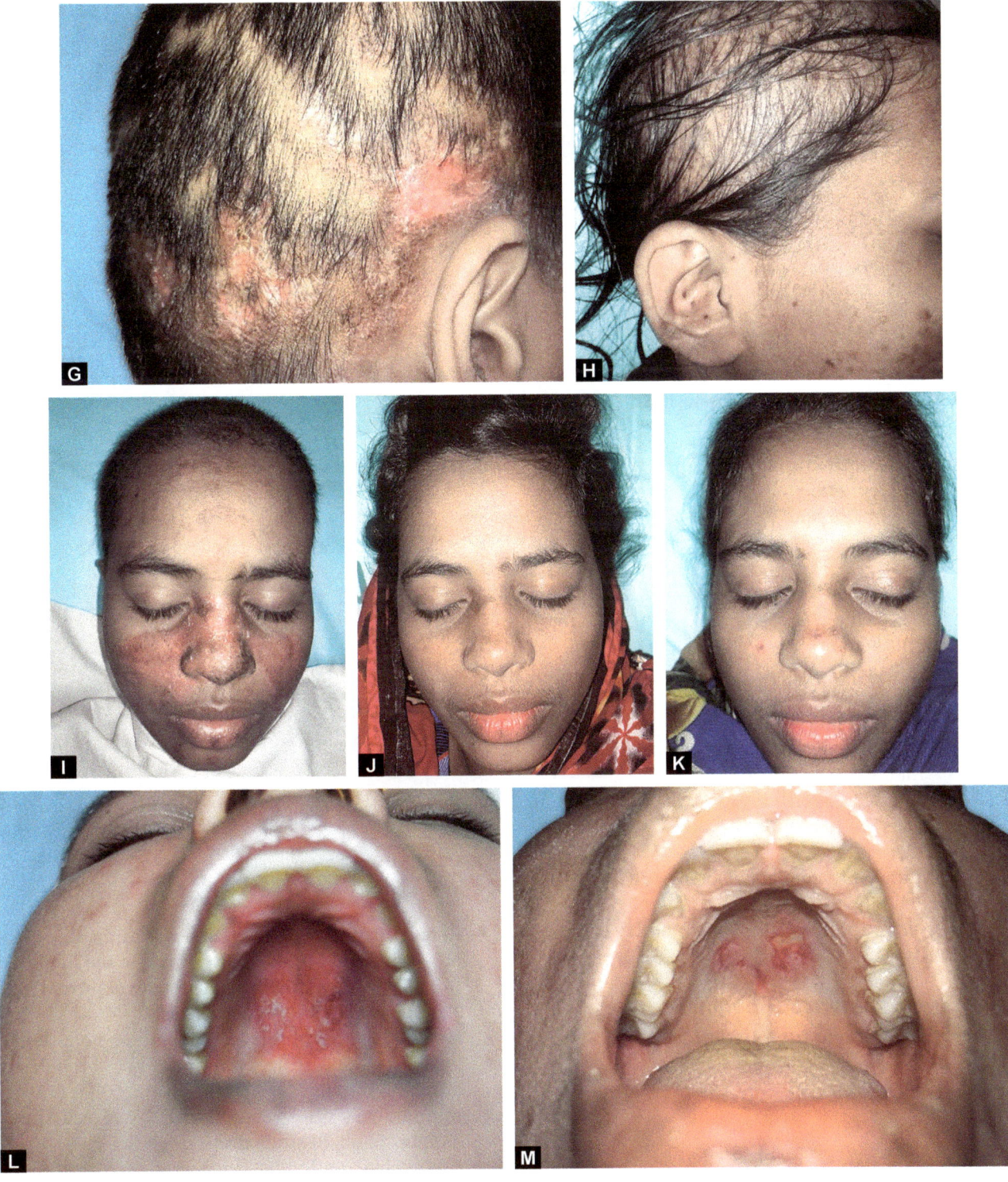

FIGS. 2A TO O: Continued

Continued

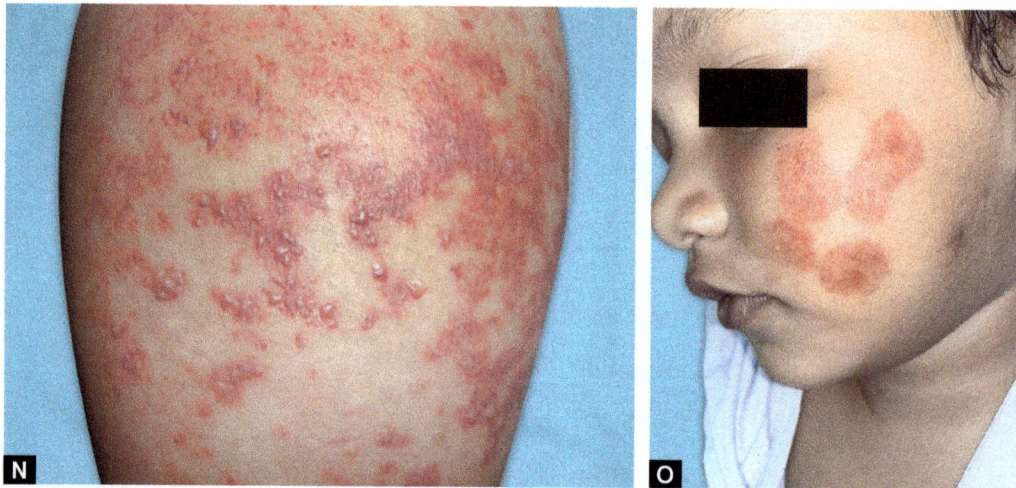

FIGS. 2A TO O: Systemic lupus erythematosus (SLE).

- o Topical calcineurin inhibitor
- o Topical retinoids
- o Topical imiquimod 5%
- *Systemic*:
  - o *First line*:
    - *Hydroxychloroquine*: Adult—6-6.5 mg/kg/day and children <5 mg/kg/day.
    - Chloroquine
    - Quinacrine
  - o *Second line*:
    - Methotrexate 7.5-25 mg/week
    - Mycophenolate mofetil 1-2 g/day
    - Thalidomide
    - Retinoid—acitretin
    - Dapsone 100 mg/day
  - o *Third line*:
    - Intravenous immunoglobulin (IVIG)
    - Belimumab
  - o *Life-threatening or severe inflammatory cutaneous disease*: Systemic corticosteroid (CS).

1982 Revised American Rheumatism Association Criteria for Systemic Lupus Erythematosus

- Malar rash—fixed erythema, flat or raised over malar eminences.
- Discoid lupus—typical DLE lesion.
- Photosensitivity—skin rash due to an unusual reaction to sunlight.
- Oral ulcer—oral or nasal ulceration, usually painless.
- Arthritis—nonerosive arthritis involving two or more peripheral joints characterized by tenderness, swelling, or effusion.
- Serositis—pleuritis or pericarditis.

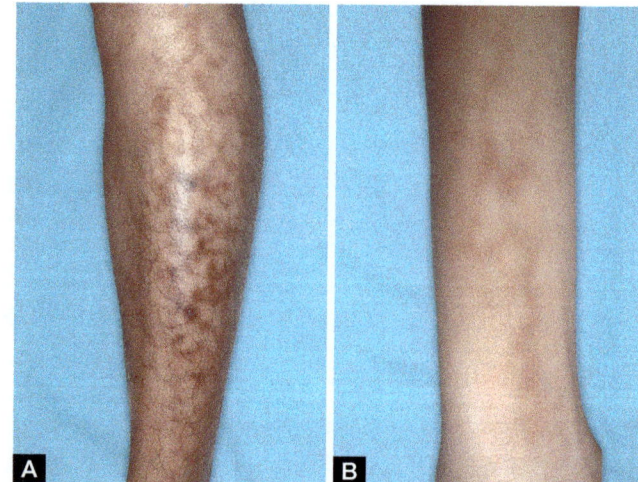

FIGS. 3A AND B: Livedo reticularis.

- Renal disorder—persistent proteinuria 0.5 g/day or +++ in urine, cellular casts [may be red blood cell (RBC), hemoglobin, granular, tubular, or mixed].
- Neurological—seizures or psychosis.
- Hematologic disorders—hemolytic anemia, leukopenia (<4,000/μL), lymphopenia (<1,500/μL), thrombocytopenia (<100,000/μL), and ESR is raised.
- Immunologic disorder—anti-dsDNA or anti-Sm-OE antiphospholipid antibodies.
- Antinuclear antibody—abnormal ANA titer in the absence of drug-induced SLE.

Livedo Reticularis (Figs. 3A and B)

Livedo reticularis is a mottled bluish discoloration of the skin that occurs in a net-like pattern. It is not a diagnosis in itself but a reaction pattern.

Raynaud Phenomenon (Figs. 4A to C)

Raynaud phenomenon is digital ischemia that occurs on exposure to cold and/or as a result of emotional stress, it may occur in persons using vibratory tools.

- Secondary RP
- Connective tissue diseases—scleroderma, SLE, and dermatomyositis.
- Vasculitis
- Obstructive arterial disease—atherosclerosis, thromboembolism.
- Drugs/Toxins—β-blocker, ergotamine, and bleomycin.
- Neurologic disorder—carpal tunnel syndrome.
- Occupational/environmental exposure—vibration injury, vinyl chloride.
- Hyperviscosity disorders—cryoproteins and cold agglutinins.

SYSTEMIC SCLEROSIS AND SCLERODERMOID DISORDERS

Scleroderma (Figs. 5A to K)

- Multisystem disorder characterized by inflammatory, vascular, and sclerotic changes of skin and various internal organs, especially the lungs, heart, and gastrointestinal tract (GIT).
- Major clinical features—skin sclerosis and RP.
- Synonyms—progressive systemic sclerosis (SSc), SSc, and systemic scleroderma.
- Age of onset—30–50 years.
- Female to male ratio—4:1.
- Etiology unknown, but pathogenesis involves vasculopathy, endothelial dysfunction, tissue fibrosis, and immune system activation.

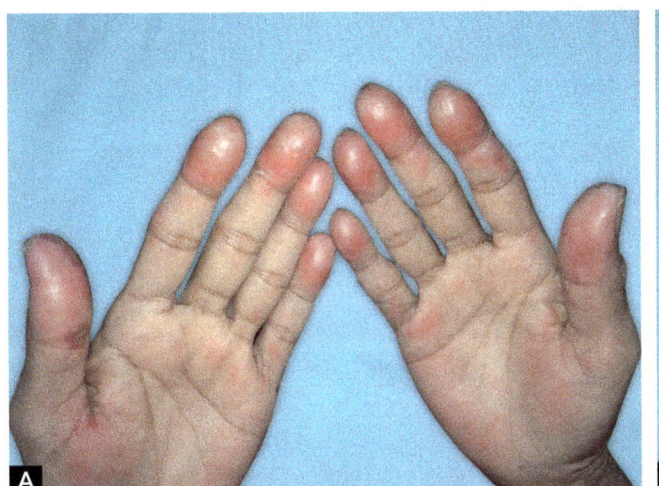
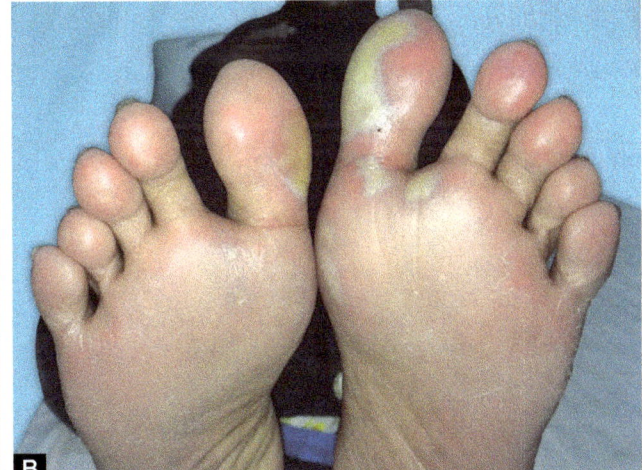
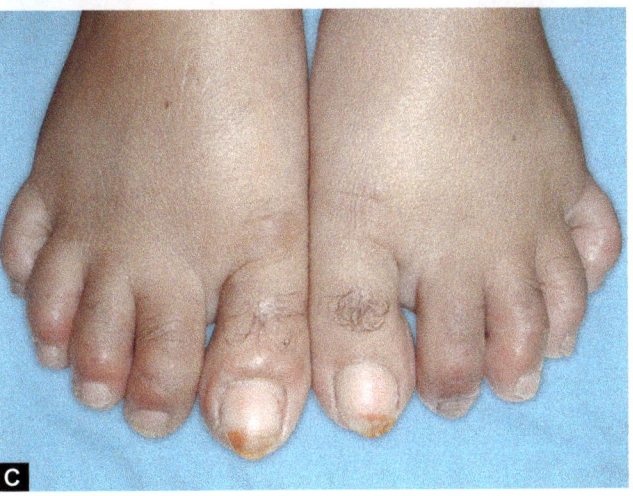

FIGS. 4A TO C: Raynaud phenomenon.

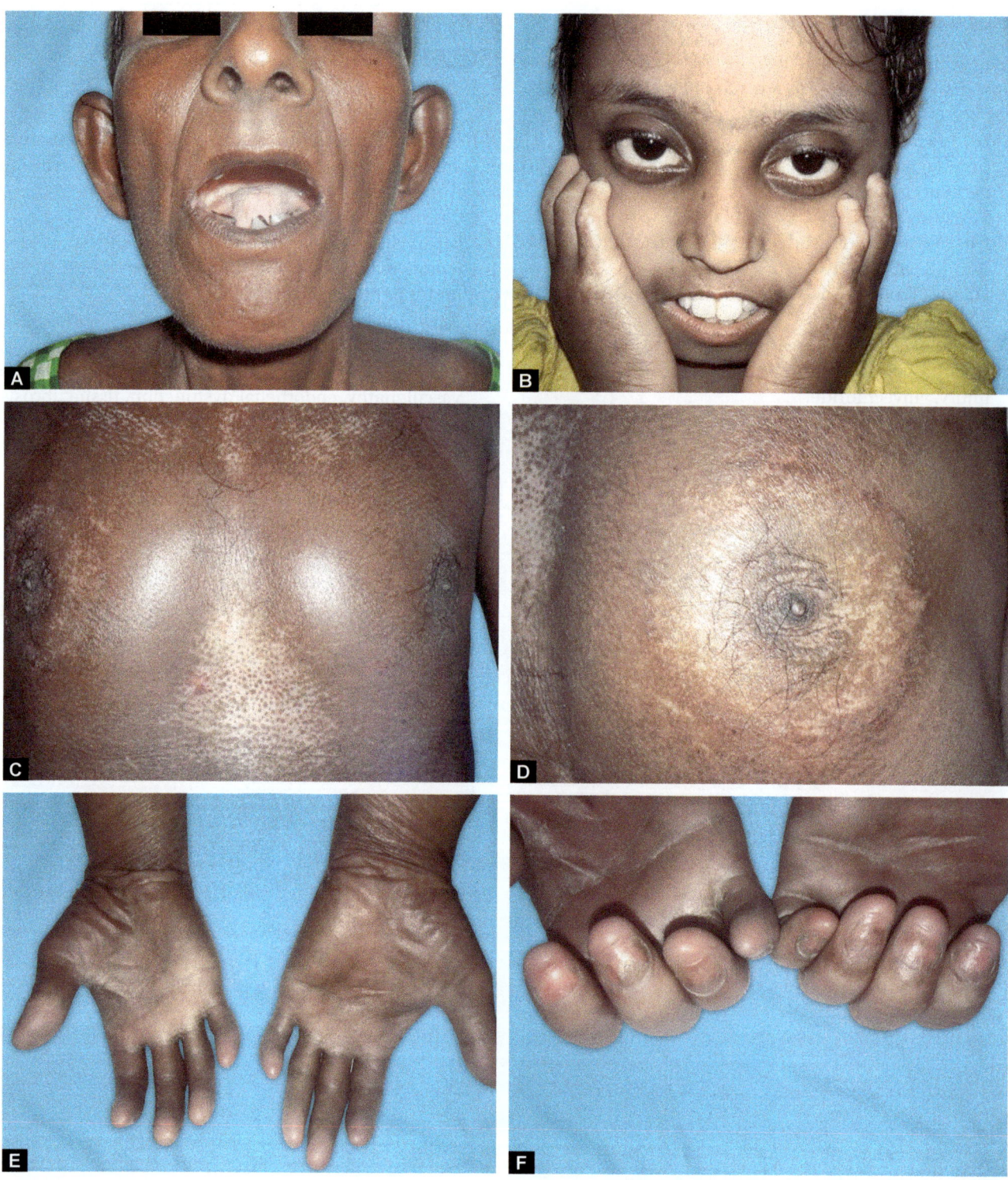

FIGS. 5A TO K: *Continued*

Continued

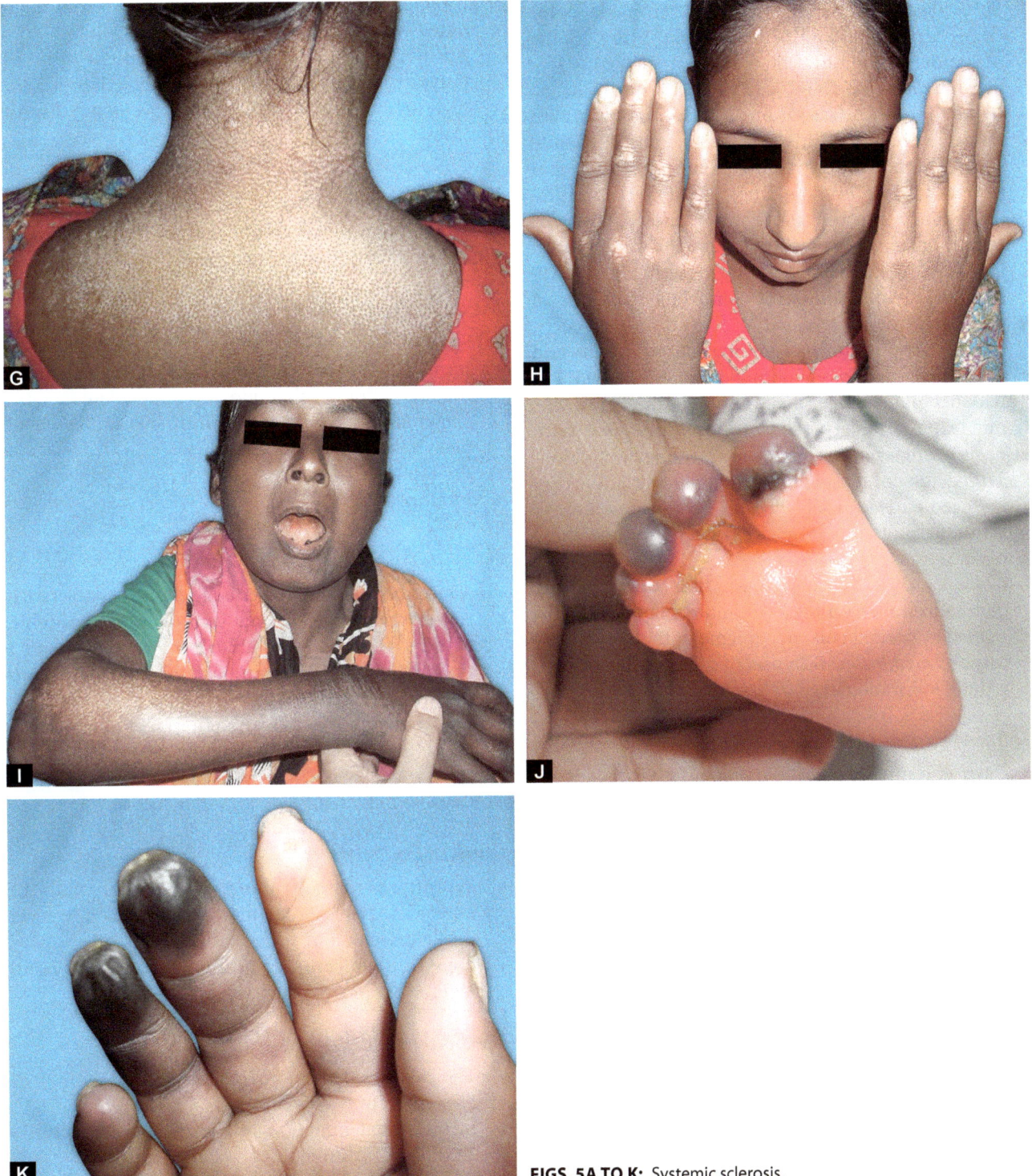

FIGS. 5A TO K: Systemic sclerosis.

Clinical Features

- *Skin*: Hands/feet, early RP with triphasic color change, pallor, cyanosis, rubor, nonpitting edema of hands/feet, painful ulceration at fingertips (rat bite necrosis), knuckles, and heal with pitting scars. In late presentation, there is sclerodactyly with tapering fingers with waxy, shiny, and hardened skin, which is tightly bound down and does not permit folding or wrinkling, leathery crepitation over joints, flexion contractures, and periungual telangiectasia. Bony resorption and ulceration result in loss of digital phalanges, loss of sweat glands with anhidrosis, and thinning or complete loss of hair on distal extremities.
- *Face*—Early: Periorbital edema. Late: Edema and fibrosis result in loss of normal facial lines, mask-like patients look younger than they are, thinning of lips, microstomia, radial perioral furrowing, beak-like sharp nose, telangiectasia, and diffuse hyperpigmentation.
- *Trunk*: The chest and proximal upper extremities are involved early. Tense, stiff, and waxy appearance of skin as a result of impairment of respiratory movement of chest wall and joint mobility.
- *Color change*: Hyperpigmentation that may be generalized and on the extremities may be accompanied by perifollicular hypopigmentation.
- *Mucous membrane*: Sclerosis of sublingual ligament, painful induration of gums and tongue.

General Examinations

- Gastrointestinal system—small intestine involvement may produce constipation, diarrhea, bloating, and malabsorption.
- Esophagus—dysphagia and reflex esophagitis.
- Lung—pulmonary fibrosis and alveolitis.
- Heart—conduction defect, heart failure, and pericarditis.
- Musculoskeletal—carpal tunnel syndrome, muscle weakness.

Laboratory Findings

Biopsy for Histopathology

- In SSc, ANA is positive in >90% of cases.
- In case of nucleolar antigen, ribonucleic acid (RNA) polymerase and fibrillarin are present. Diffuse sclerosis, generalized telangiectasia, and internal organ involvement are seen.
- Patients with antibodies to Scl-70 tend to have diffuse truncal involvement; pulmonary fibrosis and digital pitted scar are seen.
- Antibody to nRNP is found in patient with RP, polyarthralgia, arthritis, and swollen hands. Very high RNP indicates mixed connective tissue disorder (MCTD).
- Anti-dsDNA positive in linear scleroderma.

Radiographic Findings

Bony resorption and ulceration may result in loss of digital phalanges with flexion contractures.

Medical Prescription

- Systemic CS.
- Immunosuppressive drugs—cyclosporine, methotrexate, cyclophosphamide, mycophenolate mofetil—shown improvement of skin score but limited benefit for systemic involvement.
- Photopheresis
- Immunoablation

Morphea (Figs. 6A to E)

- A localized and circumscribed sclerosis characterized by early violaceous, later ivory-colored, hardening of skin, subcutaneous tissues and may extend to underlying bone and can be associated with central nervous system (CNS) abnormalities.
- May be solitary, linear, generalized, and rarely accompanied by atrophy of underlying structures.
- Unrelated to SSc.
- Cause is unknown.

Clinical Features

- Symptoms—usually none. No relation with RP. Linear and pansclerotic morphea can result in severe disfigurement.
- Signs—circumscribed, indurated, hard, and poorly defined plaque.

Medical Prescription

- Topical CS and tacrolimus preparation
- Phototherapy
- Intralesional injection of triamcinolone acetonide 3–5 mg/mL in strength.
- Fractional erbium laser followed by platelet-rich plasma (PRP) or human fibroblast.

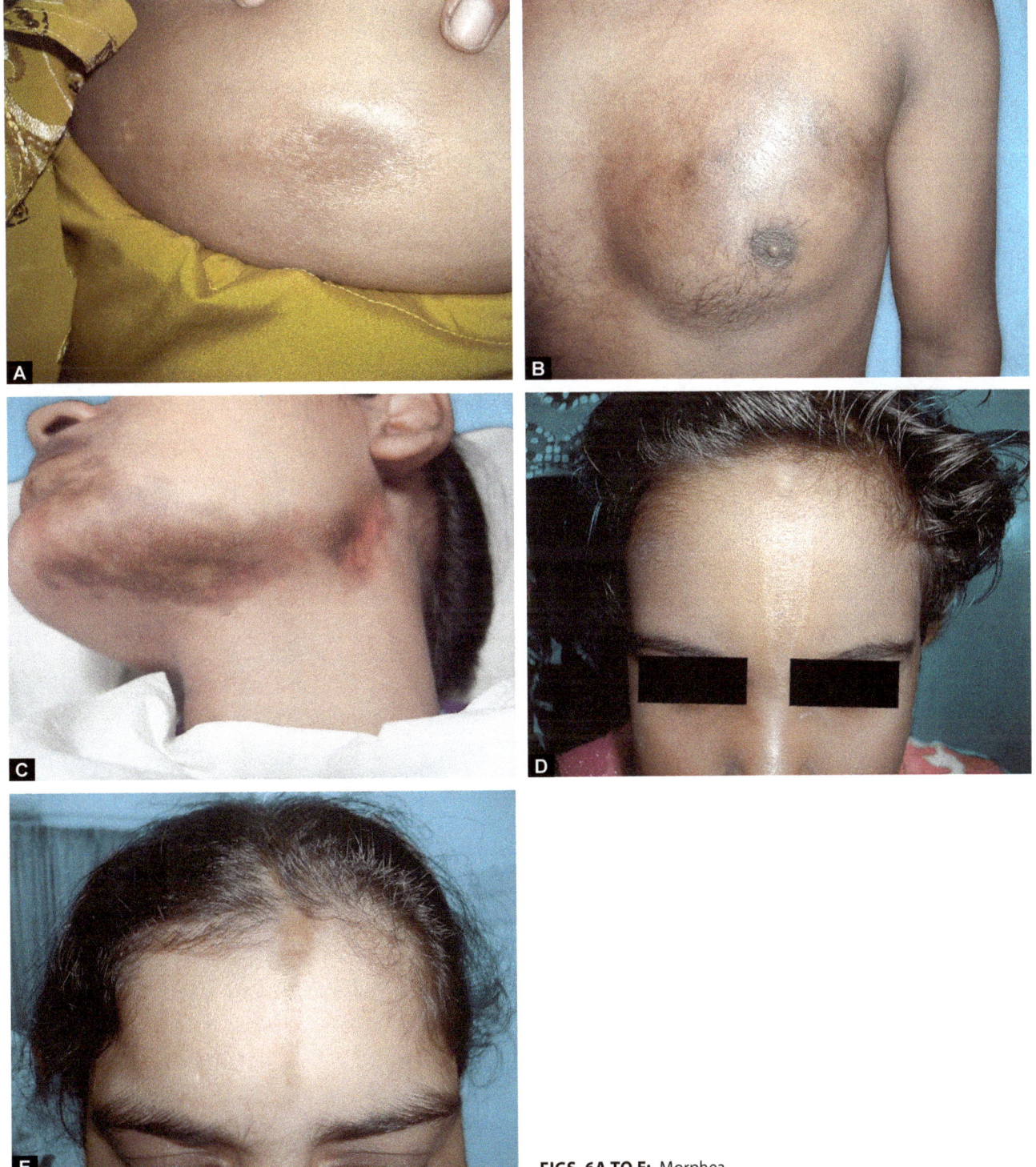

FIGS. 6A TO E: Morphea.

Lichen Sclerosus (Lichen Sclerosus et Atrophicus) (Figs. 7A to F)

Lichen sclerosus is a chronic inflammatory disease of skin and mucosa characterized by:
- *Females*—flat-topped papules, plaques, or atrophic patches surrounded by erythematous to violaceous halo. Skin becomes smooth, atrophied, soft, and white and often bullae, hemorrhagic, telangiectasia, and purpura may be seen. These result in loss or obliteration of normal anatomic structure with loss of the labia minora, clitoral hood, and urethral meatus. Introital stenosis or fusion may occur. Vaginal or cervical mucosa is not involved by lichen sclerosus.

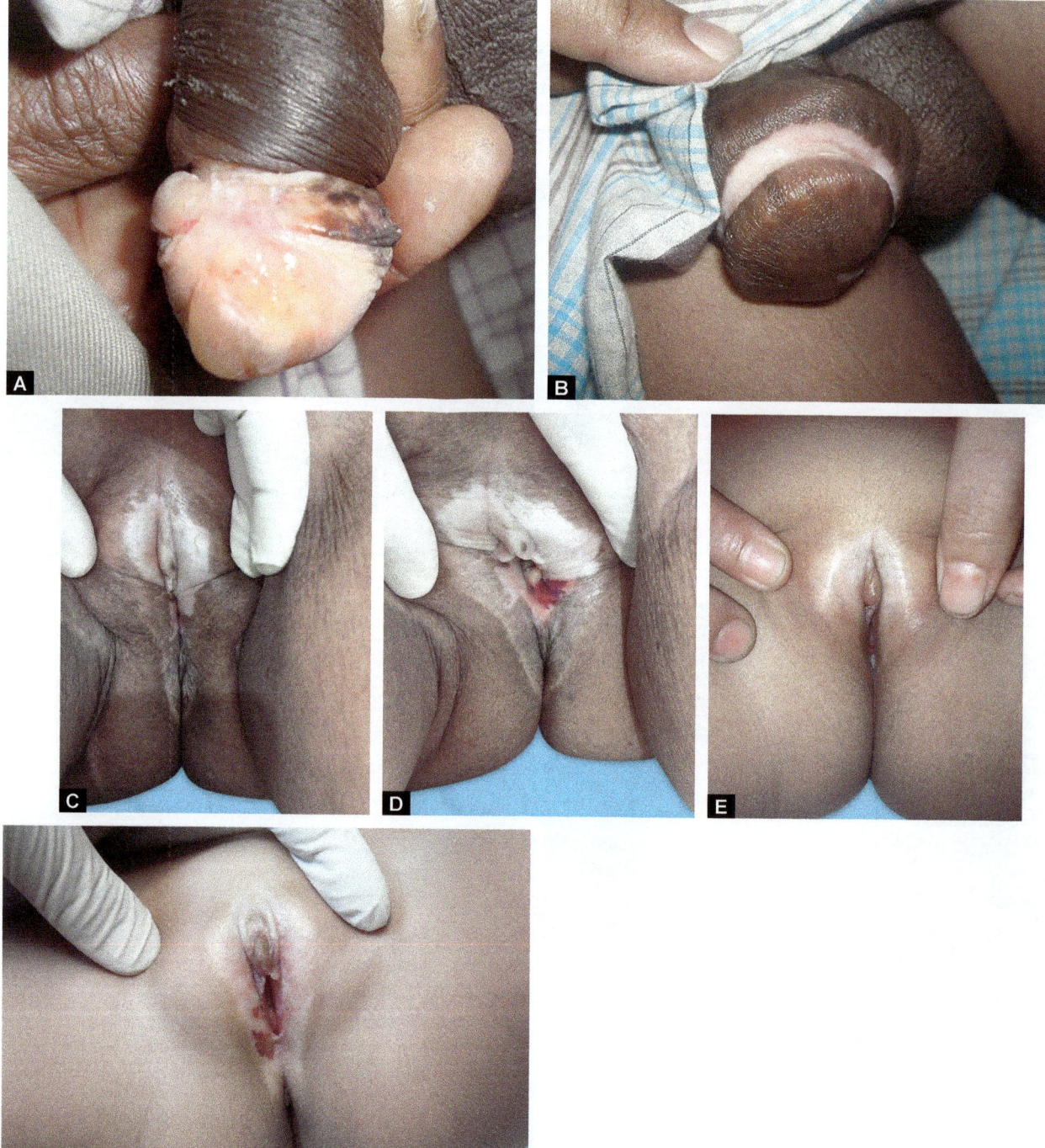

FIGS. 7A TO F: Lichen sclerosus et atrophicus (LSA).

About 40% patients are asymptomatic. Patients come to specialist with the complain of itching, burning sensation, especially during micturition, pain when fissuring erosion develops, vaginal discharge and dyspareunia. Perianal involvement may produce constipation, stool holding, or rectorrhagia due to rectal fissure.

- *Males*—involve usually on glans penis, inner foreskin of the uncircumcised male. Lesions are atrophic and hypopigmented patches may extend on scrotum. Hemorrhage, erosion, and ulceration are usual presentations. Most cases are asymptomatic, but may present with burning, pain, and itching. Phimosis, paraphimosis, and destruction of structures are the common complications.

Extragenital involvement may occur in 6–20% in upper back, chest, breasts, tongue, and oral mucosa and usually asymptomatic.

There is a higher risk of development of squamous cell carcinoma (SCC) in both male and female.

Doctor's Prescription
Biopsy for histopathological examination.

Medical Prescription
- Superpotent topical CS once or twice weekly with topical tacrolimus 0.1% rest of the days.
- Fractional erbium followed by application of injection of triamcinolone acetonide or PRP brings excellent outcome due to regeneration of normal structures.

■ Dermatomyositis (Figs. 8A to F)

Dermatomyositis (DM) is a genetically determined autoimmune disease involving skin and/or skeletal muscles characterized by violaceous (heliotrope) changes ± edema of the eyelids and periorbital area; erythema of face, neck, and upper trunk; and flat-topped violaceous papules over the knuckles, associated with polymyositis, interstitial pneumonitis, and myocardial involvement **(Figs. 9A and B)**.

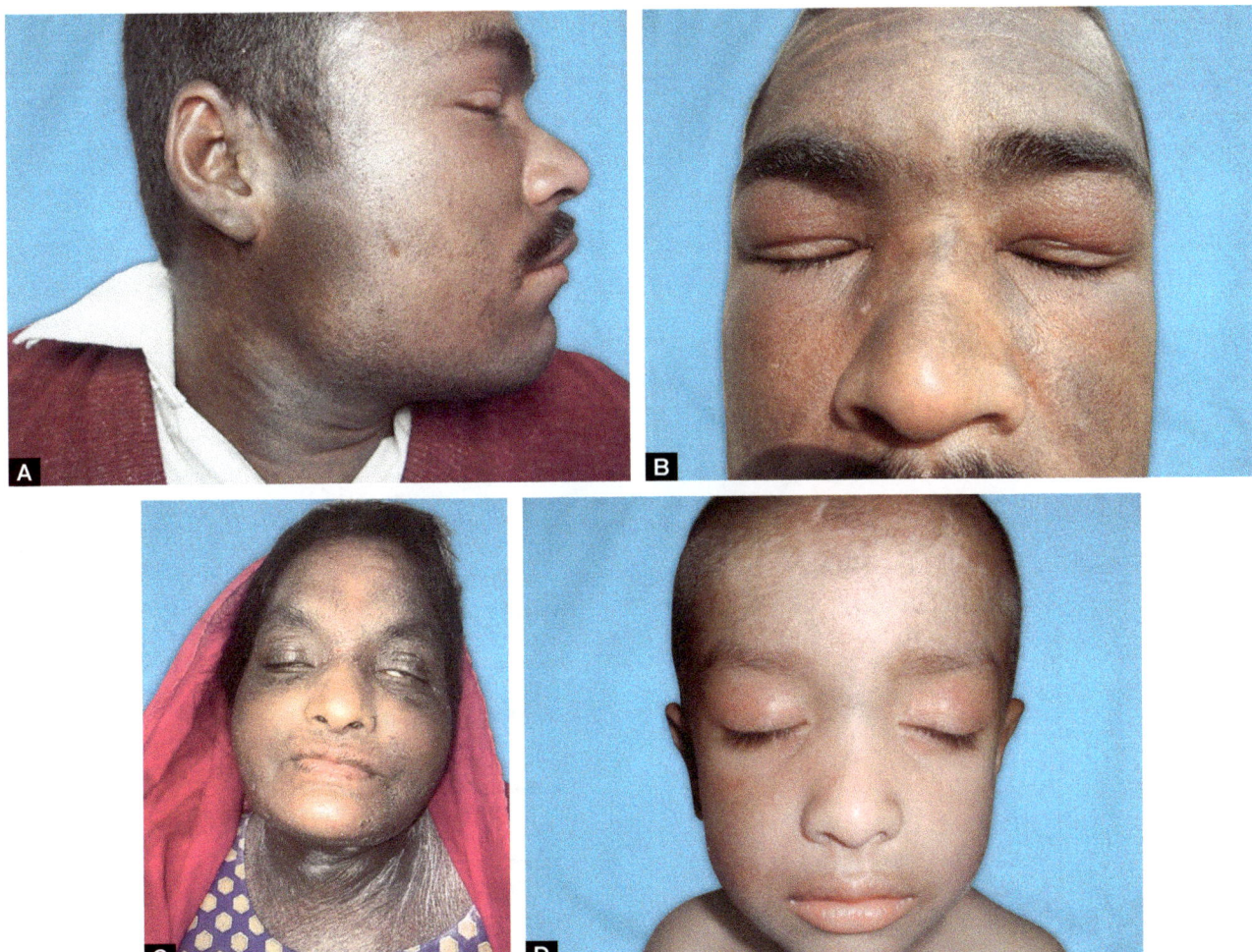

FIGS. 8A TO F: *Continued*

Continued

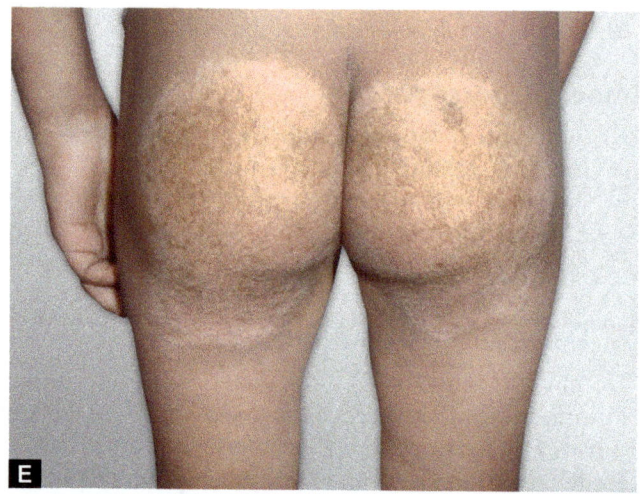
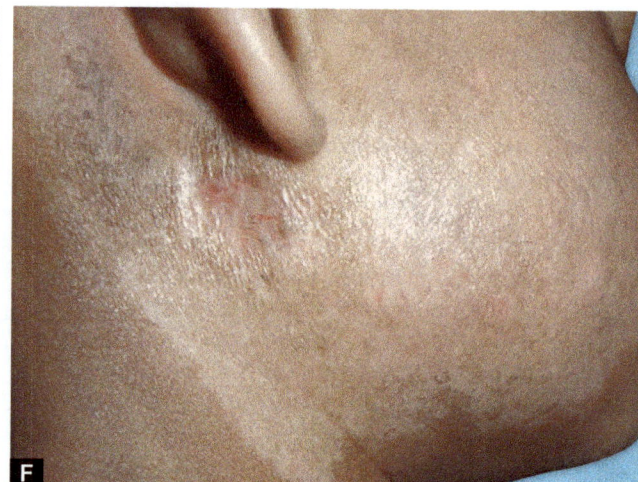

FIGS. 8A TO F: Dermatomyositis (DM).

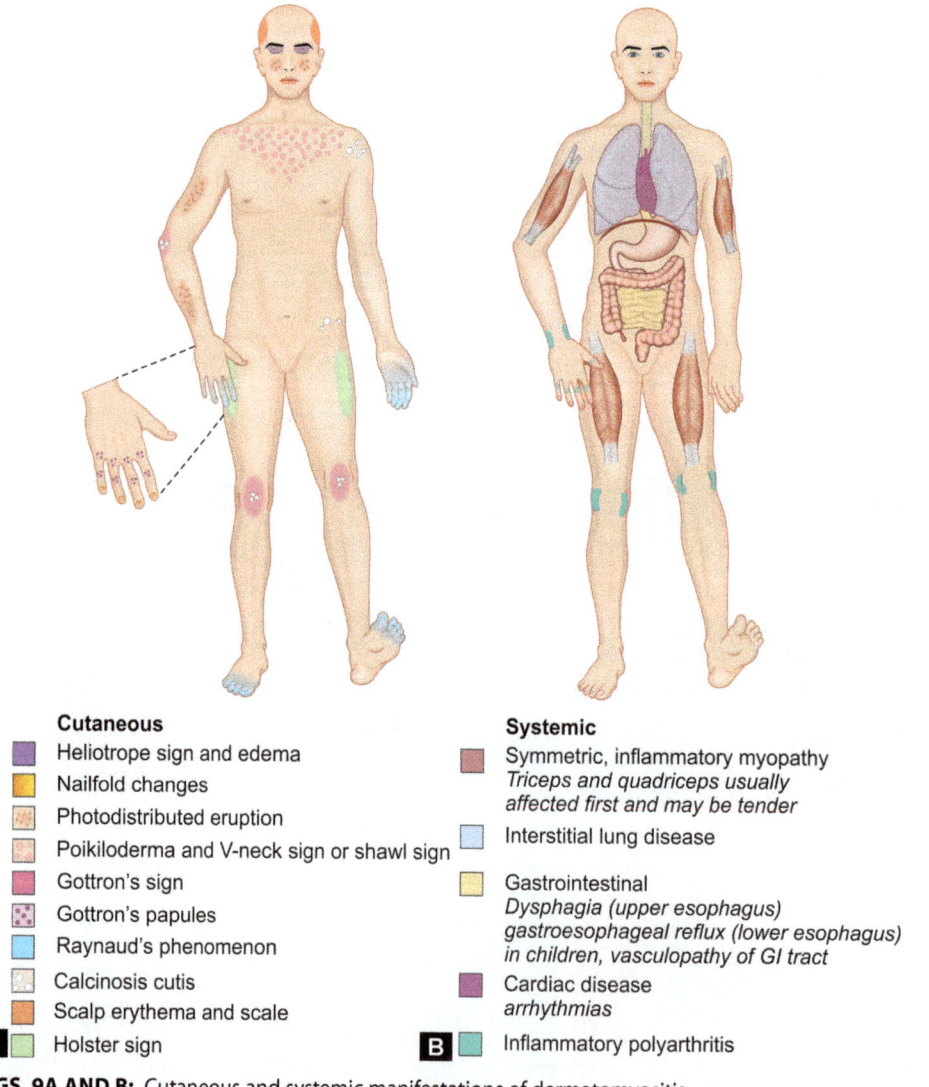

FIGS. 9A AND B: Cutaneous and systemic manifestations of dermatomyositis.

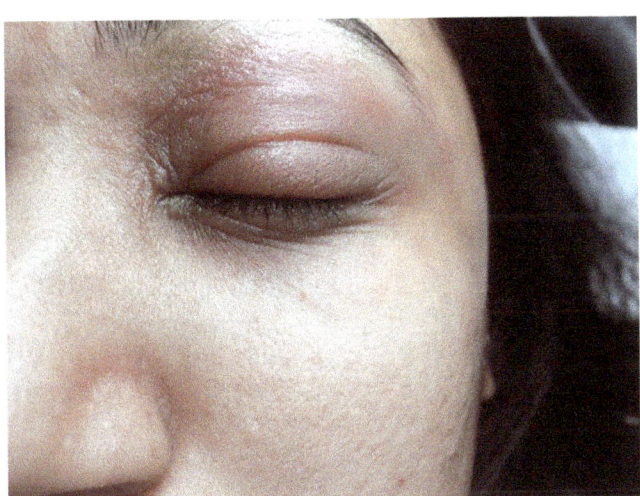

FIG. 10: Heliotrope (reddish papule) erythema.

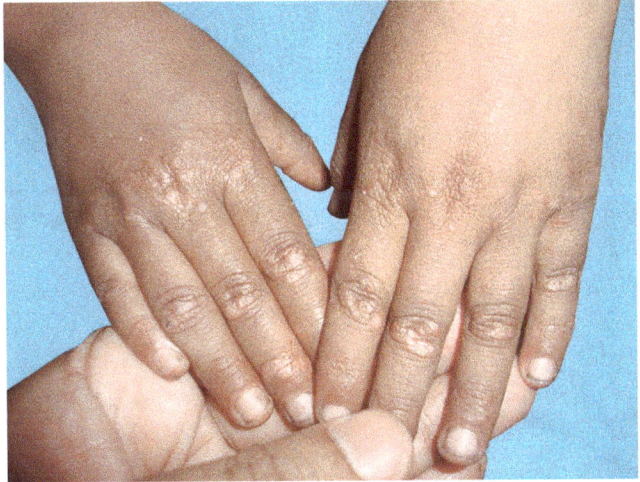

FIG. 11: Violaceous erythema and Gottron's papules.

Adult onset may be associated with internal malignancy.

■ Poikiloderma

Clinical Features Symptoms
- Muscle weakness, difficulty in rising arms from supine position, climbing stairs, rising arms over head, or turning on bed.
- Dysphagia
- Burning and pruritus

■ Skin Lesions
- Periorbital heliotrope (reddish purple) flush, usually associated with some degree of edema. It may extend to scalp, face, upper chest, and arms **(Fig. 10)**.
- Nonscarring alopecia may develop.
- Violaceous erythema may be seen in same site **(Fig. 11)**. Flat-topped, violaceous papules and varying degree of atrophy on the nape of neck, shoulders, knuckles, and interphalangeal joints. Long-standing lesions produce poikiloderma (mottled, reticular brownish pigmentation, and telangiectasia plus small white scars). Calcification in the subcutaneous or facial tissue is common in later stages of juvenile DM over bony prominences.
- Progressive muscle weakness, especially proximal limb girdle muscles with muscle atrophy seen.

Doctor's Prescription
- Creatine phosphokinase—raised 65%.
- Aldose—raised 40%.
- Antibody serum 80% positive, Jo-1 20%, and ANA 40%.
- Electrocardiogram (ECG)
- MRI
- X-ray of chest
- Biopsy from skin and muscle for histopathology

Treatment
- Prednisolone—0.5–1 mg/kg/day along or in combination with azathioprine 2–3 mg/kg/day.
- Alternate regimens—methotrexate, cyclophosphamide, cyclosporine, anti-tumor necrosis factor (TNF)-α agents, and immunoglobulin.

CHAPTER 15

Neutrophilic Dermatosis

INTRODUCTION

This is characterized by infiltration of neutrophils within the skin, but lack of any infectious etiology.

SWEET'S SYNDROME (FIGS. 1A AND B)

- Acute onset of erythematous edematous painful nonpruritic papules and plaques that often giving the appearance of vesiculation (pseudovesiculation).
- Accompanied by fever, malaise, arthralgia, and peripheral leukocytosis.
- Associated with infection, malignancy, or drugs.
- Treatment with systemic glucocorticoids, potassium iodide, dapsone, or colchicine.

ERYTHEMA NODOSUM SYNDROME (FIG. 2)

- The most common type of panniculitis characterized by the appearance of painful nodules on the lower legs.
- Lesions are bright red and flat but nodules on palpation.
- Accompanied by fever, malaise, and arthralgia.

Etiology—Infections

- Bacterial—streptococcal, tuberculosis, *Salmonella*, and *Mycoplasma*.
- Fungal—coccidioidomycosis, blastomycosis, histoplasmosis, sporotrichosis, and dermatophytosis.

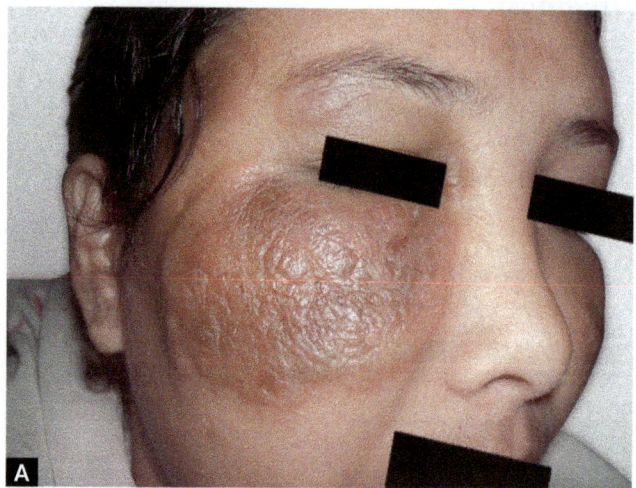
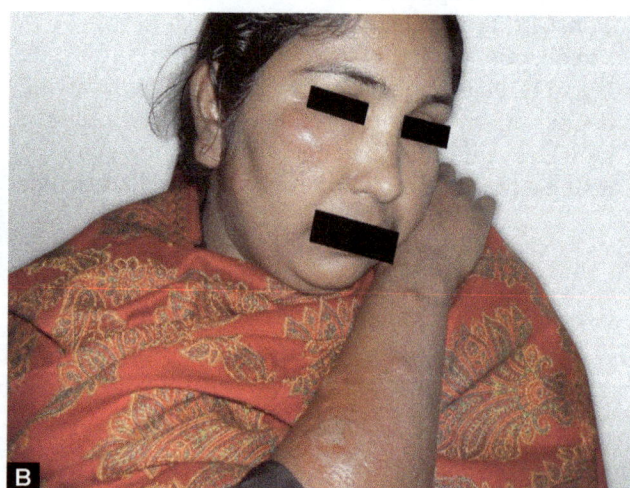

FIGS. 1A AND B: Sweet's syndrome—erythematous papules and plaques.

- Viral—infectious mononucleosis, hepatitis B, Orf, and herpes simplex.
- Others—amebiasis, giardiasis, and ascariasis.
- Drugs—sulfonamides, bromides, iodides, oral contraceptives, minocycline, gold salt, penicillin, and salicylate.
- Malignancy—Hodgkin's and non-Hodgkin's lymphoma, leukemia, and renal cell carcinoma.
- Others—sarcoidosis, inflammatory bowel disease, ulcerative colitis, Crohn's disease, and pregnancy.

■ Doctor's Prescription

- Hematology—elevated erythrocyte sedimentation rate (ESR), C-reactive protein, and leukocytosis.
- Bacterial culture
- Radiology—X-ray of chest and gallium scan to rule out sarcoidosis.
- Dermatopathology—to establish diagnosis. It is a septal panniculitis.

■ Medical Prescription

- Bed rest, compressive bandages, and wet dressing
- Salicylates
- Nonsteroidal anti-inflammatory drug (NSAID).
- Systemic corticosteroid
- Treatment of the cause.
- Erythematous nodules on the lower legs.

PYODERMA GANGRENOSUM (FIGS. 3A TO D)

- Idiopathic, either acute or chronic, severely debilitating skin disorder characterized by neutrophilic infiltration, destruction of tissue, and ulcer formation.
- May occur alone, usually associated with systemic disease, especially arthritis, inflammatory bowel disease, hematologic dyscrasias, and malignancy.
- Pyoderma gangrenosum (PG) is characterized by the presence of painful, rapidly enlarging regular, boggy, blue-red ulcers with undermined borders, and purulent necrotic bases.
- Ulcer may occur at lower extremity, face, upper extremity, and trunk.

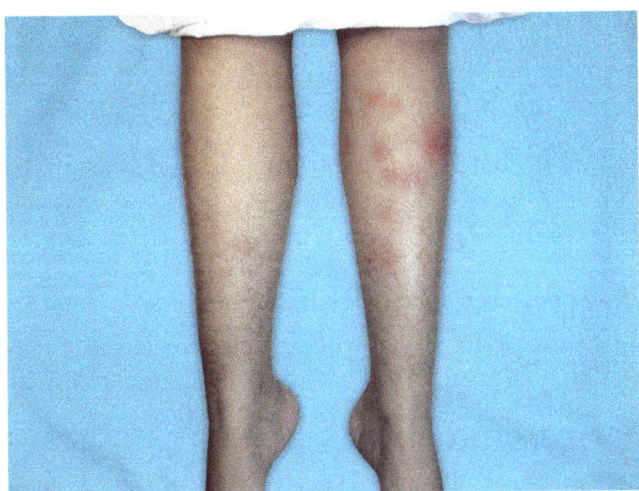

FIG. 2: Erythema nodosum (EN).

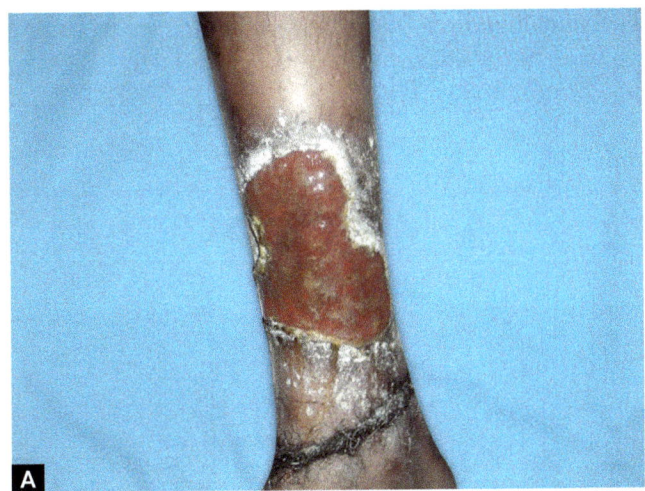

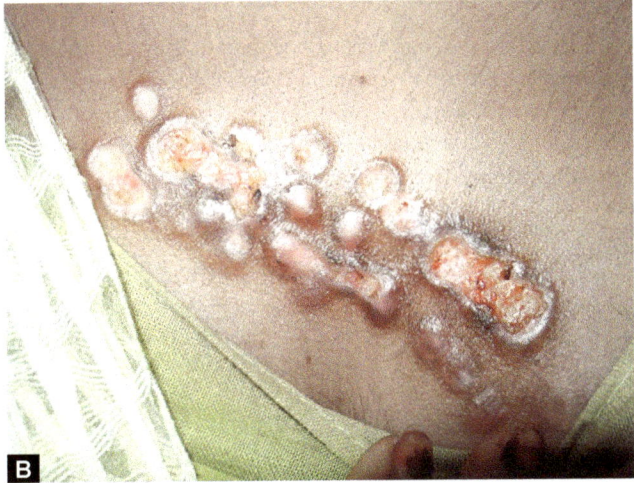

FIGS. 3A TO D: *Continued*

Continued

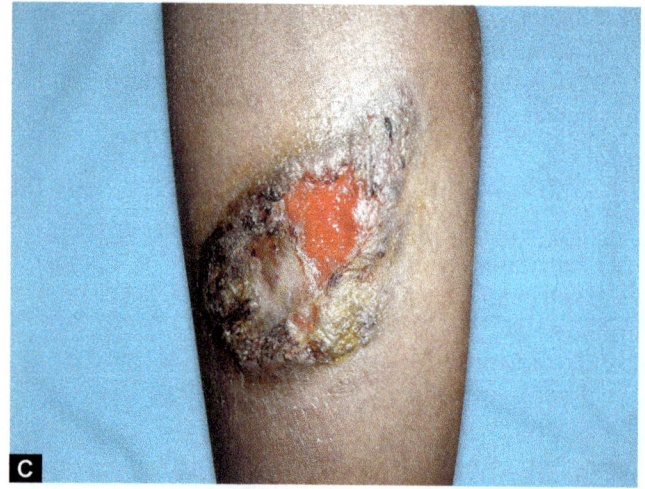
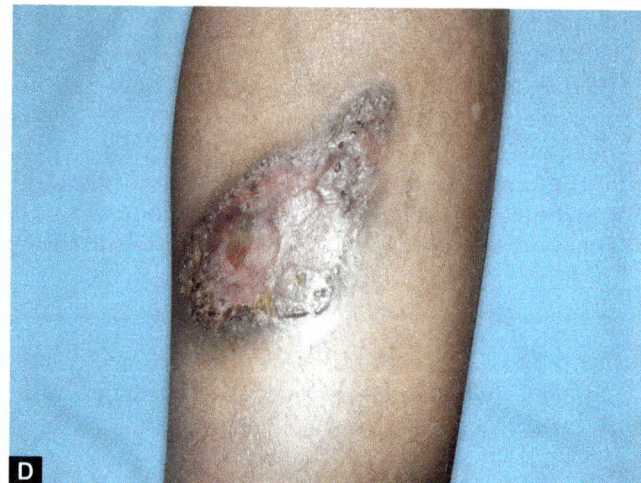

FIGS. 3A TO D: Pyoderma gangrenosum.

■ Doctor's Prescription
No laboratory test that establishes diagnosis.

■ Medical Prescription
- Treatment of underlying disease
- Topical tacrolimus or intralesional triamcinolone acetonide (5–10 mg/mL)
- High dose of oral glucocorticoid (1 mg/kg/day) or intravenous (IV) glucocorticoid pulse therapy.
- Cyclosporin, minocycline, dapsone, or clofazimine may be tried.

BEHÇET'S DISEASE (FIGS. 4A TO C)

A multisystem disease with the mucocutaneous findings of painful aphthous orogenital ulcers, sterile pustules, erythema nodosum, superficial thrombophlebitis, iridocyclitis, posterior uveitis, and palpable purpura due to small vessels vasculitis.

Additional symptoms may include arthritis, epididymitis, ileocecal ulcerations, vascular, and central nervous system lesions.

■ Doctor's Prescription
- Dermatopathology—leukocytoclastic vasculitis with fibrinoid necrosis of blood vessel walls in acute lesions and lymphocytic vasculitis in late lesions.
- Pathergy test is positive.

■ Medical Prescription
- Potent topical glucocorticoid.
- Intralesional triamcinolone acetonide 3–10 mg/mL.
- Thalidomide 50–100 mg/day
- Colchicine 0.6 mg two to three times a day
- Dapsone 100 mg/day

CHAPTER 15 Neutrophilic Dermatosis

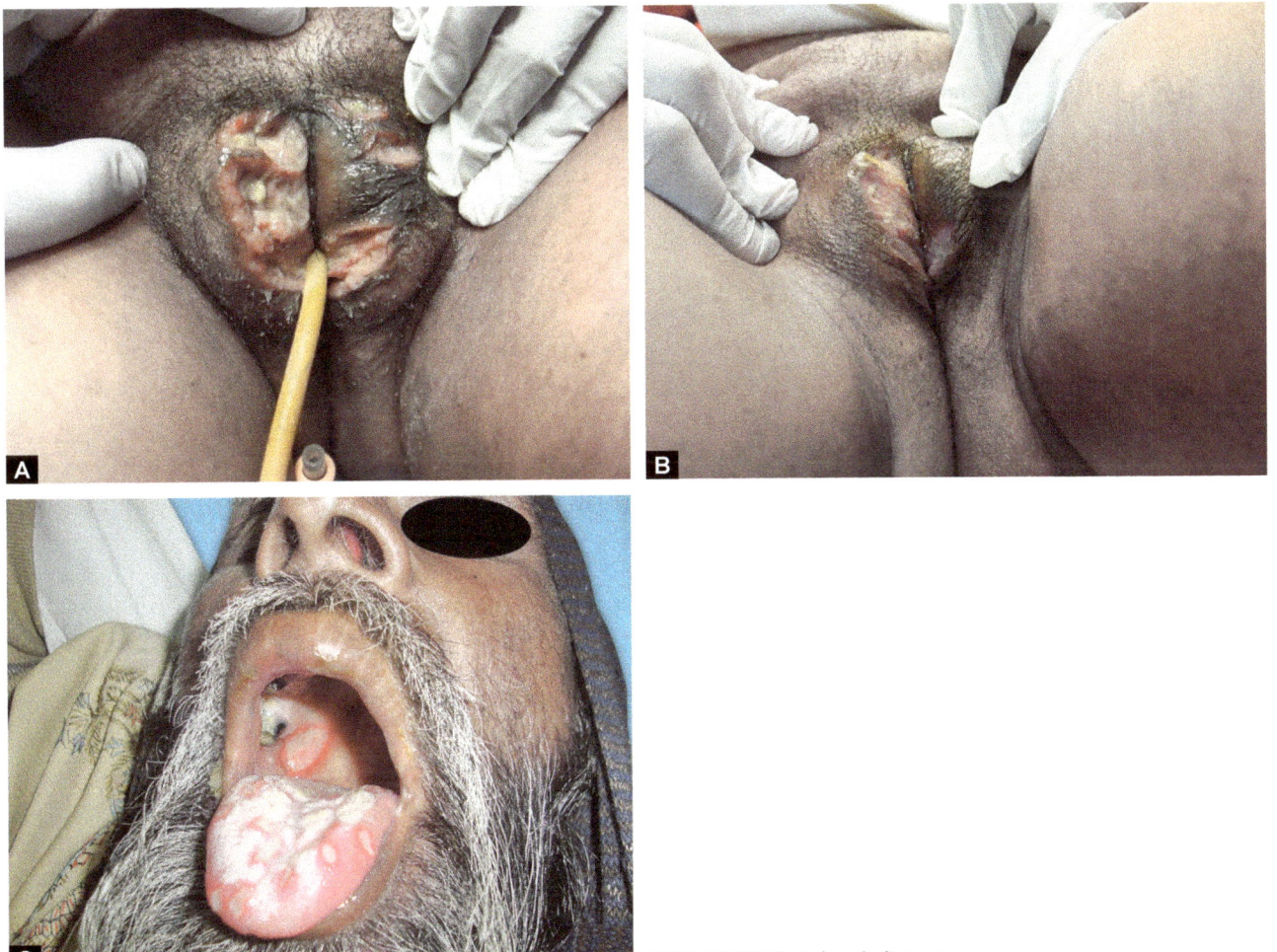

FIGS. 4A TO C: Behçet's disease.

CHAPTER 16

Disorders of Sebaceous, Eccrine, and Apocrine Glands

ACNE VULGARIS (COMMON ACNE) AND CYSTIC ACNE (FIGS. 1A TO D)

- An inflammation of pilosebaceous units, characterized by papule, pustule, pathognomonic comedo, nodule, and cyst.
- Appears on the face, trunk, and rarely on buttocks.
- Occurs in 85% of individuals having 12–24 years of age and 15–35% of adults, especially women in their 30–40 years.

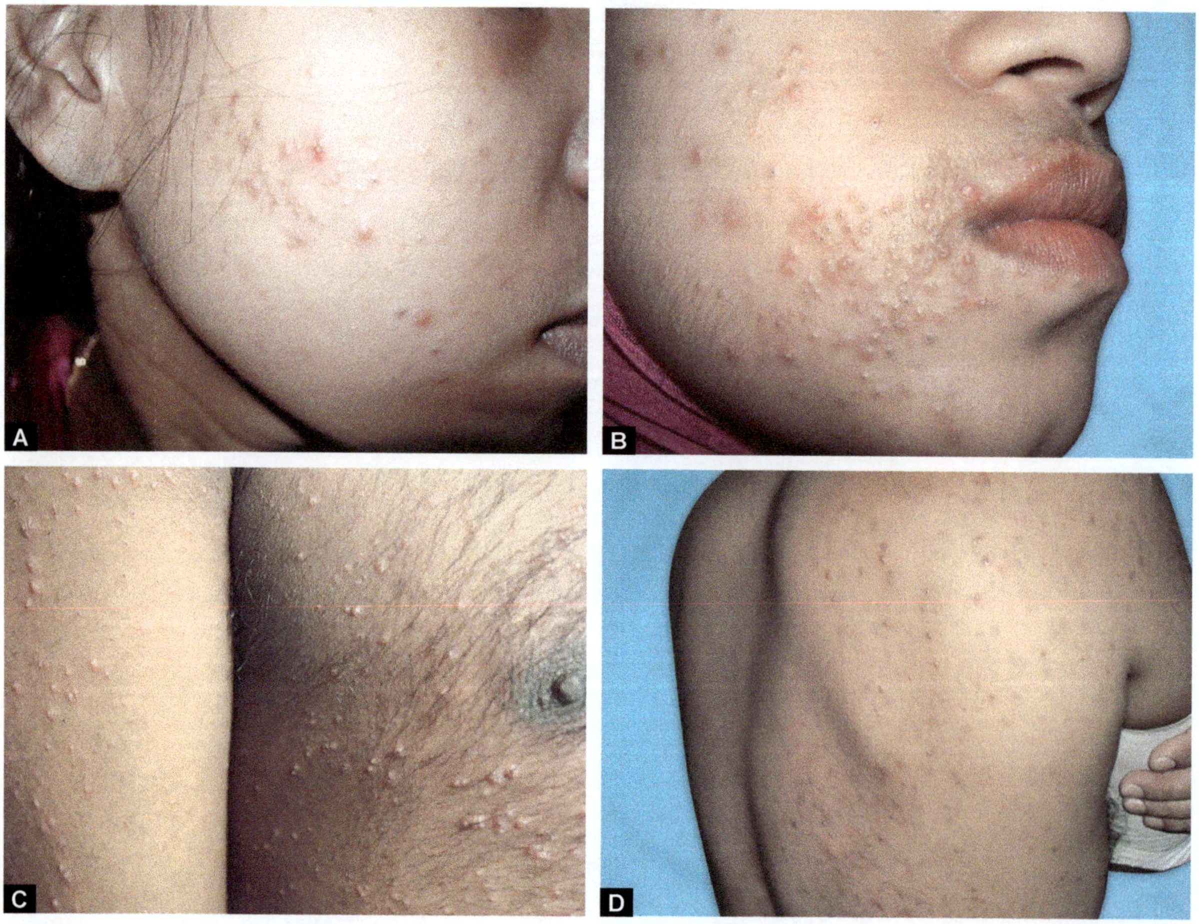

FIGS. 1A TO D: Acne vulgaris.

- In untreated or maltreated cases, there are scarring and psychological outbreak such as anxiety, depression, and social withdrawal.

Clinical Features

Noninflammatory Acne
- Closed comedones (whiteheads) are skin color papules without an obvious follicular opening.
- Open comedones (blackheads) have a dilated follicular opening filled with a keratin plug. This black color is due to oxidized lipids and melanin.

Inflammatory Acne
- Erythematous papule and pustules
- Nodules and cysts filled with pus or serosanguinous fluid may coalesce and form sinus tracts.
- Acne conglobata (severe nodulocystic acne)

- Inflammatory acne commonly results in postinflammatory hyperpigmentation, especially in patients with darker skin, which fades slowly over time; pitted scar or hypertrophic scar or keloid **(Figs. 2A to H)**.

Doctor's Prescription

No laboratory examination is required for diagnosis. Clinical presentation is enough for diagnosis. If endocrine disease is suspected, serum-free testosterone, follicle-stimulating hormone (FSH), luteinizing hormone (LH), and dehydroepiandrosterone sulfate (DHEAS) to exclude hyperandrogenism and polycystic ovary syndrome (PCOS). Recalcitrant acne can also be related to congenital adrenal hyperplasia (11b or 21bhydroxylase deficiency). If systemic isotretinoin treatment is planned, determine transaminases [alanine aminotransferase (ALT) and aspartate aminotransferase (AST)], triglyceride, and cholesterol levels.

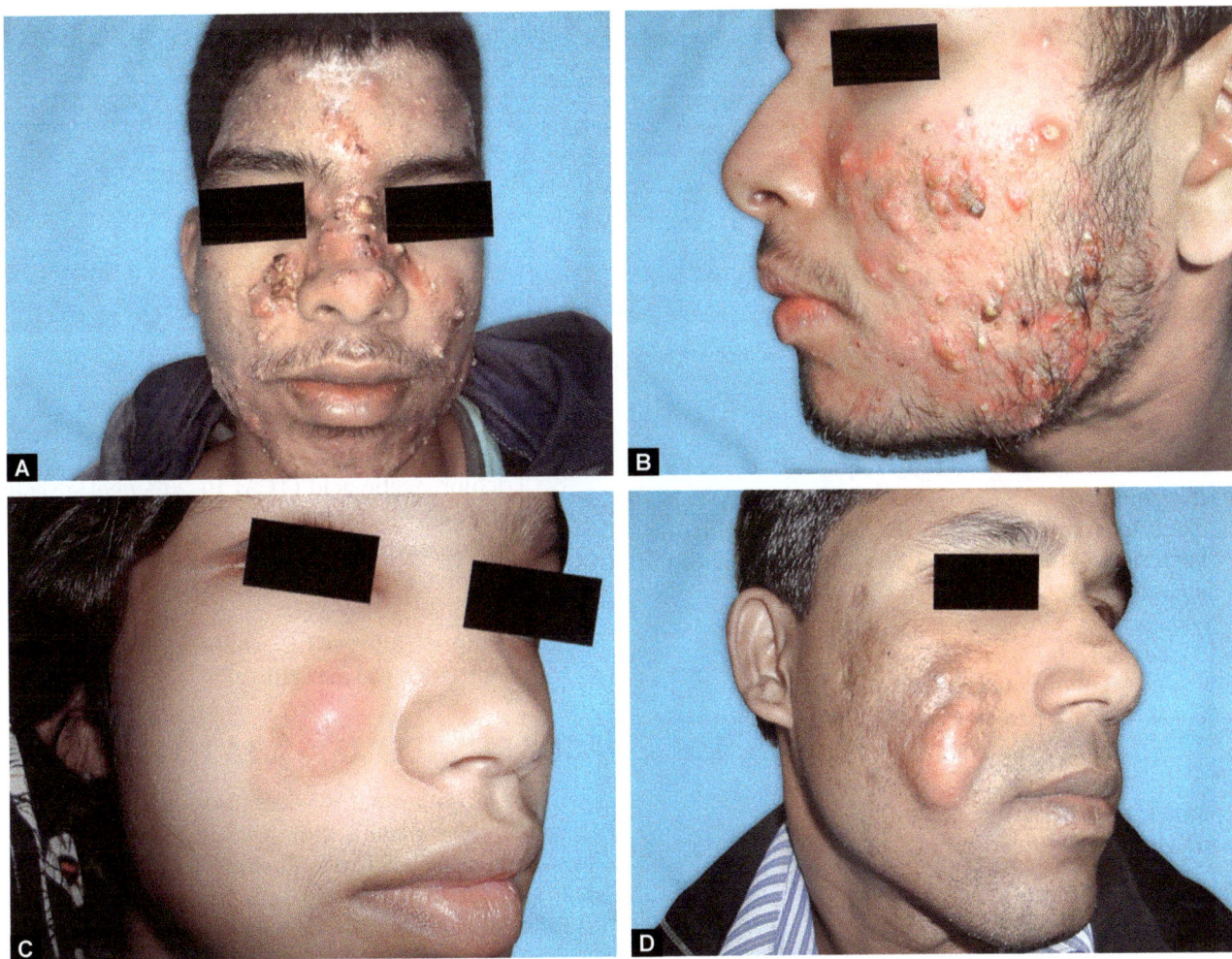

FIGS. 2A TO H: *Continued*

Continued

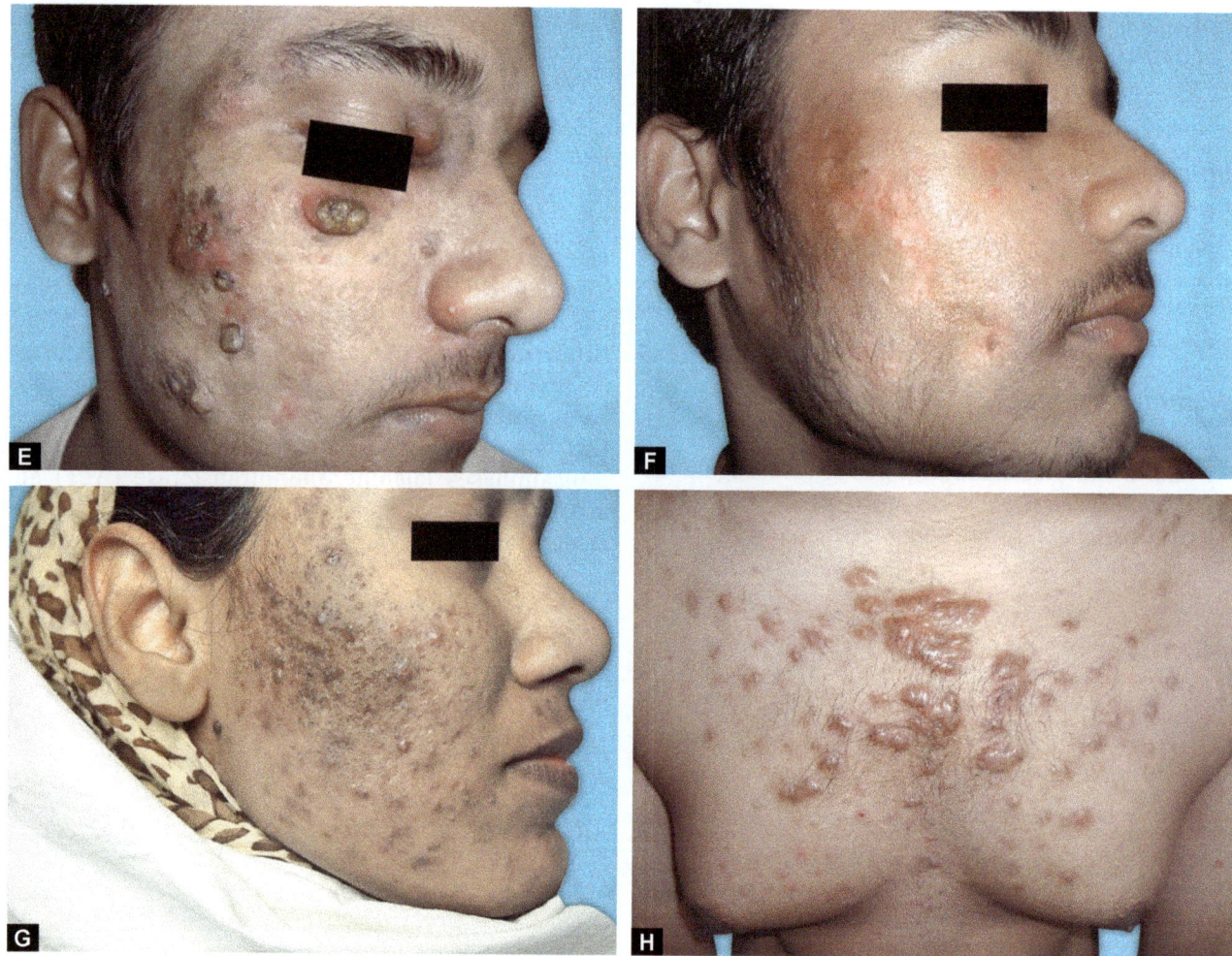

FIGS. 2A TO H: Cystic acne. Complications of acne—atrophy, hypertrophy, and keloid.

■ Medical Prescription

- Substantial benefit typically requires 6-8 weeks of treatment.
- Goal of treatment—reduces sebum production, bacterial colonization, and removes plugging of the pilar drainage.
- *Mild acne*:
  - Topical antibiotics:
    - Clindamycin/Erythromycin
    - Benzoyl peroxide gel (2%, 5%, or 10%).
    - Topical retinoids (retinoic acid, adapalene, or tazarotene)
- *Moderate-to-severe acne*:
  - Add oral antibiotic:
    - Minocycline 50-100 mg/day—most effective
    - Doxycycline 50-100 mg/day
    - Oral isotretinoin 10-20 mg/day—most effective to prevent.
    - Scarring
- *For remission of postinflammatory hyperpigmentation or scar*:
  - Trichloroacetic acid (TCA) 10-20% peel/glycolic acid peel
  - Fractional erbium laser
  - Fractional carbon dioxide (CO_2) laser
  - Subcision
  - Fractional erbium/CO_2 followed by 10% TCA/platelet-rich plasma (PRP)

ACNE ROSACEA (FIGS. 3A TO F)

- Chronic inflammatory acneiform disorder of the facial pilosebaceous units with increased reactivity of capillaries leading to flushing and telangiectasia. It may result in rubbery thickening of nose, cheeks, forehead, or chin caused by sebaceous hyperplasia.
- Commonly affecting 10% of fair-skinned people with a peak incidence between 40 and 50 years.
- With a female predominance, but rhinophyma occurs mostly in males.

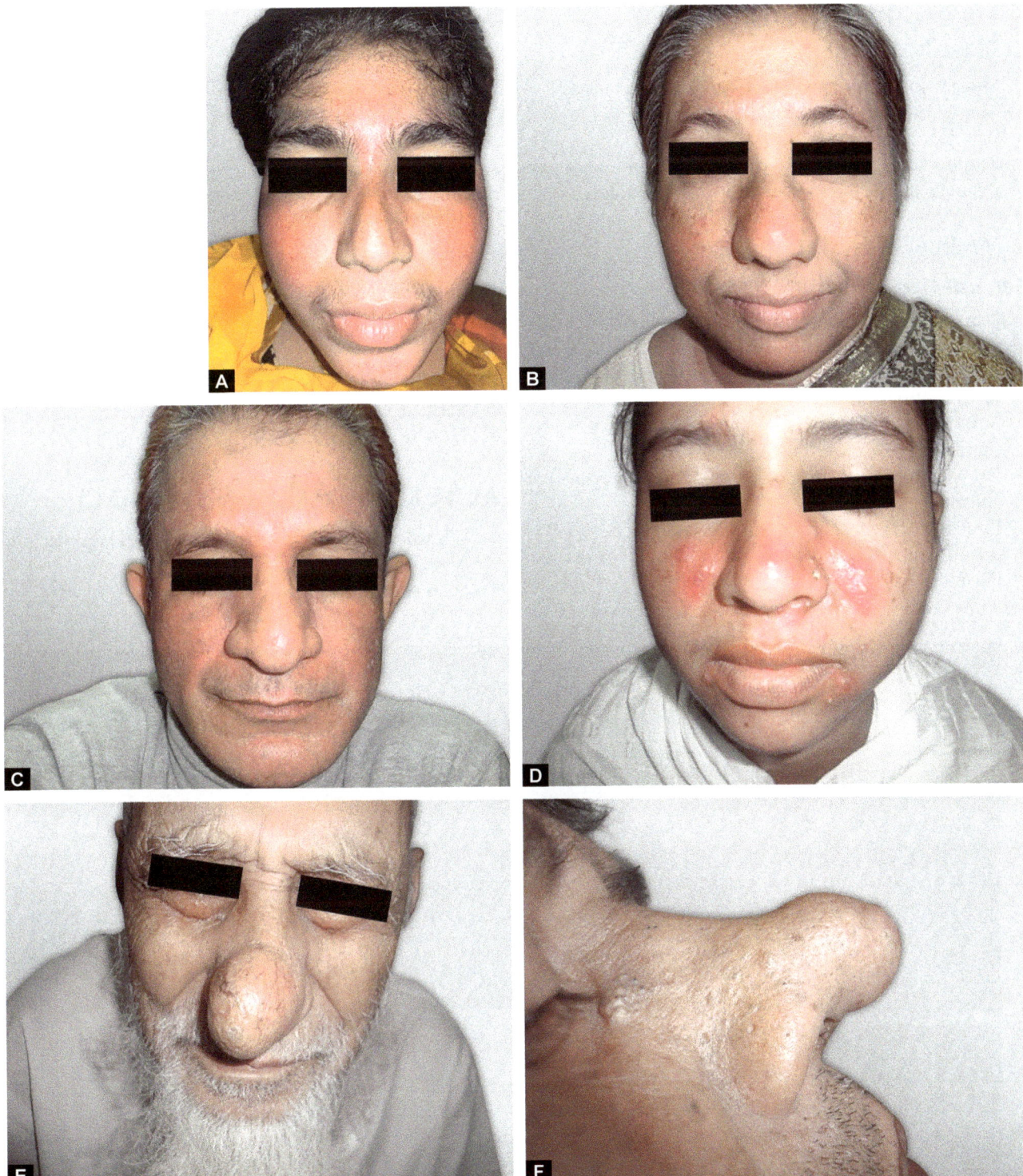

FIGS. 3A TO F: Acne rosacea.

Staging (Plewig and Kligman Classification)

- Stage I—persistent erythema with telangiectasias.
- Stage II—persistent erythema, telangiectasias, papules, and tiny pustules.
- Stage III—persistent deep erythema, dense telangiectasias, papules, pustules, and nodules.

Medical Prescription

General Measures

- Use soap-free cleansers that are pH balanced.
- Use sunscreens with both ultraviolet A (UVA) and ultraviolet B (UVB) protection and a sun protection factor (SPF) = 15.
- Sunscreen containing the physical barriers such as titanium dioxide and/or zinc oxide
- Use cosmetic and sunscreens that contain protective silicones.
- Educate on the importance of sun avoidance.
- Avoid procedures such as glycolic peels or dermabrasion.

Specific Measures

Papulopustular Rosacea

- Topical—metronidazole (0.75-1%), azelaic acid, benzoyl peroxide (5%), clindamycin (1%), and erythromycin (2%).
- Systemic—tetracycline 500 mg BD, doxycycline 100 mg BD, minocycline 100 mg BD, or isotretinoin 10-40 mg/day.

Erythematotelangiectatic Rosacea

- Vascular laser or intense pulsed light (IPL)/calibrated pulsed light (CPL)
- Fractional erbium

Phymatous Rosacea

- Surgical excision
- Electrosurgery

ACNE KELOIDALIS (FIGS. 4A TO C)

- Chronic folliculitis of the posterior neck and occipital scalp, with time keloidal papules and plaques develop.
- Seen almost exclusively in male patients.

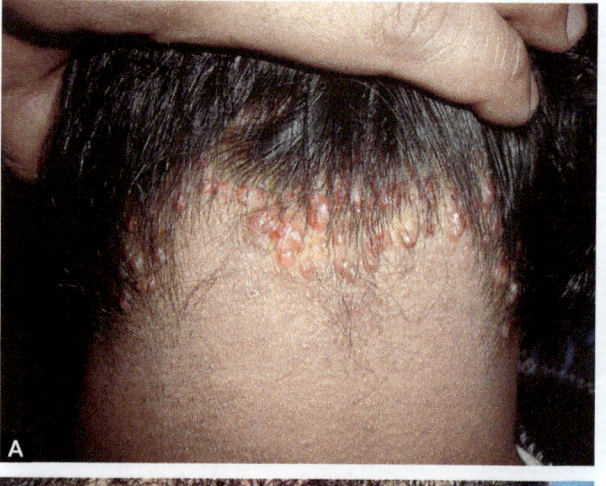
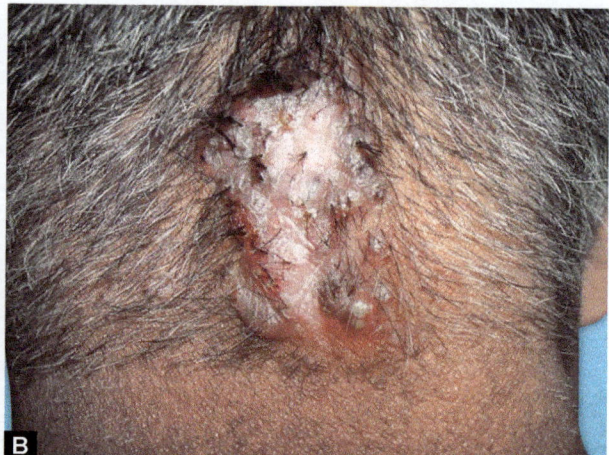
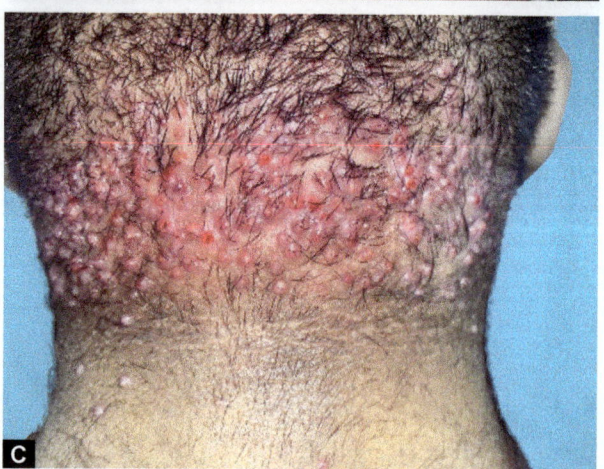

FIGS. 4A TO C: Acne keloidalis.

- Lesions are usually pruritic, painful, and disfiguring.
- Sometimes, subcutaneous abscesses with malodorous draining sinuses and alopecia are seen.

▪ Doctor's Prescription

Bacterial culture and sensitivity.

▪ Medical Prescription

- Topical—tretinoin gel, potent corticosteroid (CS).
- *Systemic*:
  - Antibiotic according to culture and sensitivity
  - Isotretinoin
- Surgery—fractional erbium followed by intralesional triamcinolone acetonide (TA) given intermittently.

HIDRADENITIS SUPPURATIVA (FIGS. 5A TO D)

- A chronic suppurative disorder of apocrine gland bearing skin (axillae, groin, buttock, perianal region, nape of neck, behind ears, and inframammary folds).
- A chronic case characterized by recurrent boils and draining sinus tracts with subsequent scarring.
- Etiology is unknown. Predisposing factors are obesity, smoking, and genetic predisposition to acne. It favors females than males.
- Complications may include anemia of chronic disease, secondary amyloidosis, lymphedema, fistula, arthropathy, and squamous cell carcinomas (SCCs) within the chronic scars.

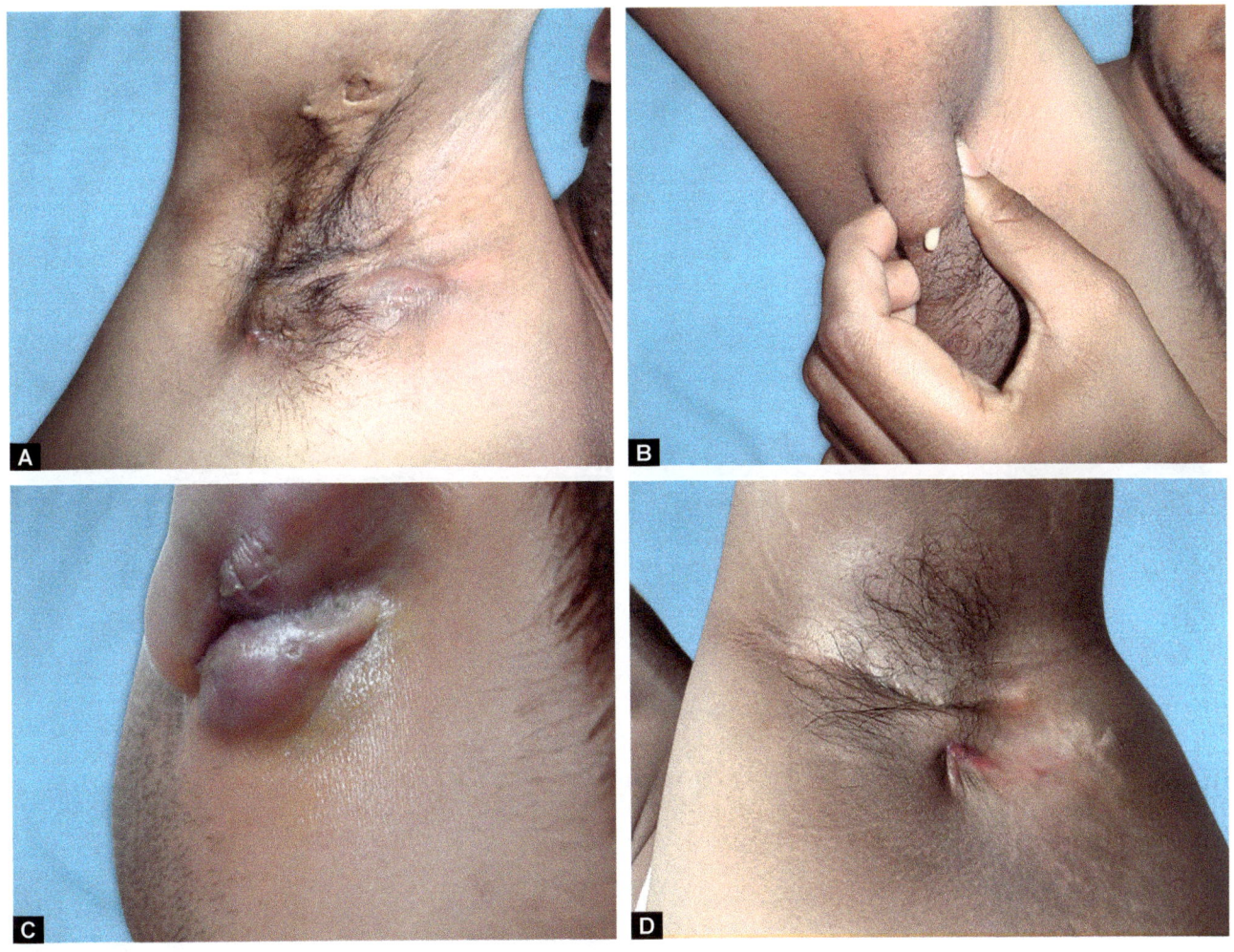

FIGS. 5A TO D: Hidradenitis suppurativa.

Medical Prescription

Combination of:
- Antibiotics—erythromycin, tetracycline, minocycline, combination of clindamycin with rifampin 300 mg BD, and azithromycin. Treatment may continue for weeks or months.
- Oral isotretinoin—useful in early condition to prevent follicular plugging.
- Prednisone—if pain and inflammation are severe, 70 mg daily for 2-3 days then tapered over 14 days.
- Intralesional TA 3-5 mg/mL into the wall followed by incision and drainage of abscess.
- Nd-Yag, Diode laser for removing hair—fractional erbium followed by laser-guided injection of TA.

PERIORIFICIAL DERMATITIS (FIGS. 6A TO D)

- This is referred to as perioral dermatitis, but lesions can surround other orifices, hence the term periorificial.
- Female predominance is seen in adult.
- Lesions around mouth and nose, even the eye.
- Monomorphic pink papules and pustules with eczematous patches and plaques, sometimes with fine scale.

Medical Prescription
- Avoid topical glucocorticoid
- Metronidazole gel (0.75%) and erythromycin (2%)
- Systemic—minocycline or doxycycline or tetracycline (500 mg BD until clear then 500 mg daily for 1 month then 250 mg daily for another month) bring outstanding result.

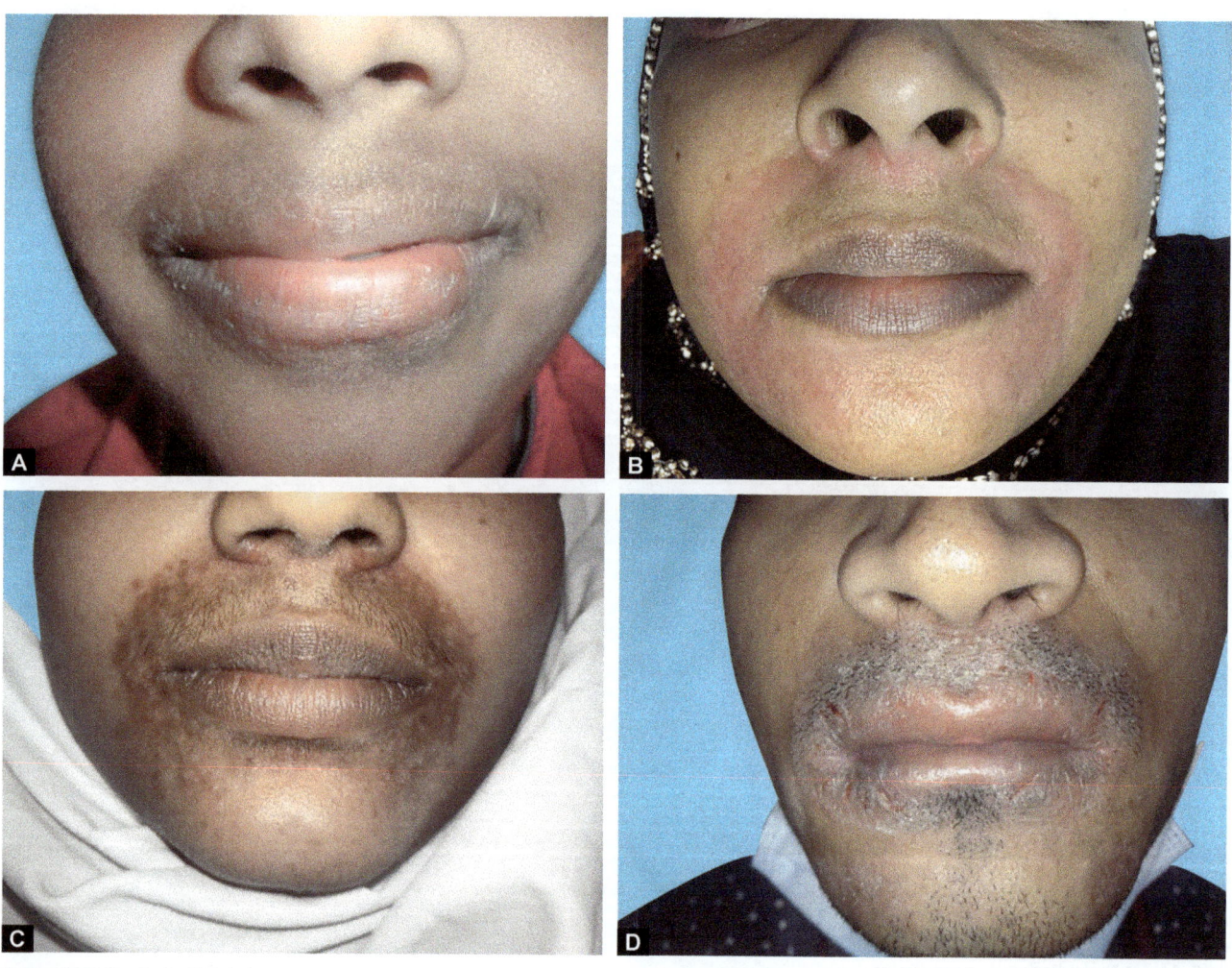

FIGS. 6A TO D: Periorificial dermatitis.

CHAPTER 17

Hair, Nail, and Mucous Membrane

HAIR

Normal hairs can be classified according to cyclic phases of growth.

Anagen hairs (Fig. 1): Growing hair and they grow for about 1,000 days (3 years), with a range between 2 and 6 years. The follicular matrix cells grow, divide, and become keratinized to form growing hairs. As the matrix produces the hair shaft, it incorporates substances.

Catagen hair (Fig. 1): Transition phase hair from growing to the resting hair. This phase lasts about 1-2 weeks, in which all growth activity ceases, with the eventual formation of telogen club hair.

Telogen hair (Fig. 1): Resting hair. This remains in follicle for variable lengths of time before they fall out (teloptosis). This phase lasts about 100 days (3-5 months) before they are released.

Kenogen: Lag period between loss of the telogen hair and growth of a new anagen hair.

In normal individual, about 85-90% anagen hairs, catagen about <1% and 10-15% are telogen hairs.

It has been estimated that the scalp normally contains about 100,000 hairs and average number of hairs shed daily about 100-150.

Hair is also designated as lanugo, vellus, or terminal hair.

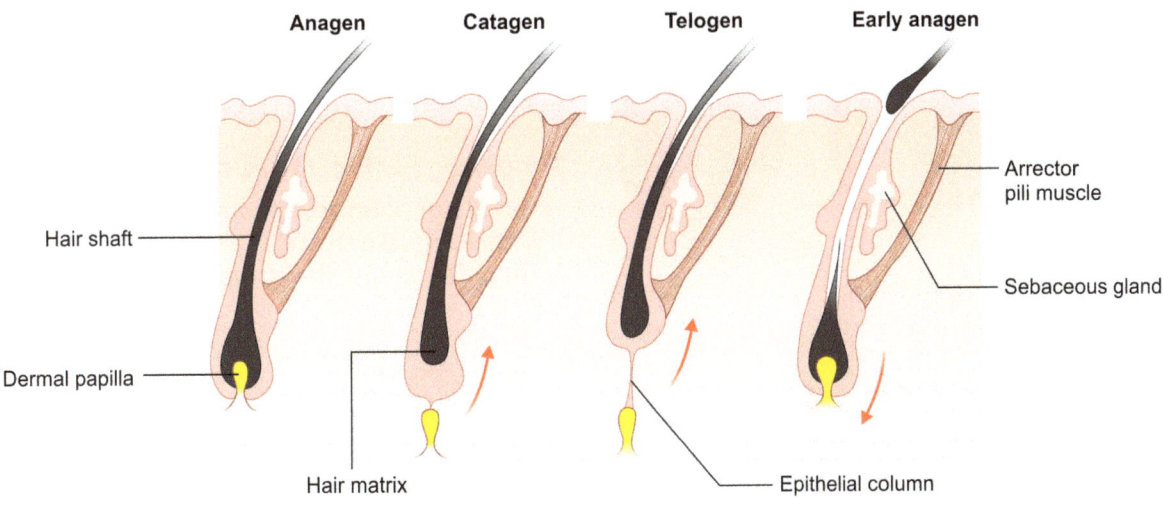

FIG. 1: Hair growth cycle.

Lanugo hair: Fine hair that is grown in utero covers the fetus and is normally shed either in utero or during the first few weeks of life.

Vellus hair: Short, non- or lightly pigmented hair that covers most areas of the body.

Terminal hair: Course thick hair on scalp, and around under arms pubic area. Also found on face trunk and extremities in mail.

■ Alopecias

- In a normal scalp, 90–95% of hairs are in anagen phase, 5–10% in telogen phase.
- About 50–100 hairs normally shed daily.

■ Androgenic Alopecia (Male and Female Pattern of Hair Loss, Figs. 2A to C)

- Sensitivity of scalp hair to androgen hormone causes gradual miniaturization of hairs on the frontal/vertex regions of men and midline and crown of women.
- Related to hormonal effects of dihydrotestosterone (DHT), converted from testosterone by 5-α reductase.
- In women, the frontal hairline is spared (except in the setting of virilization) and a Christmas tree pattern of widening of hair may be seen.

Should exclude hyperandrogenism in younger women or in women with signs of virilization.

Treatment

- *Topical minoxidil 2% or 5% solution* or foam for both genders
- *Finasteride (inhibits 5-α reductase)* for male
- *Spironolactone* in women
- *Platelet rich plasma (PRP)* does not block the production of DHT, but rather reverses its effect on it. Since DHT miniaturizes the hair follicles, PRP restores them to normal size. Recommended platelet concentration in PRP for androgenic alopecia should be 1–1.5 million platelets/μL and dose 0.05–0.1 mL/cm^2.
- More effective than minoxidil or finasteride or spironolactone alone. Combination with minoxidil brings excellent result within 6 months.
- Hair restoration with PRP is not a permanent solution for all forms of hair loss, but comparatively it is safe and long lasting one.
- Recommended dose three times every 4–6 weekly and maintenance is done every 4–6 months.

Hair Transplantation

Permanent treatment for androgenic alopecia with combination of PRP brings excellent outcome.

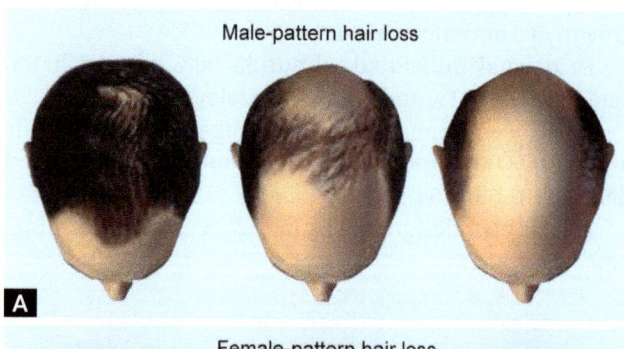
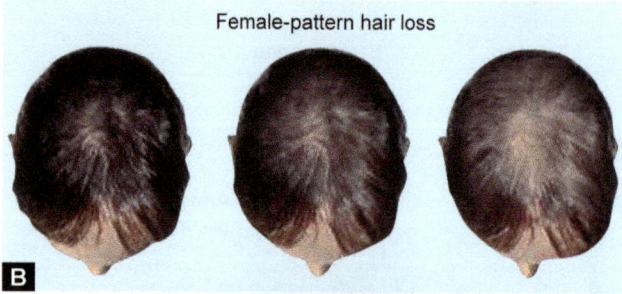
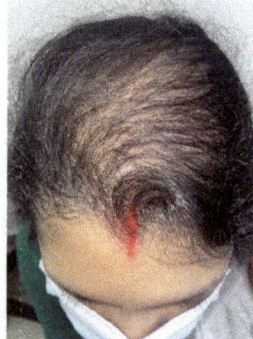

FIGS. 2A TO C: Androgenic alopecia: (A) Male pattern of hair loss; (B and C) Female pattern of hair loss.

■ Telogen Effluvium

One of the most common causes of temporary hair loss due to excessive shedding of resting or telogen hair after some shock to the system **(Figs. 3A and B)**.

Triggering Factors for Telogen Effluvium

- *Childbirth*: Postpartum hair loss.
- Physiological neonatal hair loss
- Acute or chronic illness, especially if there is fever
- Surgical operation
- Accident
- Psychological stress
- Weight loss, unusual diet or nutritional deficiency
- *Drugs*: Retinoids (acitretin and isotretinoin), discontinuing the contraceptive pill, anticoagulants (heparin), antidepressants, lithium, antithyroid (propylthiouracil and methimazole), anticonvulsants (e.g., phenytoin, valproic acid, carbamazepine), interferon-α-2b, and β-blockers (e.g., propranolol).

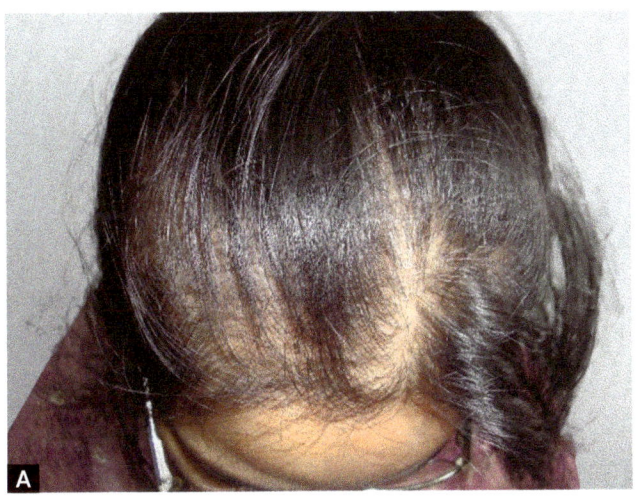
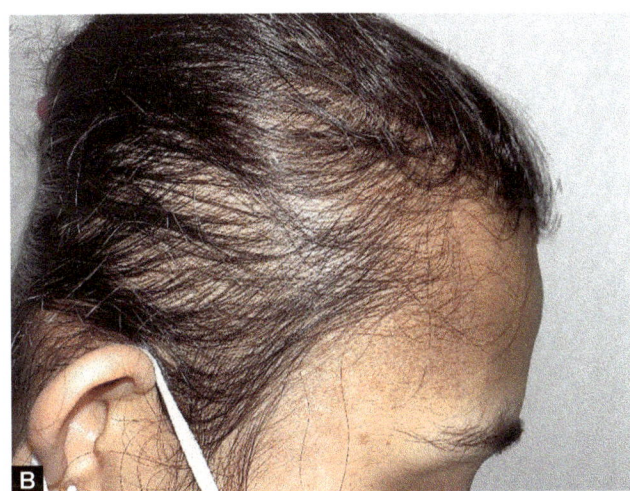

FIGS. 3A AND B: Telogen effluvium.

- Endocrine disorders (e.g., hypothyroidism and hyperthyroidism)
- Overseas travel resulting in jetlag
- Skin disease affecting scalp
- Excessive sun exposure—
  - Can affect people of all age groups and both sexes.
  - Is a nonscarring form of diffuse hair loss with no clinical or histological evidence of inflammation and can affect up to 50% of the scalp hair.

Treatment
Identification and elimination of cause.

■ Alopecia Areata (Figs. 4A to E)

- Autoimmune disease with increased T cells presents in the hair matrix.
- Associated with atopy and other autoimmune diseases (e.g., autoimmune thyroid disease, vitiligo, inflammatory bowel disease, and autoimmune polyendocrinopathy syndrome type 1)
- Average lifetime risk for developing alopecia areata is 1–2%.
- Circular to oval areas of alopecia that progresses to total scalp loss (alopecia totalis) or total body hair loss (alopecia universalis).
- Positive pull test (easily extractable telogen hairs at periphery of oval areas of loss) correlates with active stage.
- Ophiasis pattern is a band-like pattern of loss along the temporal/occipital scalp that may be less responsive to therapy.
- Associated nail findings—nail pitting, trachyonychia > brittle nails, onycholysis, koilonychia, and onychomadesis.

Treatment
- Treatment of underlying disease
- High potency topical steroid
- Topical irritants (e.g., anthralin or tazarotene)
- Topical immunotherapy (e.g., squaric acid dibutyl ester)
- Topical minoxidil 5%
- Oral corticosteroids for short period (2–3 months)
- Platelet rich plasma

■ Trichotillomania (Figs. 5A and B)

- Self-induced twirling, pulling, and/or breaking of hair.
- May be related to a psychological disorder or stress.
- Plucking of scalp hair results in patchy >> diffuse alopecia, sometimes in a wavelike pattern or centrifugally, hairs tend to be different lengths.

Treatment
Counseling and treat underlying psychiatric illness.

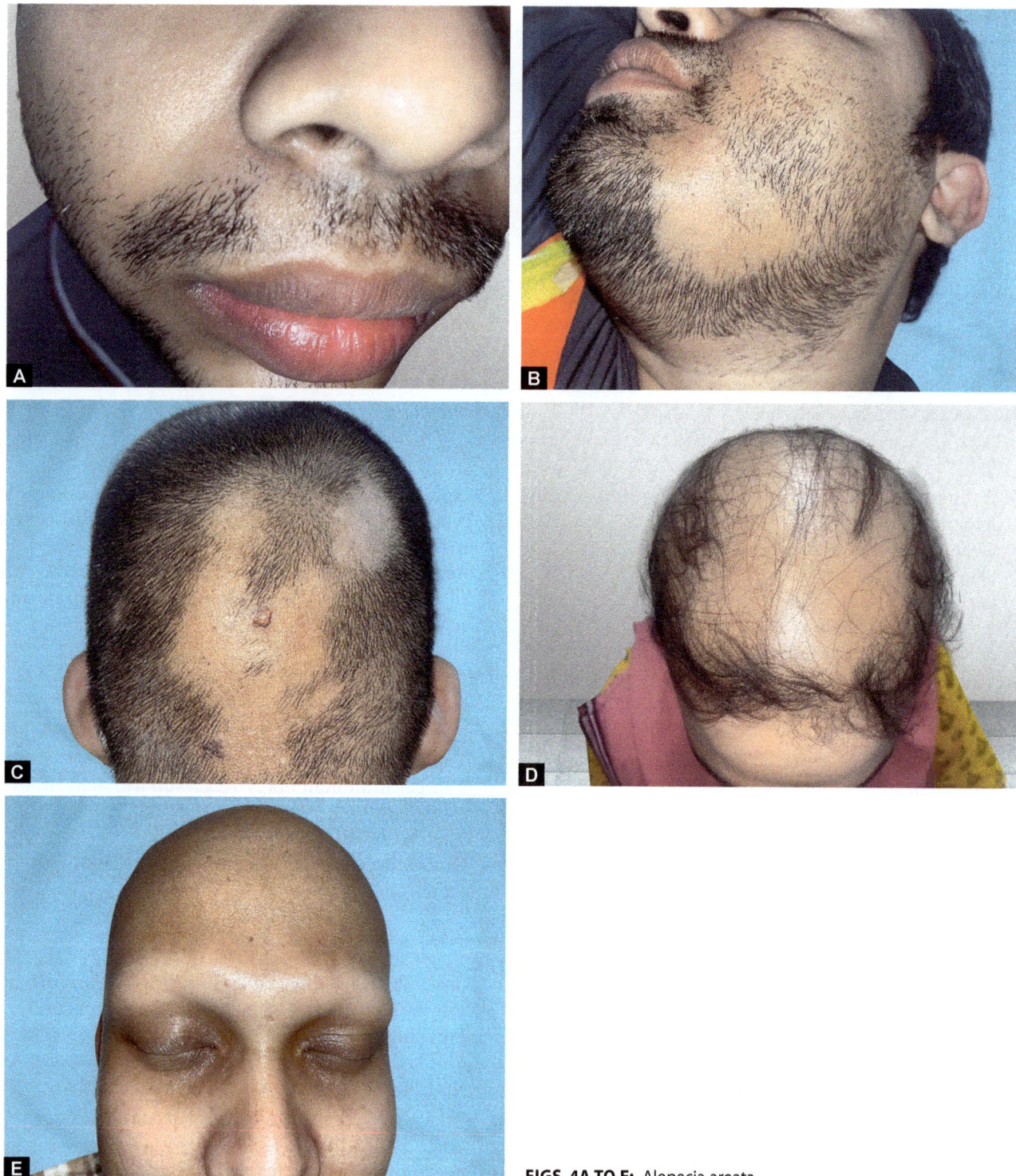

FIGS. 4A TO E: Alopecia areata.

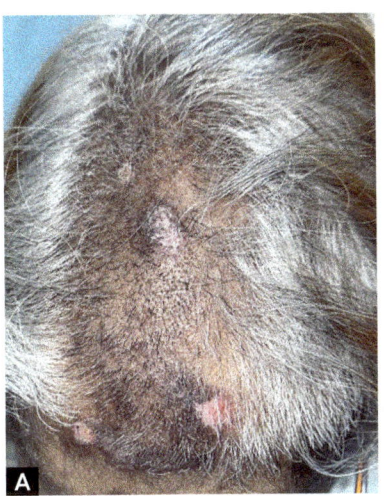 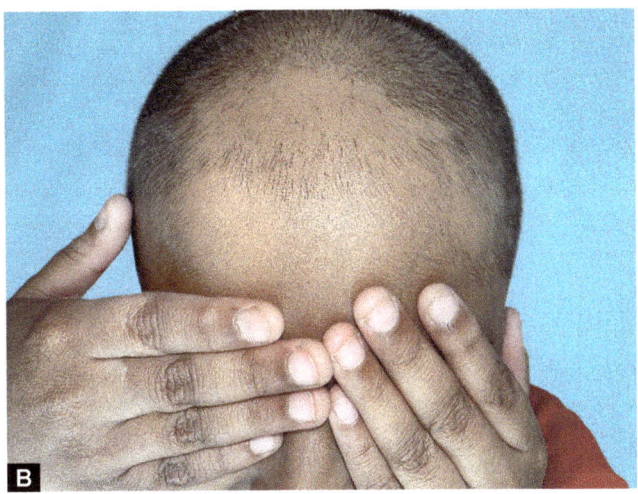

FIGS. 5A AND B: Trichotillomania.

Drug-induced Alopecia (Fig. 6)

- Chemotherapeutic agents (e.g., cyclophosphamide, doxorubicin, paclitaxel, and etoposide) are common causes of anagen effluvium.
- Anagen effluvium can also be secondary to exposure to metals, e.g., arsenic and gold.
- Telogen effluvium can be drug-induced.

Scarring (Cicatricial) Alopecia

Classically defined as loss of hair follicles with scarring (e.g., lupus erythematosus, lichen planopilaris) or an alopecia in which hair does not grow back (e.g., chronic and long-standing traction alopecia) **(Figs. 7A to J)**.

In secondary scarring alopecia, the hair is destroyed nonspecifically, i.e., secondary to burns, radiations dermatitis, cutaneous malignancy, morphea, sarcoidosis, necrobiosis lipoidica, kerion, hypertrophic or atrophic scar, and cicatricial pemphigoid.

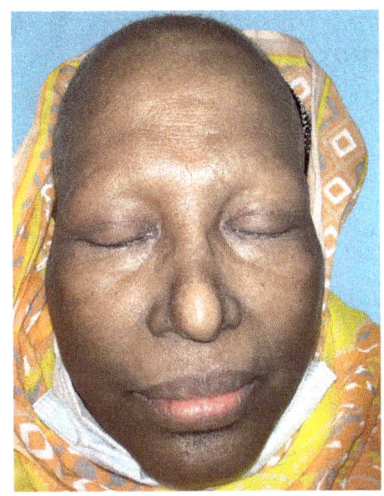

FIG. 6: Drug-induced alopecia.

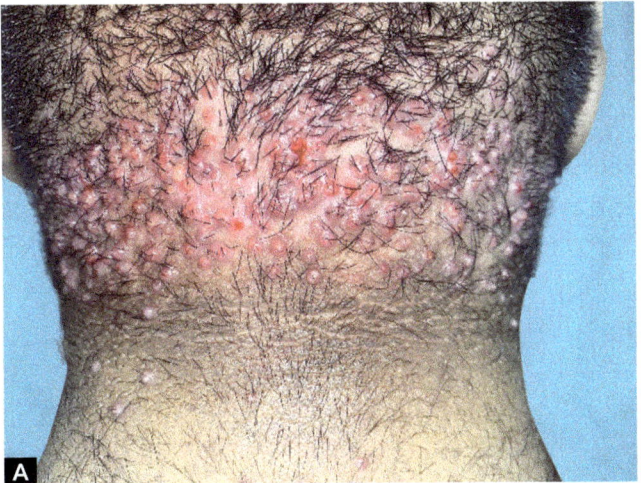 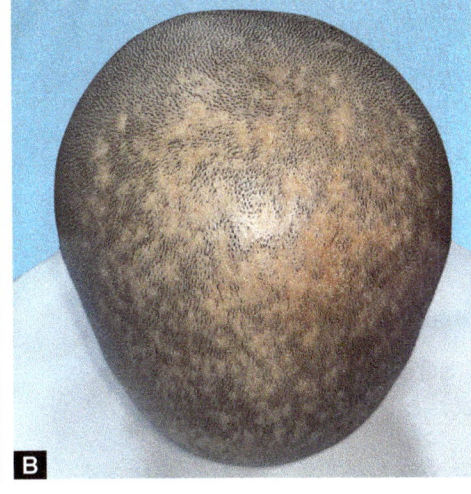

FIGS. 7A TO J: *Continued*

Continued

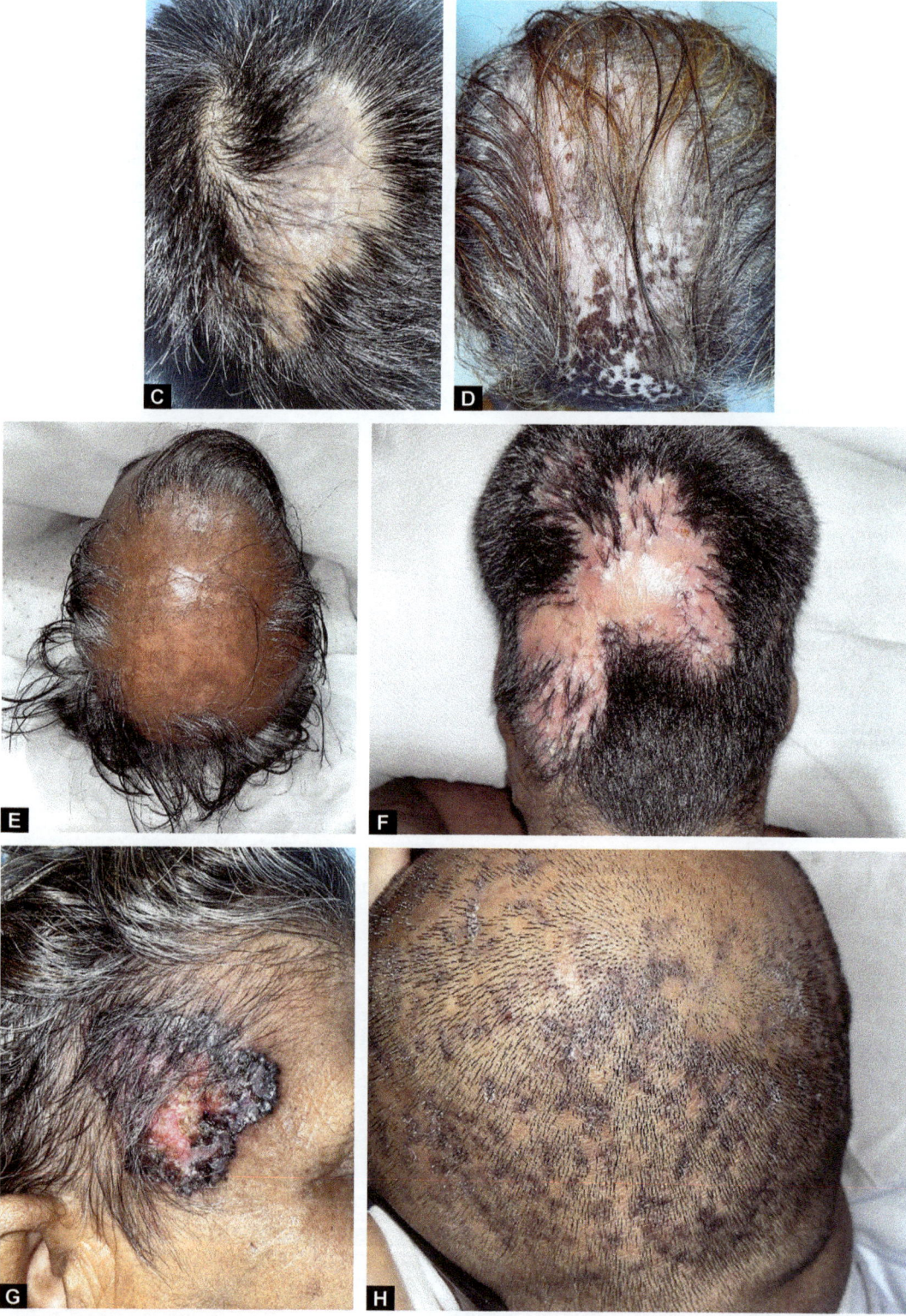

FIGS. 7A TO J: *Continued*

Continued

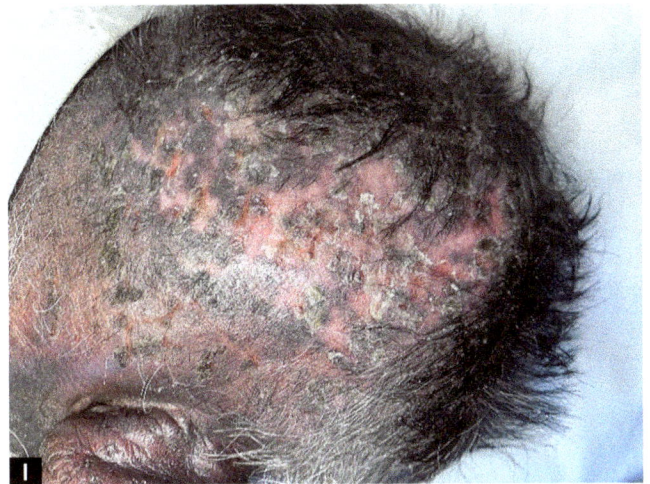
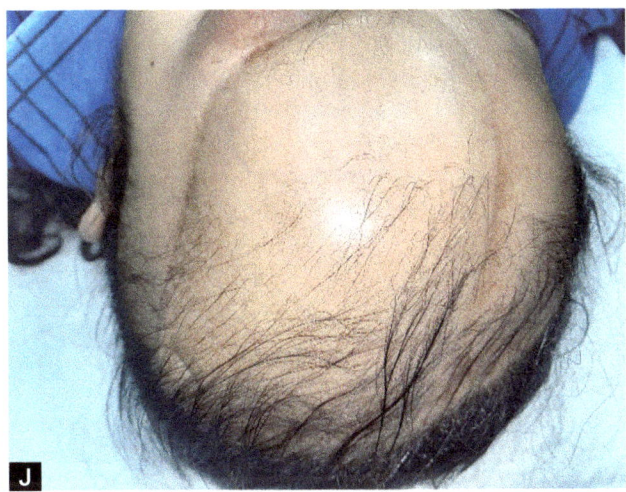

FIGS. 7A TO J: Scarring (Cicatricial) Alopecia.

HYPERTRICHOSIS AND HIRSUTISM

Hypertrichosis

- Excessive hair growth on any area of body.
- Can be classified based on the distribution—generalized versus localized
  - Age of onset: Congenital versus acquired
  - Type of hair: Lanugo versus vellus versus terminal
- Three mechanisms of hypertrichosis are recognized:
  i. Conversion of vellus to terminal hair (due to chronic rubbing or scratching)
  ii. Changes of hair growth cycle (e.g., Intranasal and ears hairs grow in older males due to prolongation of anagen phase.
  iii. Increase in hair follicle density beyond normal for a given site (e.g., Congenital melanocytic nevus)

Hirsutism

Affects 5-10% of females of reproductive age, can also affect postmenopausal women.

Due to hyperandrogenism (exogenous or endogenous) or increased sensitivity of the hair follicle to normal androgen levels is the most commonly used clinical criteria of androgen excess.

The modified Ferriman–Gallwey (mFG) hirsutism scoring system—nine sites of assessment **(Fig. 8)**:
- *Score 0*: No hair to score 4 frankly virile
- For Asian women total score ≥6 define hirsutism.

Etiologies of hyperandrogenism and hirsutism in premenopausal women includes **(Fig. 9)**:
- Polycystic ovary syndrome (PCOS), idiopathic
- Less commonly nonclassic congenital adrenal hyperplasia, tumoral

- Must exclude—pregnancy, drugs-androgens, anabolic steroids, and valproic acids
- Etiology of postmenopausal women (new onset) is most likely ovarian hypertrichosis or tumoral hirsutism.

Polycystic Ovary Syndrome

Diagnosed by the presence of ≥2 of the following criteria and exclusion of other possible etiology:
- Oligo or anovulation (<8 menses/year or cycle >35 days)
- Clinical and/or biochemical signs of hyperandrogenism:
  - Central obesity
  - Acanthosis nigricans
  - Signs of virilization (excess body or facial hair, baldness, acne, increased muscularity and an increase sex drive)
  - Infertility
  - Galactorrhea
- Early morning plasma total testosterone (best 4-10th day of a menstrual cycle):
  - If normal total testosterone—check free testosterone
    - Normal free testosterone: Idiopathic hirsutism
    - Free testosterone elevated: Hyperandrogenemia
  - Increased total testosterone—Hyperandrogenemia
  - Total testosterone > 200 ng/dL—Tumoral hirsutism
- *Polycystic ovaries*:
  - Luteinizing hormone (LH): Follicle stimulating hormone (FSH) ratio is >3 in 90% of cases.
- Occurs only during the reproductive years, and although the majority of patients are obese, some are normal weight.

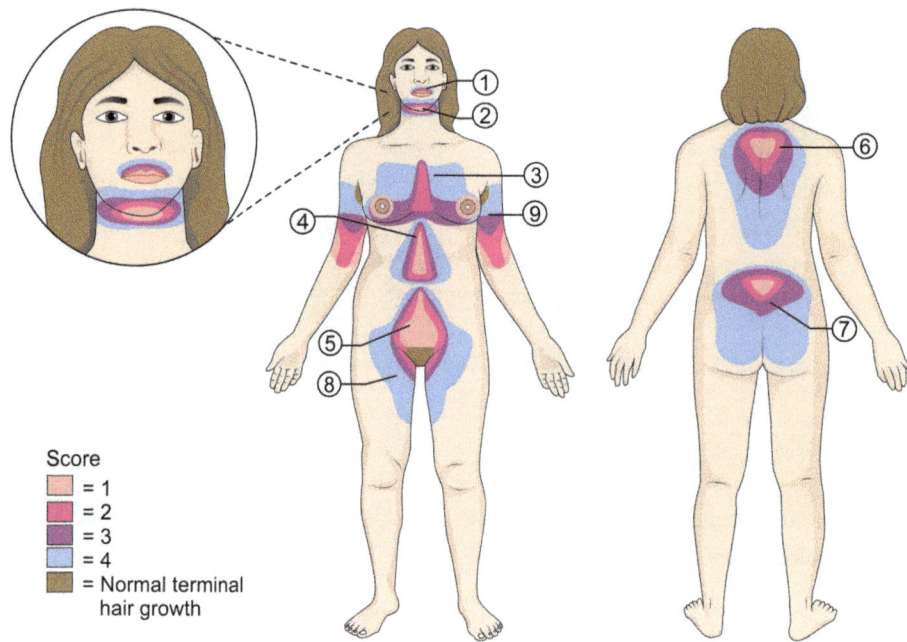

FIG. 8: Modified Ferriman–Gallwey (mFG) hirsutism scoring system—nine sites of assessment.

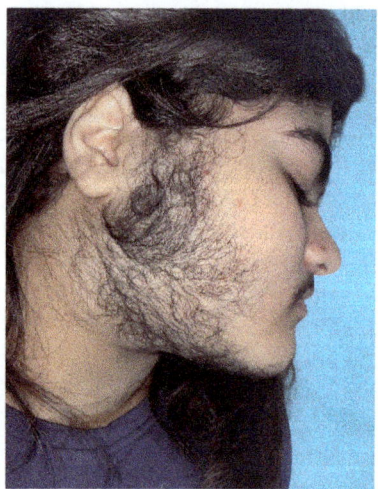

FIG. 9: Hirsutism in premenopausal women.

- Others associated findings may include insulin resistance, infertility, obstructive sleep apnea, endometrial carcinoma, and anxiety.

Treatment Options for Hypertrichosis and Unwanted Hairs

- Camouflage—make-up, lightening of hair color with commercial bleach or 6–12% hydrogen peroxide.
- Hair removal:
  - *Depilation*—Chemical-barium sulfate cream, calcium thioglycolate cream
  - *Mechanical*—Hair trimming and shaving
  - *Epilation:* Lasers—neodymium-doped yttrium aluminum garnet (Nd:YAG), diode, alexandrite, IPL, and CPL
    - Electrolysis
    - Thermolysis
    - Waxing/Threading
- Retardation of hair growth—Eflornithine hydrochloride cream

Treatment of Hirsutism and Hyperandrogenism

Systemic Agents

Oral contraceptive pills (OCPs): All OCPs appear to be equally effective for treating hirsutism.

If relatively higher risk for venous thromboembolism (e.g., obesity or age >39 years), then choose an OCP with lowest effective dose of ethinyl estradiol 20 µg and a low-risk progestin (e.g., norethindrone, levonorgestrel, and norgestimate)

Antiandrogens

- Spironolactone 100–200 mg/day
- Cyproterone acetate (CPA); given on days 5–15 of menstrual cycle
- Finasteride > flutamide; not recommended because of potential hepatotoxicity.
- *Insulin-lowering agents* (e.g., metformin: improves metabolic syndrome and reproductive function but not hirsutism as a single agent.)

NAIL DISORDERS

Nail Unit Anatomy (Figs. 10A and B)

The nail matrix has two components, proximal and distal. The nail matrix forms the underside of nail plate, therefore, biopsies of the distal matrix are less likely to produce a deformity of the surface of the nail plate.

- Fingernails grow 1-3 mm per month and are replaced every 6 months.
- Toenails grow 0.5-1 mm per month and are replaced every 12 months.

Ingrowing Nail (Figs. 11A to D)

- Painful inflammation of lateral nailfold with growth of granulation tissue.
- Due to ill defect nail trimming
- Due to horizontal over curvature of the nail plate with aging
- Most commonly involves the great toes
- Overgrowth of granulation tissue

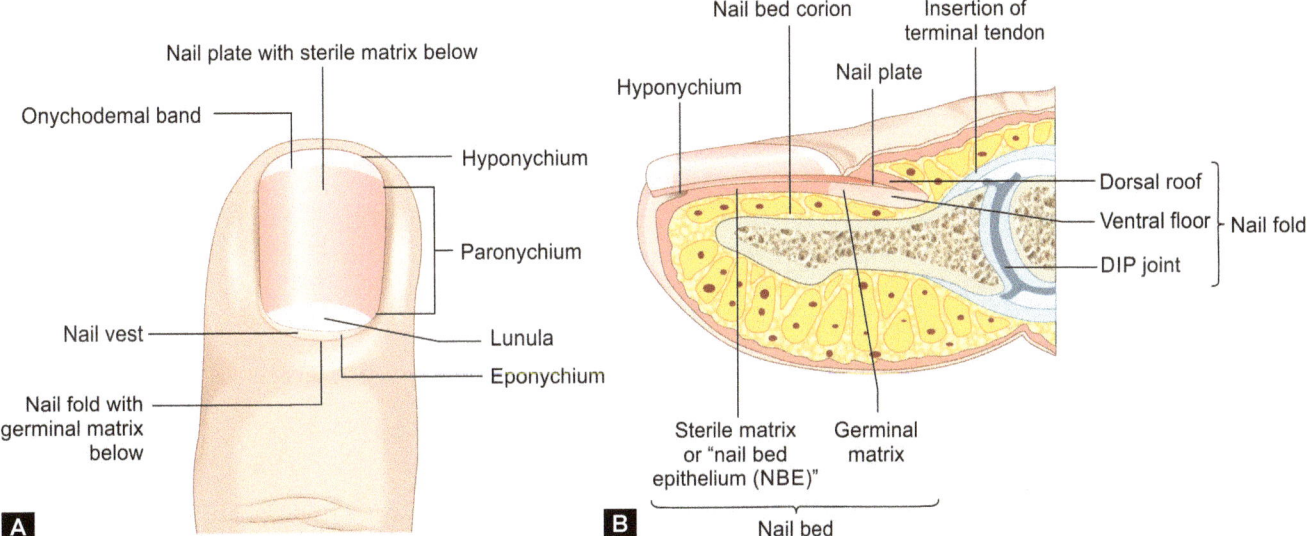

FIGS. 10A AND B: Nail anatomy.

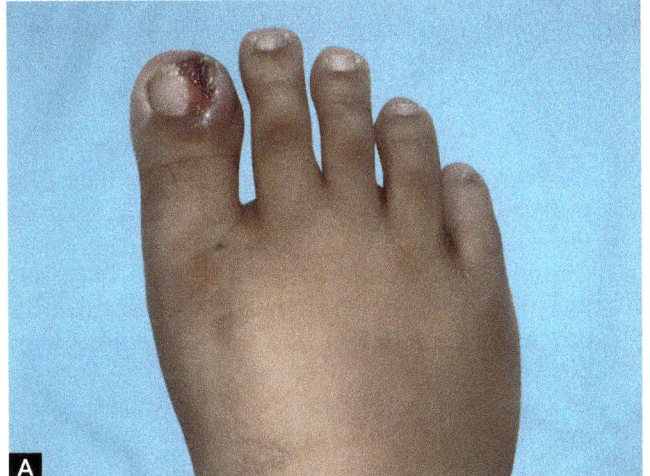
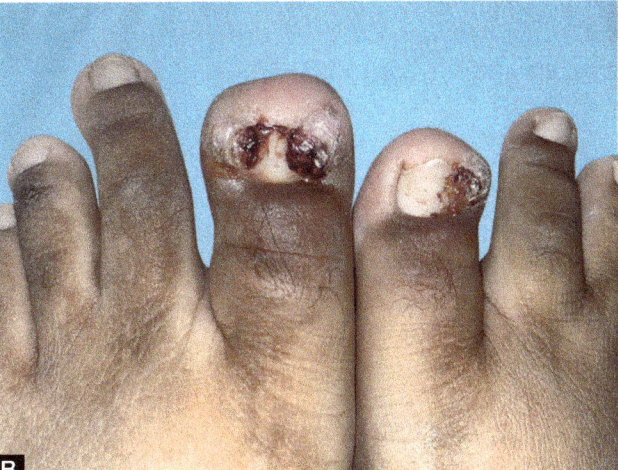

FIGS. 11A TO D: *Continued*

Continued

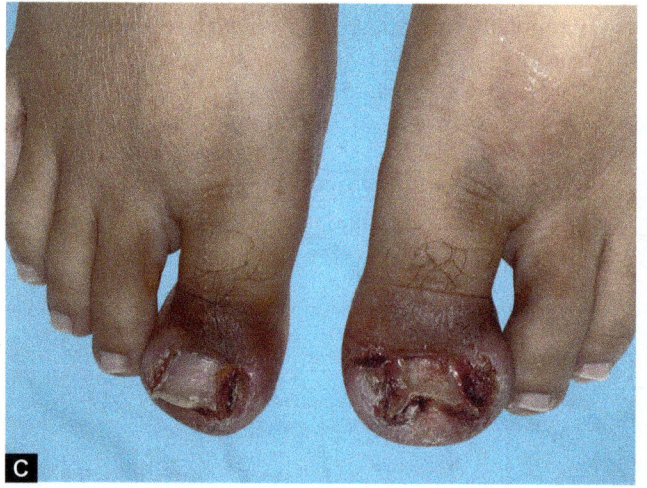
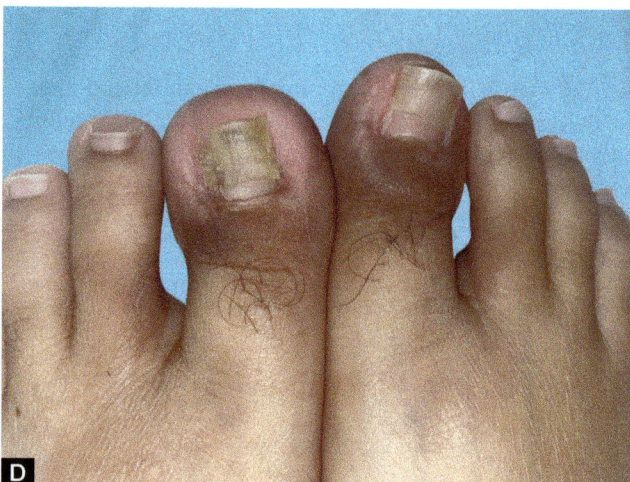

FIGS. 11A TO D: Ingrowing nail.

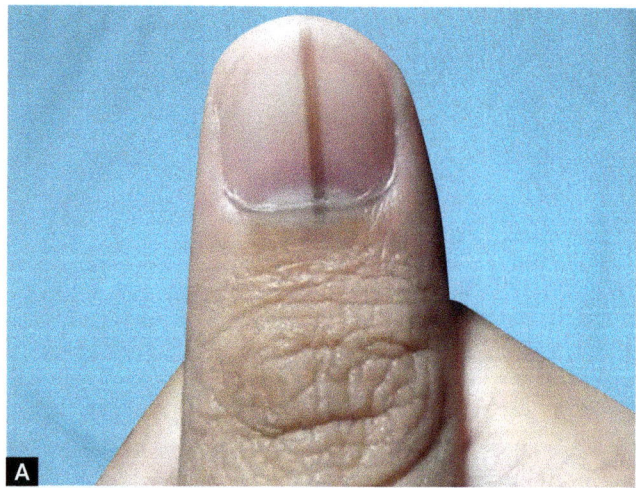
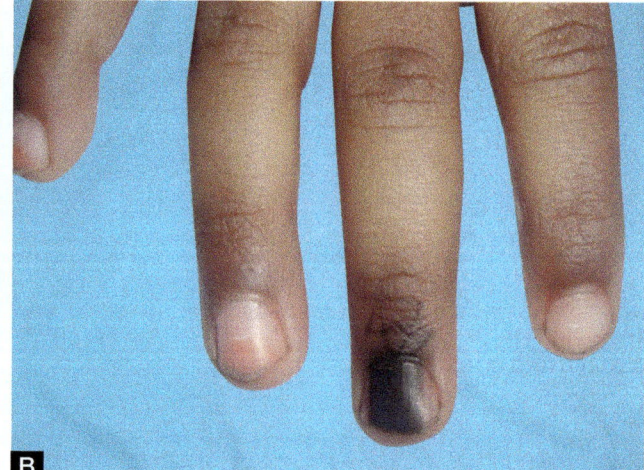

FIGS. 12A AND B: Longitudinal melanonychia.

Longitudinal Melanonychia (Figs. 12A and B)

- Longitudinal brown to black band.
- Multiple bands common in darker skin type; also, it can be due to trauma.
- Single band may be sign of nail melanoma.

Onycholysis (Figs. 13A and B)

- Distal nail plate detachment, causing nail look white to yellow-white.
- Exogenous pigments beneath the nail plate (e.g., pyocyanin from *Pseudomonas*) may cause yellow to green black coloration.
- Chronic exposure to water and irritants (e.g., soap and detergents) is a common cause of fingernail onycholysis whereas onycholysis of the great toe is often due to biomedical forces.
- Associated with psoriasis, onychomycosis, hyperthyroidism, and medications.

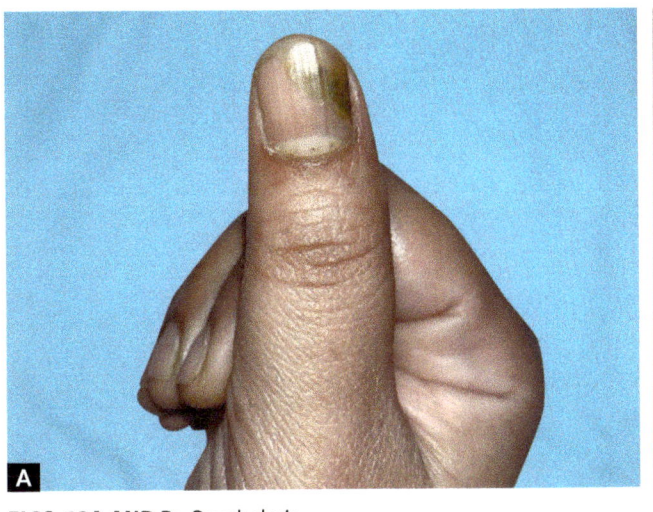
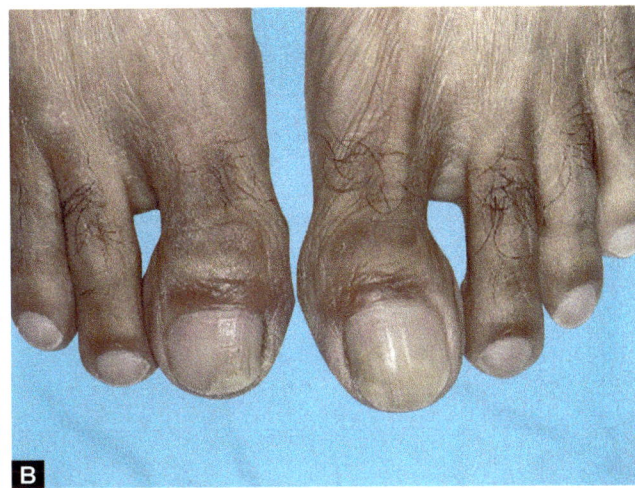

FIGS. 13A AND B: Onycholysis.

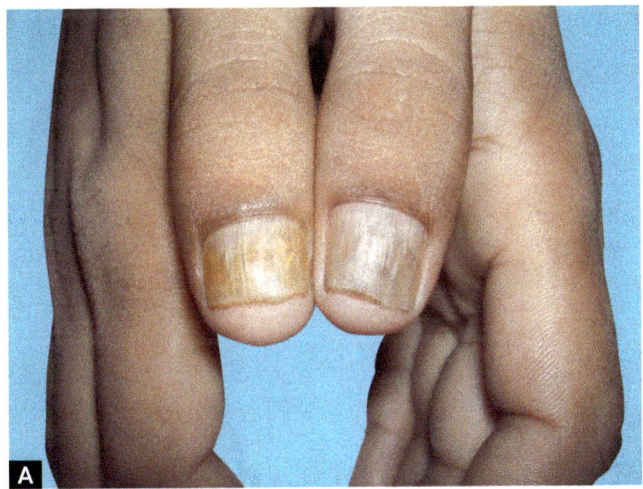
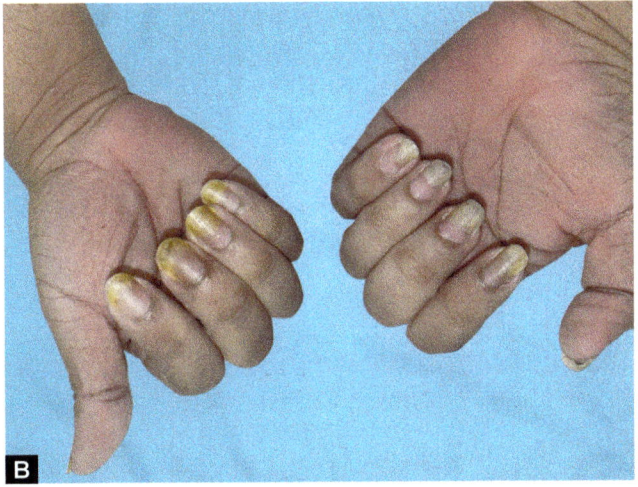

FIGS. 14A AND B: Distal subungual onychomycosis.

■ Onychomycosis

Distal Subungual Onychomycosis
See **Figures 14A and B.**

White Superficial Onychomycosis
See **Figure 15**.

Proximal Subungual Onychomycosis
See **Figure 16**.

Candida Onychomycosis
See **Figure 17**.

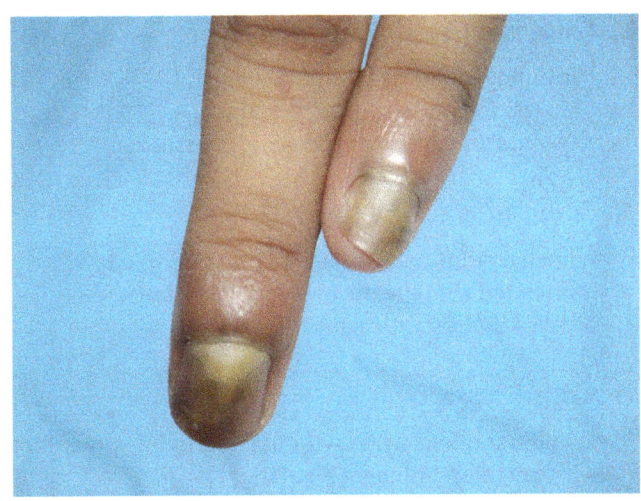

FIG. 15: White superficial onychomycosis.

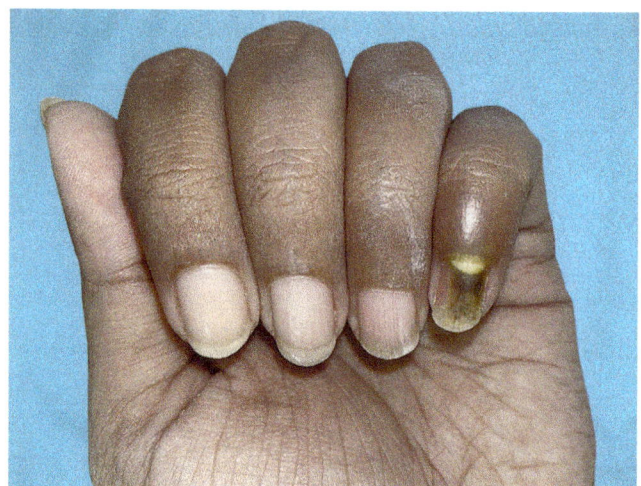

FIG. 16: Proximal subungual onychomycosis.

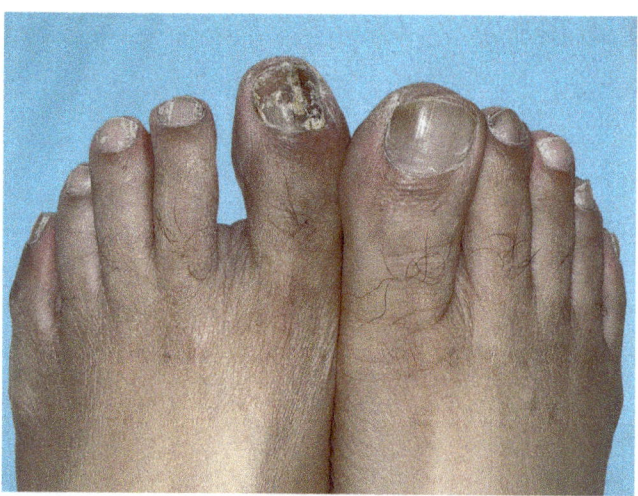

FIG. 17: Condition of nail due to *Candida* onychomycosis.

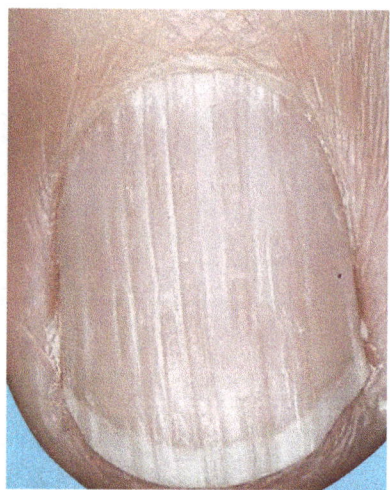

FIG. 18: Condition of nail due to thinning and longitudinal ridging.

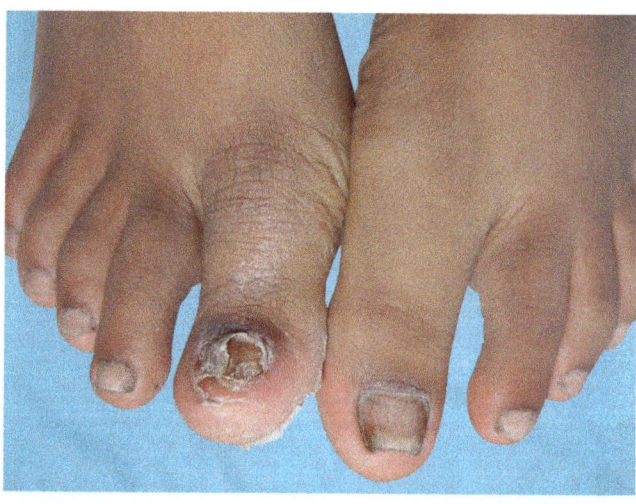

FIG. 19: Lamellar splitting of distal nail into multiple layers.

Onychorrhexis (Fig. 18)
- Thinning and longitudinal ridging
- May develop fissuring or notching.
- Trauma and aging are two major causes.

Onychoschizia (Fig. 19)
- Lamellar splitting of distal nail into multiple layers.
- Associated with the use of soap and irritants.
- Normal finding with aging.

Acute Paronychia
- Swollen nailfold with erythema and pain, sometimes with pustular drainage **(Fig. 20)**.
- Caused usually by *Staphylococci*.

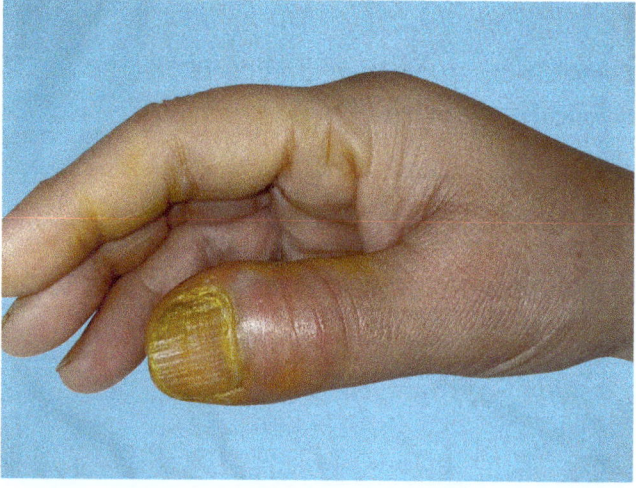

FIG. 20: Swollen nailfold with erythema and pain.

Chronic Paronychia

- Chronic proximal nailfold inflammation with loss of cuticle **(Figs. 21A and B)**.
- Exacerbation by exposure to water and irritants or overaggressive nail grooming.

Subungual Hematoma

- Purple-red to black color beneath nail plate due to hemorrhage **(Fig. 22)**.
- Secondary to trauma.

True Leukonychia

White discoloration of nail that persists when pressure is applied **(Fig. 23)**.

Beau's Lines (Fig. 24)

- Transverse depression of nail plate.
- Often secondary to trauma, especially when limited to a single digit.
- Consider systemic insult (e.g., high fever, chemotherapy) if multiple nails involved.

Dorsal Pterygium

- Triangular extension of proximal nailfold into the nail bed.
- Loss of nail plate **(Fig. 25)**
- Most commonly associated with lichen planus.

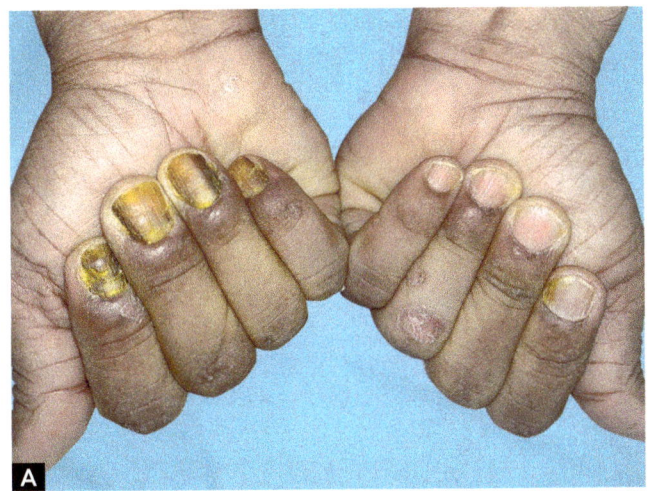
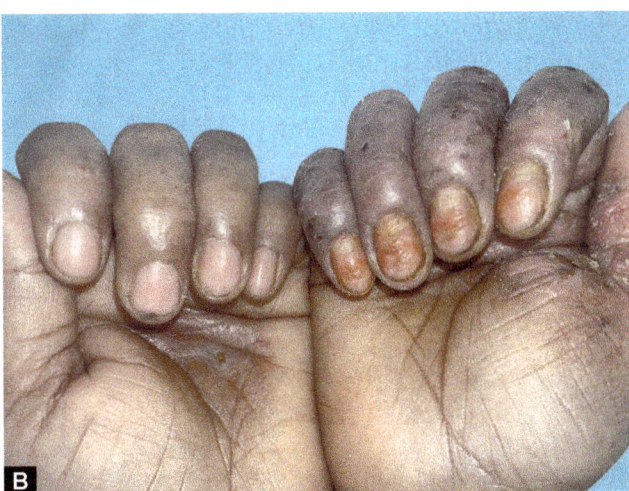

FIGS. 21 A AND B: Chronic proximal nailfold inflammation with loss of cuticle.

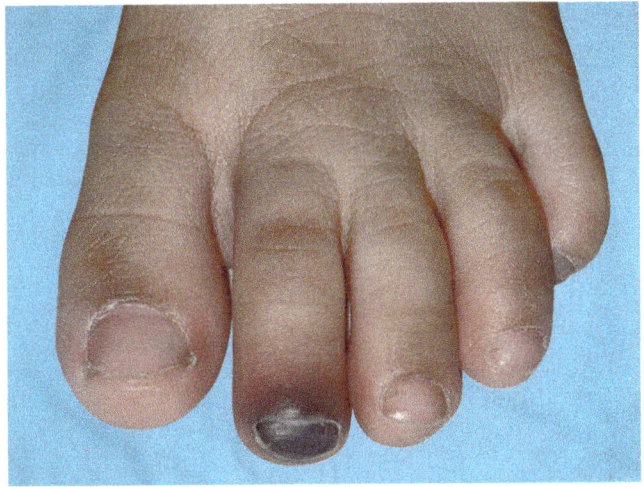

FIG. 22: Purple-red to black color beneath nail plate due to hemorrhage.

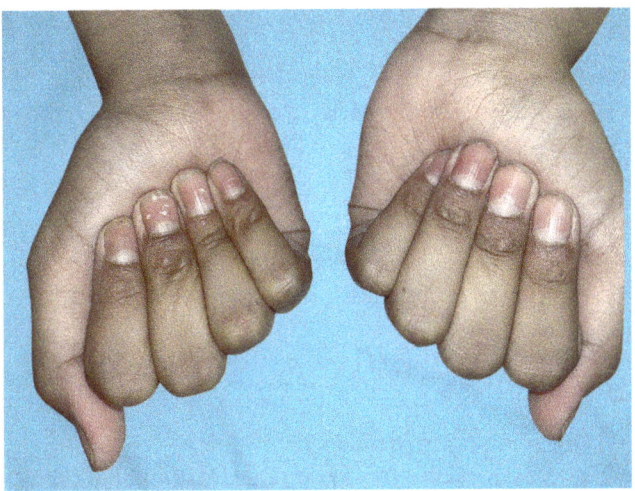

FIG. 23: White discoloration of nail.

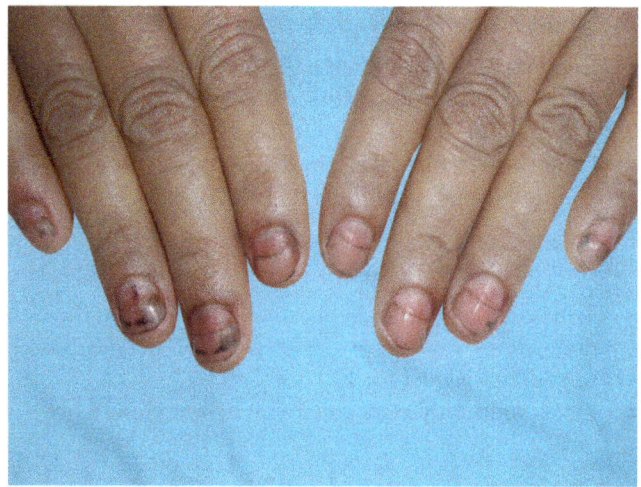

FIG. 24: Beau's lines—transverse depression of nail plate.

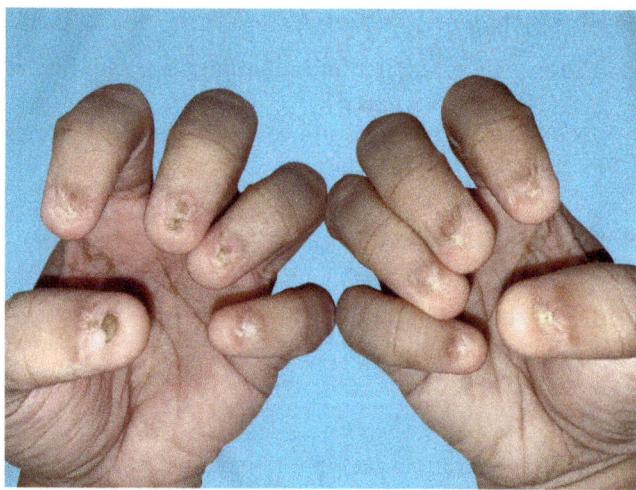

FIG. 25: Loss of nail plate—dorsal pterygium.

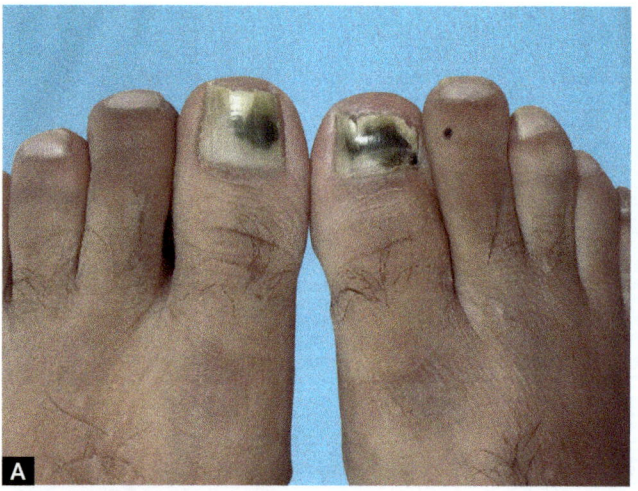

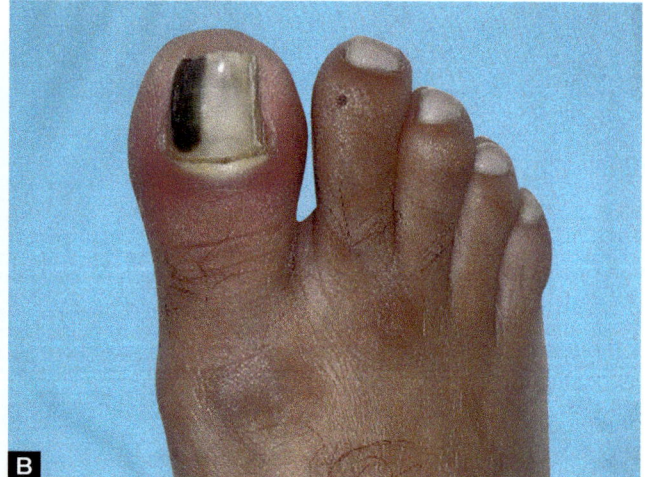

FIGS. 26A AND B: Blue-green to green-black discoloration.

■ Green Nail

Blue-green to green-black discoloration secondary to pyocyanin produced by *Pseudomonas aeruginosa* (Figs. 26A and B).

■ Alopecia Areata (Fig. 27)

- Pitting in nail plate (punctate depression in nail plane).
- Compared to psoriasis, pits, and smaller and more numerous.

■ Dariers Disease (Fig. 28)

- Digital fissuring (notches)
- Alternating longitudinal red and white streaks (i.e., longitudinal erythronychia and leukonychia)

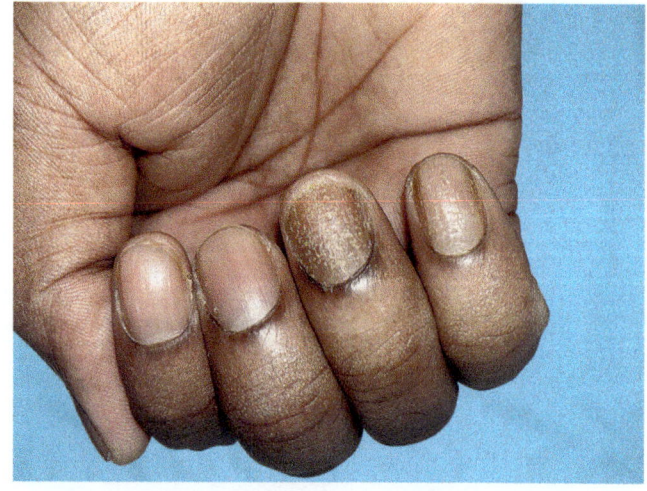

FIG. 27: Alopecia areata—pitting in nail plate.

Psoriasis (Figs. 29A and B)

- Pitting, punctate depressions in the nail plate, irregular in size and distribution.
- Yellow-orange discoloration of nail plate due to oil spot changes.
- Additional changes include yellowing, thickening, onycholysis, subungual debris, splinter hemorrhages, paronychia, and rarely pustules.

Pustular Psoriasis (Fig. 30)
- Pustules can form under the nail plate.
- Psoriatic lesions may be found on the tip of the digit.

Yellow Nail Syndrome (Fig. 31)

- Yellow coloration of all or most of fingernails > toenails.
- Associated with lymphedema and bronchopulmonary disease.

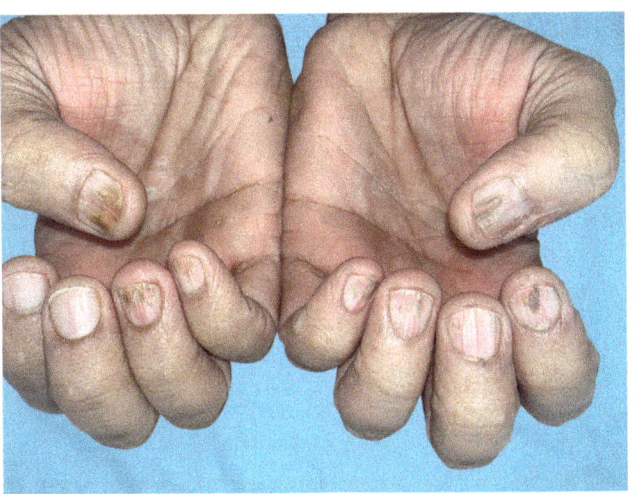

FIG. 28: Dariers disease.

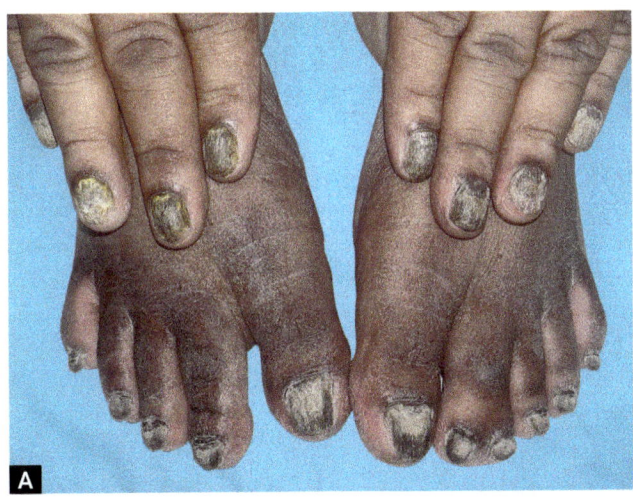
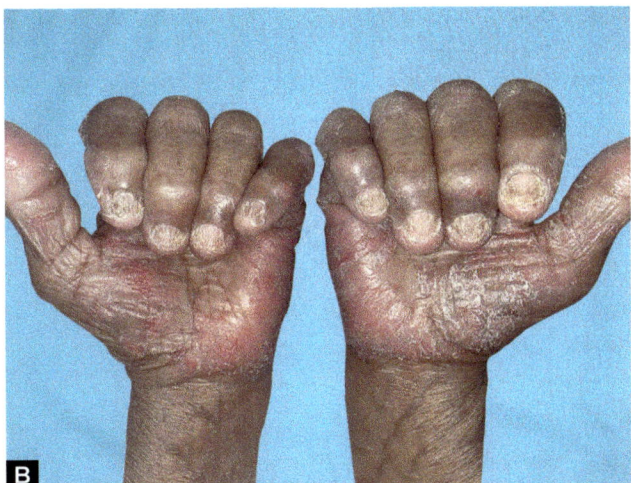

FIGS. 29A AND B: Psoriasis: Pitting, punctate depressions in the nail plate, irregular in size and distribution.

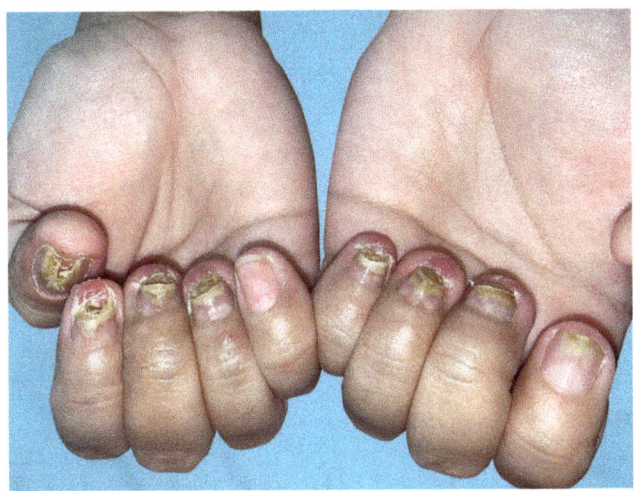

FIG. 30: Pustular psoriasis.

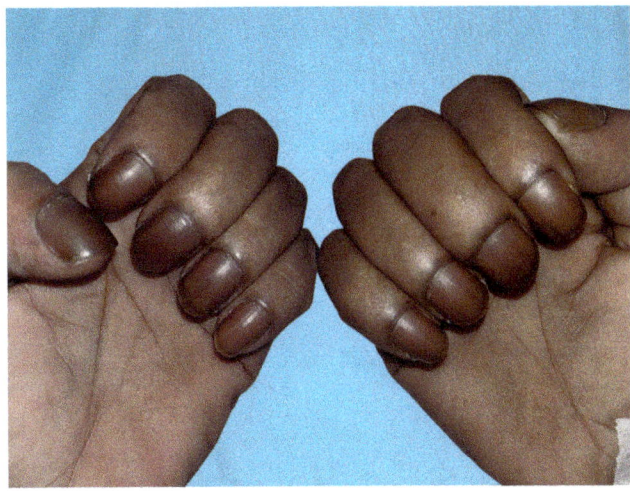

FIG. 31: Yellow nail syndrome.

Periungual Fibroma
See **Figure 32**.

Myxoid Cyst
See **Figure 33**.

Glomus Tumor
See **Figure 34**.

Periungual Pyogenic Granuloma
See **Figure 35**.

MUCOSAL DISEASES

- Oral manifestations of infectious diseases are covered in Chapter 12.
- Common oral mucosal findings

Fordyce Granules

- Free sebaceous gland (i.e., not associated with hair follicle)
- Evidence in as many as 75% of adults

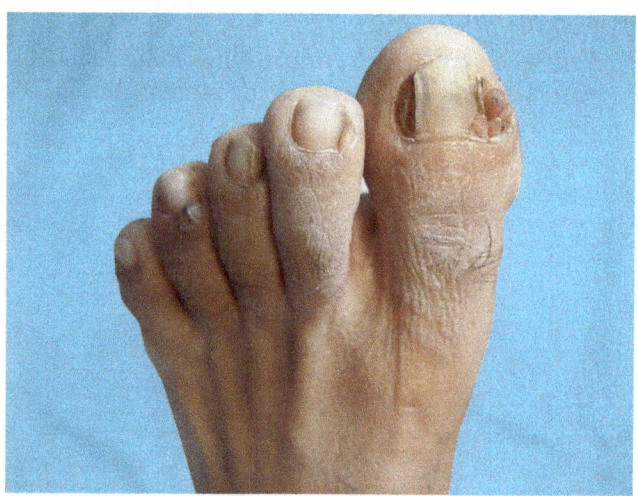

FIG. 32: Periungual fibroma.

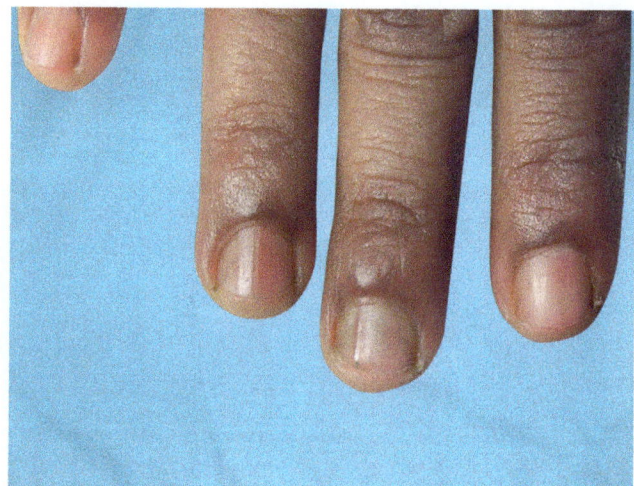

FIG. 33: Myxoid cyst.

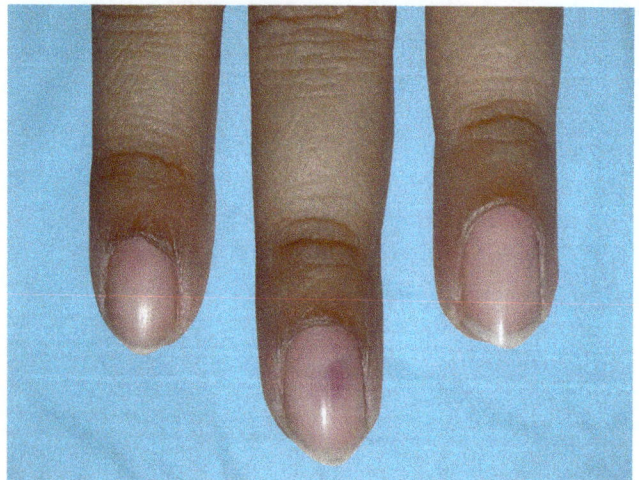

FIG. 34: Glomus tumor.

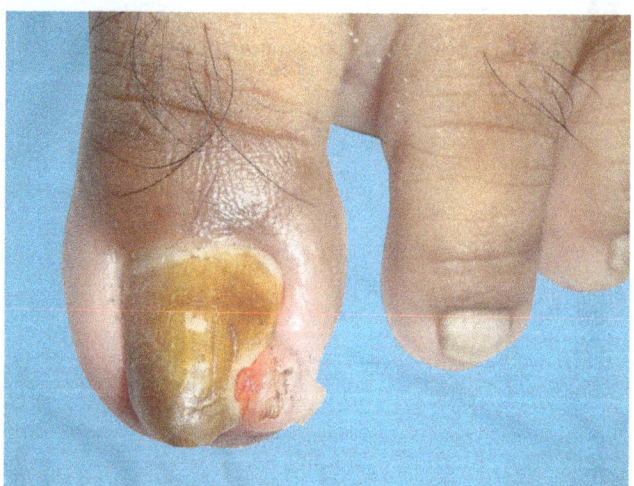

FIG. 35: Periungual pyogenic granuloma.

Geographic Tongue

Well-demarcated areas of erythema and atrophy of the filiform papillae, surrounded by a whitish, hyperkeratotic serpiginous border, lesions tend to migrate over time, may affect other oral sites and are occasionally associated with a burning sensation **(Fig. 36)**.

Scrotal Tongue (Fig. 37)

Multiple grooves or furrows are present on dorsal tongue.

Mucocele

Translucent to bluish papule due to disruption of minor salivary duct **(Fig. 38)**.

Aphthae (Figs. 39 to 42)

Common condition characterized by recurrent oral ulcers, with peak prevalence during second and third decade of life; outbreaks may be triggered by trauma, psychological stress or hormonal fluctuations.

Minor Aphthae

It is the most frequent form. Painful, round to oval, shallow ulcers that are usually <5 mm in diameter characterized by yellow-white to gray pseudomembranous base, well-defined border and prominent erythematous rim; favor buccal or labial mucosa and typically heal in 1-2 weeks without scarring.

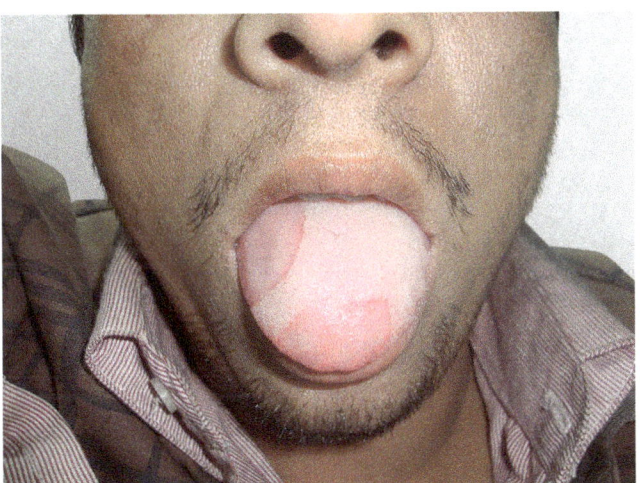

FIG. 36: Geographic tongue.

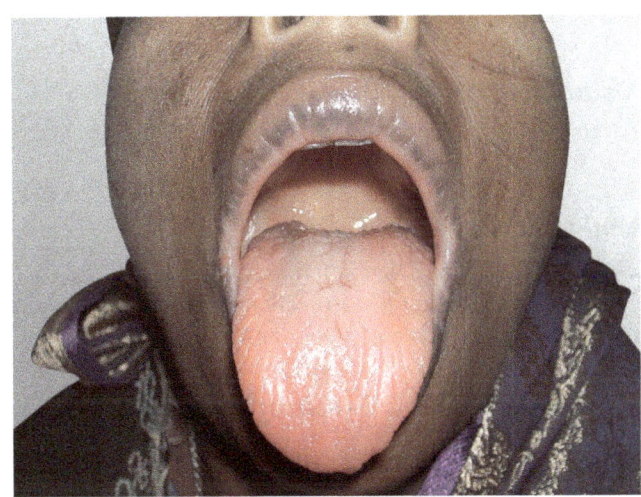

FIG. 37: Scrotal tongue.

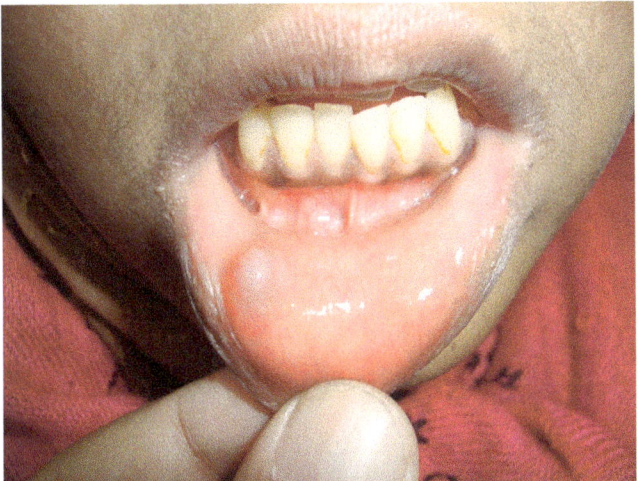

FIG. 38: Translucent to bluish papule due to disruption of minor salivary duct.

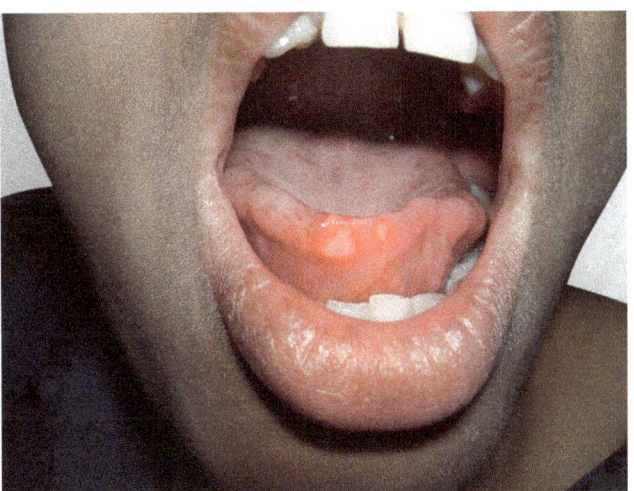

FIG. 39: Minor aphthae.

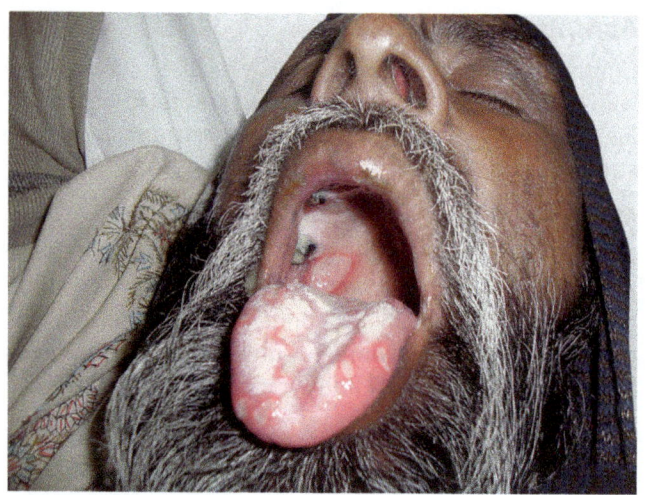

FIG. 40: Major aphthae.

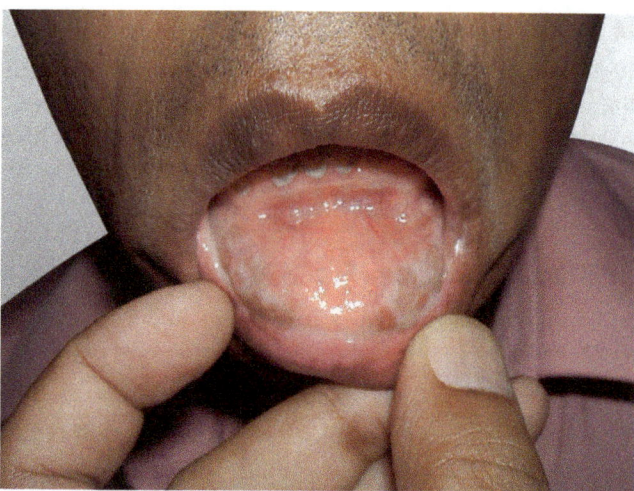

FIG. 41: White patch or plaque on oral mucosa.

Major Aphthae (Fig. 40)
Larger (>1 cm), deeper ulcer that persists for up to 6 weeks; may heal with scarring.

Leukoplakia (Fig. 41)
White patch or plaque on oral mucosa.

Fractional erbium laser excellent outcome; symptom free and for prevention of malignancy.

■ Squamous Cell Carcinoma (Fig. 42)
It is the most common malignancy of oral cavity.

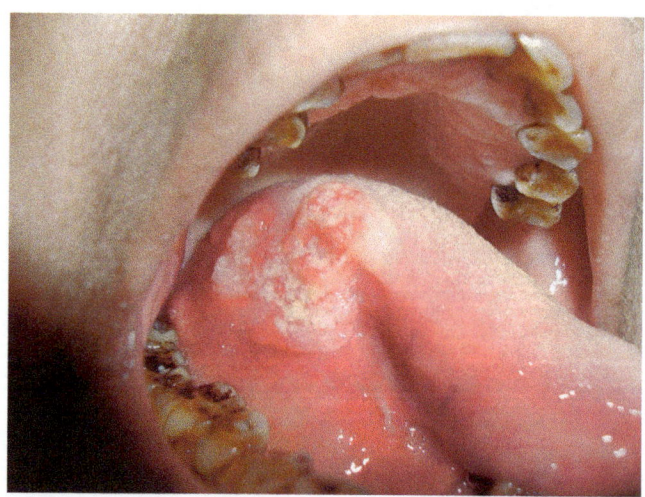

FIG. 42: Squamous cell carcinoma.

Index

Page numbers followed by *f* refer to figure.

A

Abdomen 69*f*
Abscess 100, 101*f*
 prostatic 112
 staphylococcus 101*f*
 sterile 101*f*
Acantholysis 96
Acanthosis nigricans 72, 72*f*, 203
Acitretin 19, 198
Acne 5*f*
 complications of 192*f*
 conglobata 191
 inflammatory 191
 keloidalis 194, 194*f*
 mild 192
 nodulocystic 4*f*
 noninflammatory 191
 rosacea 192, 193*f*
 severe nodulocystic 191
 vulgaris 190, 190*f*
Acquired immunodeficiency
  syndrome 84, 108
Acroangiodermatitis 38
Acrochordons 71*f*
Acrodermatitis enteropathica 78
Actinomycosis 159
Acupuncture 12
Acyclovir 124, 128
Adalimumab 20
Adapalene 192
Addison's disease 72, 77, 77*f*
Adenosine triphosphate 63
Adenovirus 55
Alanine aminotransferase 191
Alcohol 11
Allergens 41
Allergic contact dermatitis 35, 38, 41,
  46, 47
Allopurinol 55
Alopecia
 areata 95, 198, 199, 200*f*, 210, 210*f*
 drug-induced 201, 201*f*
Alström syndrome 70
American Rheumatism Association
  Criteria 176
Aminolevulinic acid plus photodynamic
  therapy 65

Amitriptyline 12
Amyloidosis 80
 localized cutaneous 80
 macular 80*f*
 secondary 195
Ancylostoma braziliense 137
Androgenic alopecia 198, 198*f*
Anemia 195
 severe 21
Anetoderma 171
Angioedema 52, 53*f*
 hereditary 54
Angiofibromata, facial 90
Angioid streaks 91
Angiotensin-converting enzyme
  inhibitors 28
Angular cheilitis 157
Anorectum 111
Anthralin 19
Antiandrogens 204
Antibiotics 196
 oral 87, 96
 topical 87, 96, 192
Anticoagulants 198
 use 7
Anticonvulsants 198
 antipruritic 12
Antidepressants 198
 tricyclic 12, 54
Antifungal
 oral 157
 systemic 146
Antigen detection 128
Antihistamine 12, 35, 54
 long-acting nonsedative 53
 nonsedative 12
 oral 11
Anti-inflammatory agents
 systemic 35
 topical 35
Antimalarials 28
 drugs 13
Antinuclear antibody 53, 167, 173, 176
Antioxidant 92
Antiphospholipid antibody syndrome,
  cutaneous signs of 171
Anti-tumor necrosis factor-alpha
  agents 185

Anus 111
Anxiety 13
Aphthae 213
 major 214, 214*f*
 minor 213, 213*f*
Apocrine glands 190
Arsenate inhibits 63
Arsenic poisoning, chronic 63, 64
Arsenicosis, chronic 2*f*, 63
Arthralgias 56
Arthritis 19, 176
 gonococcal 111
 reactive 19
Arthropathy 195
 psoriatic 18, 19*f*
Aspartate aminotransferase 191
Aspirin 11, 53, 54
Asthenia 56
Atenolol 54
Athlete's foot fungus 147
Atopic dermatitis 11, 31, 34, 35, 38
 diagnostic features of 31
 triggers of 31
Atopic eruption 68
Atrophic blanche 171
Atrophic scar 7*f*, 201
Atrophy 7, 113, 126*f*, 192*f*
Auricular nerve 117*f*
Autoimmune disease 163, 199
Autoimmune polyendocrinopathy
  syndrome 199
Autosomal-recessive genetic disorder 78
Axilla 84*f*
Azathioprine 167
Azelaic acid 194
Azithromycin 113
Azole 158

B

Bacillus Calmette-Guérin 132
Bacteria 132
Balanitis 157
Balanoposthitis 157
Bandages, compressive 187
Barbiturates 55, 62
Bardet–Biedl syndrome 70
Bartholin gland abscess 112

Basal cell
  carcinoma 65, 65f, 80, 92
  epithelioma 64
Beau's lines 209, 210f
Becker's nevus 2f
Behçet's disease 188, 189f
Belimumab 176
Benzoyl peroxide 192, 194
Beta-blockers 13, 28
Biopsy 22, 53, 180
Black dot tinea 153
Blaschko lines 18
Blood 173
  count, complete 52
  pressure, high 20
  vessels
    permanent dilatation of cutaneous 10f
    poor dermal support of 7
Body
  mass index 70
  surface area 57
Borrelia burgdorferi 132
Botulinum toxin 106
Bovine serum albumin 20
Bowel disease, inflammatory 187, 199
Bowen's disease 65, 65f
Brain, computed tomography of 109f
Breastfeeding 20
Breasts, eczema of 38
Brugia
  malayi 137
  timori 137
Bullae 4, 43, 44f, 61f, 69f
  diabetic 75, 75f
Bullosa, epidermolysis 161
Bullous disease 161
  autoimmune 168, 169
  chronic 96
Bullous impetigo 98f
Bullous pemphigoid 5f, 168, 168f
Burns 5f, 7f, 8f, 201
  chemical 40
Butenafine 146
Butterfly rash 171

C

Café-au-lait
  macules 89f
  patches 89f
Calcification, dystrophic 81f
Calcineurin inhibitor 19
  topical 12, 40
Calcinosis cutis 81
Calciphylaxis 73, 73f
Calcipotriene 19
Calcitriol 19
Camphor 12

Cancer 20
Candida 53
  albicans 88, 102, 154
  leukoplakia 157
  onychomycosis 207, 208f
Candidiasis 75f, 154, 156f
  chronic mucocutaneous 88, 88f
  control chronic mucocutaneous 88
  cutaneous 154
  follicular 155
  genital 157, 158f
  pseudomembranous 155
Cantharidin 132
Carbamazepine 198
Carbon dioxide 92, 132
Carbuncles 73f, 100
Carcinoma, terminal 108
Cellulitis 38, 74f, 103, 104f
  staphylococcal 101f
Central nervous system 90, 125, 180
Cerebellar ataxia 124
Cervix 111
Cetirizine 53, 54, 67
Chancre 109, 143f
Chancroid 109, 110f
Cheilitis 40
Chemosis 111
Chemotherapy 62, 209
Chickenpox 122
Chikungunya 133, 134f
Chilblain lupus 171
Chills 103, 108
Chlamydia 55
Chlamydophila 55
Chloroquine 54, 176
Cholestasis, intrahepatic 11
Cholesterol, high 20
Cicatricial alopecia 201, 203f
Cicatricial pemphigoid 201
Ciclopirox 35, 146
Cidofovir, topical 132
Cimetidine, oral 132
Ciprofloxacin 61f, 62
Cirrhosis 94
  primary biliary 95
Cleavage, Langer's lines of 21, 21f
Clindamycin 192, 194
Clobetasol propionate 19
Clofazimine 120
Clotrimazole 106, 146
Codeine 11, 48f, 53
Colchicine 54
Cold hemolysins 53
Colitis, ulcerative 187
Concomitant immunosuppressive therapy 167
Condyloma accuminata 132
Condylomata lata 144f
Conjunctiva 122

Conjunctivitis 19, 57, 59, 63, 111, 120
Connective tissue
  disease, autoimmune 11, 81
  hereditary disorder of 91
Contact dermatitis 38, 63
  irritant 11, 35, 40, 40f
Contraceptive pill 198
  oral 62, 204
Coronal sulcus 25f
Coronavirus disease 2019 (COVID-19) 135, 136f
Corticosteroids 18
  low-potency topical 12
  mild topical 38
  oral 199
  systemic 13, 40, 176, 187
  topical 19, 40, 87
Corynebacterium minutissimum 105
Coryza 120
Cough 120
Coxsackievirus 122, 132
C-reactive protein 187
Crohn's disease 187
  metastatic 94
Crusts 4, 122
Cryofibrinogen 53
Cryoglobulin 53
Cryosurgery 132
Cryotherapy 132
Cushing disease 70, 72
Cushing syndrome 70, 76
Cutaneous leishmaniasis
  new world 135
  old world 135
Cyclophosphamide 167, 185, 201
Cyclosporine 19, 20, 168, 185
Cyproterone acetate 204
Cystic acne 101f, 190, 192f
Cytomegalovirus 55, 132
Cytopenia 57, 59

D

Danazol 54
Dapsone 54, 120, 168, 170, 176
Dariers disease 86, 210, 211f
Dehydroepiandrosterone sulfate 191
Delusional infestation 51
Dengue 133
  hemorrhagic fever 9f
Dennie–Morgan sign 34, 35f
Deoxyribonucleic acid 92, 128
  anti-double-stranded 173
Dermatitis 31, 36f, 47
  acute 42f
  asteatotic 35
  chronic 42f
  factitious 48
  herpetiformis 169, 169f

periorificial 196, 196f
pruritic 36
seborrheic 11, 35, 41, 105
Dermatofibroma 80
Dermatological diseases 11
Dermatology, rheumatologic 171
Dermatomal vesiculobullous eruption 125f
Dermatomyositis 11, 84, 183, 184f
cutaneous manifestations of 184f
systemic manifestations of 184f
Dermatopathology 35, 146, 187, 188
Dermatophytes 55, 74f, 144
infections 145f
Dermatophytosis 144
Dermatosis 11
neutrophilic 186
pregnancy-induced 67
Dermopathy 76
diabetic 72
Dextran 11
Diabetes mellitus 11, 35, 72, 75, 95, 103
type 1 75
type 2 75
Diaper dermatitis 155, 156f
Digital gangrene 171
Dihydrotestosterone 198
Diphtheria 132
Direct fluorescent antibody 128
Discoid lupus erythematosus 171, 173f, 176
generalized 171
hypertrophic 171
lichenoid 171
mucosal 171
verrucous 171
Distal nail, lamellar splitting of 208f
Dorsal pterygium 209, 210f
Doxepin 12, 53
oral 12
Doxicap 113
Doxorubicin 201
Doxycycline 62, 192, 196
Drug eruption 11
Ducrey's bacillus 109
Dusky macules 57, 59
Dysesthesia 11, 12
Dysphagia 185
Dyspigmentation, chemotherapy induced 62
Dystrophic epidermolysis bullosa 161, 162, 163f

E

Ecchymosis 7, 9f, 10f
Econazole 146
Ecthyma 99, 99f
gangrenosum 106, 107f

Eczema 31
asteatotic 38
chronic 15f, 37f
discoid 38
dyshidrotic 38
microbial 38
nummular 38
xerotic 35
Edema 36, 37f, 41f, 42f, 44f, 98f
Ehlers–Danlos syndrome 82
Ekbom syndrome 51
Electrocardiogram 185
Electrodesiccation 132
Electrolysis 204
Electrosurgery 194
Emollients 83
Encephalitis 124
Encephalomyelitis 120
Endocrine disease 67
Enzyme, dysfunction of 81
Epidermodysplasia verruciformis 132
Epidermolysis bullosa 161
acquisita 94
junctional 161, 162, 162f
simplex 161, 161f, 162f
subtypes 161
Epididymorchitis 112
Epstein–Barr virus 132
Erosion 4, 6f, 46f, 81f
Erysipelas 102, 103f
Erythema 18, 36f, 37f, 42f, 44f, 47f, 171, 208f
acute phase 42f
blanching 9f
dyschromicum 30
infectiosum 122
mild local 103
multiforme 55, 67, 73
major 56, 55
minor 55
nodosum 94, 187f
syndrome 186
violaceous 185, 185f
Erythematotelangiectatic rosacea 194
Erythematous plaques, edematous 122f
Erythrasma 74f, 103, 105, 105f
Erythrocyte sedimentation rate 187
Erythroderma 6f
Erythromycin 109, 192, 194, 196
Esophagus 180
Etanercept 168
Etoposide 201
Eumycetoma 159
Exanthematous eruption 73
Excoriation 4
Exudation 42f
Eyebrows 35, 51
Eyelashes 51

F

Face 180
Facial pilosebaceous units, chronic inflammatory acneiform disorder of 192
Famciclovir 128
Famotidine 53
Fasciitis, eosinophilic 84
Fat, subcutaneous 82
Ferriman-Gallwey hirsutism scoring system, modified 203, 204f
Fever 56, 57, 59, 103, 108, 109, 120, 125, 173, 198, 209
Fibroma, periungual 91f, 212, 212f
Fibrosis, pulmonary 21
Filaggrin deficiency 83
Filariasis 137, 138f
Finasteride 198, 204
Fissures 4, 6f, 86f, 94
Fistula 94, 195
Fixed drug eruption 30, 55, 60, 61f, 109
Flaccid bulla 59f
Flavivirus 133
Fluconazole 60f, 62, 146, 147, 150, 153, 158
Fluorescent treponemal antibody absorption 144
Flutamide 204
Follicle stimulating hormone 191, 203
Folliculitis 63, 99f
bacterial 155
chronic 194
eosinophilic 11
Foot
diabetic 75
dorsum of 15f
Fordyce granules 212
Fossa, popliteal 32f
Fractional carbon dioxide laser 192
Fractional erbium laser 192, 194
therapy 26f
Fungal infections
deep 144
superficial 144
systemic 144
Furuncles 73f, 100f

G

Gabapentin 12
Galactorrhea 203
Gastrointestinal system 180
Gastrointestinal tract 53, 72, 91, 122, 177
Genetic disorders 82, 161
Genital discharge 111
Genitalia 111
Genitourinary tract, lower 111
Genodermatosis 83

German measles 120
Gianotti–Crosti syndrome 95, 132, 132f
Gigantism 72
Gland, sebaceous 212
Glans penis 17f
Glomerulonephritis, acute 96
Glucocorticoid 167
Glucose-6-phosphate dehydrogenase 170
Glycolic acid peel 192
Goiter, diffuse 76
Gonococcal infection, disseminated 111, 112, 112f
Gonorrhea 111, 111f, 112
Gottron's papules 185f
Gout 80
  severe 20
Graft-versus-host disease 84
Granuloma
  inguinale 109, 112, 113f
  periungual pyogenic 212, 212f
Graves' disease 76
Griseofulvin 146, 153
Gum tissues, increased growth of 20
Guttate psoriasis 14f, 18
Gynecomastia 70f, 120f

H

Haemophilus
  ducreyi 109
  influenzae 132
Hailey–Hailey disease 87, 87f
Hair 78, 95, 173, 197
  anagen 197
  axillary 95
  catagen 197
  follicle, infection of 99f
  fungal infections of 144
  growth
    cycle 197f
    excessive 20
  lanugo 197 198
  loss
    female pattern of 198, 198f
    male pattern of 198, 198f
    physiological neonatal 198
    postpartum 198
  pectoral 95
  pubic 95
  telogen 197
  terminal 197, 198
  transplantation 198
  vellus 197, 198
Hand
  dermatitis
    acute 38
    recurrent 38

eczema 46f
  foot, and mouth disease 122, 123f
Hansen's disease 113
Hard palate involvement 25f
Head lice 143, 143f
Headache 20
Heart 90
Heliotrope
  erythema 185f
  periorbital 185
Hematologic disorders 176
Hematoma, subungual 209
Hemochromatosis 95
Hemoglobin 63
Hemorrhage 91, 209f
  cutaneous 95
  gastrointestinal 94
  multiple subungual splinter 171
  petechial 8f, 135
  purpuric 134f
  retinal 91
Hemorrhagic telangiectasis, hereditary 94
Henna, chemical component of 43f
Hepatic disease 11
Hepatitis 57, 59
  A virus 132
  B virus 95 132
  C virus 95, 132
  virus 55
Hepatology, cutaneous 94
Herpes
  progenitalis 109
  simplex 4f
    simplex infections 128f
    virus 55, 96, 125
  zoster 6f, 124, 125f
    complications of 125
Hidradenitis suppurativa 195, 195f
High bacterial index 120
Hirsutism 203, 204f
  treatment of 204
Histoplasma capsulatum 55
Hodgkin's disease 11, 84
Hodgkin's lymphoma 187
Hormone, luteinizing 191, 203
Human immunodeficiency virus 55, 108, 132
  infection 13, 83
Human papillomavirus 128
Hyperandrogenic states 72
Hyperandrogenism 191, 203
  treatment of 204
Hypercorticism 76
Hyperemia, severe 111
Hyperhidrosis 106
Hyperkeratosis 64f
  diffuse 22f, 86f
  punctate 65f

Hyperlipidemia
  primary 78
  secondary 78
Hyperpigmentation 32f, 47f, 50f, 62f, 77f, 81, 95
  cutaneous 62, 95
  post-inflammatory 30
Hyperplastic candidiasis 157
Hypertension 91
  portal 94
Hyperthyroidism 11, 76
Hypertrichosis 81, 203, 204
Hypertrophic lichen planus 3f, 25f
  lesions 28f
Hypertrophy 7, 8f, 192
Hypocalcemia 18
Hypogonadal syndrome 72
Hypopigmented face 31f
Hypotension 108
Hypothyroidism 11, 35, 72, 76, 77, 83

I

Ichthyosis 83
  acquired 83, 84
  mild 83
  vulgaris 35, 83
  X-linked 83, 84
Immunoablation 180
Immunoglobulin 185
  G 163
  intravenous 40, 168, 176
Immunologic disorder 176
Immunotherapy
  intralesional 132
  topical 132
Impetigo 96
Indomethacin 54
Infarction 109f
Infections 11, 18, 73, 96, 144, 186
  bacterial 96, 96f, 105
  chronic 149f
  fungal 96, 144
  genital 125
  primary 128
  protozoal 135
  secondary bacterial 31f, 120
  severe 21
  staphylococcal 96
  staphylococcus 98f
  streptococcal 96, 98f
Infertility 112, 203
Inflammation, nail-fold 209, 209f
Inflammatory disease 35
Infliximab 168
Influenza 132
Infraorbital fold, typical 34, 35f
Ingrowing nail 205, 206f

Insect bites 96
Insulin lowering agents 204
Interferon 13
Intertrigo 71f, 105, 106f, 154
Intradermal melanocytic nevi 80
Intralesional steroid 49
Intramuscular ceftriaxone, single dose 112
Intravascular coagulation, disseminated 9f
Intravenous immunoglobulin 40, 168, 176
  high dose of 168
Iontophoresis 106
Irritant contact dermatitis 11, 35, 40, 40f
Ischemia, acral 135
Isotretinoin 19, 198
  oral 192, 196
Itch
  neuropathic 11, 12
  postherpetic 125
  renal 12
Itraconazole 146, 147, 150, 153, 158

J

Jaundice 95
Jock itch 150
Joints 13
  involvement of 16f

K

Keloid 7, 8f, 192f
Kenogen 197
Keratitis 57, 59
Keratoderma 86
  blennorrhagicum, plantar lesions of 20f
Keratolysis, pitted 105, 107f
Keratolytic 86, 87
  agents 83
Keratosis pilaris 2f, 34
Keratotic follicular papule 34, 34f
Kerion 201
Ketoconazole 35, 146, 153, 158
Ketotifen 54
Kidney 90
  disease, chronic 35
  function 20
    test 53
Klebsiella granulomatis 112
Koebner phenomenon 13, 29, 29f
Koenen tumors 90
Koilonychia 94
Koplik spot 120
Kytococcus sedentarius 105

L

Lactation 21
Lactic acid 83
Lamellar ichthyoses 84
Langer's lines 21, 21f
Larva migrans, cutaneous 137, 138f
Laryngitis 120
Larynx 122
Lasers 204
Leishmania
  aethiopica 135
  major 135
  mexicana 135
  tropica 135
Leishmaniasis 135
  cutaneous 135, 137f
  mucocutaneous 135
Lepra reactions 116
Lepromatous leprosy 113, 116, 119f
Leprosy 83
Lesions
  bullous 57, 59
  cutaneous 70, 70f
  hypertrophic 27f
  mucosal 94
  multiple cystic 3f
  nonspecific 63
  primary 1
  secondary 4
  types of 1
  ulcerative 25f
  vascular 94
Leukemia 187
  lymphocytic 11
Leukocytes, polymorphonuclear 111
Leukocytosis 187
Leukonychia, true 209
Leukopenia 21
Leukoplakia 214
Levocetirizine 53
Lichen
  nitidus 29
  planopilaris 201
  planus 2f, 11, 23, 26f, 95
    hypertrophic 3f, 25f
    pigmentosus 30
    sclerosus 11, 47, 182
      et atrophicus 182, 182f
    simplex chronicus 11, 15f, 49
    striatus 28
Lichenification 31f-33f, 39f, 40, 42f, 46f, 47f, 49, 50f
Lichenoid
  amyloidosis 80f
  dermatoses 23
  drug eruption 28, 28f
Linear psoriasis 18

Lip licking 40, 45
  dermatitis 46f
Lipodermatosclerosis 36, 71f
  acute 38
  chronic 38
Lisch nodules 89
Lithium 13, 198
Livedo reticularis 95, 135, 171, 176, 176f
  persistent 171
Liver
  cirrhosis of 95
  disease 94
  function test 53
    abnormalities 21
Long bone cortex, thinning of 89
Lupus
  profundus 82
  tumidus 171
  vulgaris 113, 115f
Lupus erythematosus 11, 171, 201
  acute cutaneous 171
  annular subacute cutaneous 171
  cutaneous 171
  drug-induced 171
  generalized acute cutaneous 171
  subacute cutaneous 171
  systemic 84, 171, 173, 176, 176f
  urticarial plaque of 171
Lutzomyia 135
Lymphadenopathy 57, 59
Lymphedema 195
Lymphoma 11, 72, 83

M

Macular atypical lesions 57, 59
Macules 1
  hypopigmented 34f, 90
Maculopapular rash 134f, 144f
Madura foot 159
Maduromycosis 144, 159, 160f
Magnesium supplements 92
Malaise 103
Malar rash 171, 176
Malassezia 35, 144
  furfur 158
Malignancy 187
  cutaneous 201
Martin-Lewis media 111
Mastocytosis 11
Measles 120
  infection 120
Melanocytic nevus, congenital 203
Melanonychia, longitudinal 206, 206f
Melanosis 64
Meningitis 108
Meningococcal infection 10f
Meningococcemia 108, 108f

Mental retardation 90
Menthol 12
Metabolic disease 67
Metformin 204
Methimazole 198
Methotrexate 19, 20, 167, 168, 176, 185
   extravasation of 62*f*
   hypersensitivity of 21
Metronidazole 194, 196
Miconazole 106, 146
Microhemagglutination assay 144
Milia 81*f*
Minocycline 62, 192, 196
Minoxidil, topical 198
Mirtazapine 12
Mixed connective tissue
   disease 84
   disorder 180
Mohs micrographic surgery 65
Molluscum contagiosum 3*f*, 133
Moon face 76*f*
Morbilliform eruption 135
Morphea 180, 181*f*, 201
Morphine 11, 53
Mucocele 213
Mucosa
   oral 95, 214*f*
   viral diseases of 120
Mucosal diseases 212
Mucosal erosion 56*f*, 79*f*, 163
Mucous membrane 13, 23*f*, 24*f*, 78, 111, 163, 173, 180, 197
   fungal infections of 144
   scarring of 24*f*
Muehrcke's nail 94
Multisystem autoimmune disease 173
Muscle weakness 185
Myalgias 120
Mycetoma 159
Mycobacterial diseases 113
Mycobacterium
   leprae 113
   tuberculosis 55, 113
Mycophenolate mofetil 167, 176
Mycoplasma pneumoniae 55-57, 132
Mycosis fungoides 38
Myelodysplasia 11
Myeloid 11
Myeloma, multiple 11
Myxedema 77
   pretibial 76
Myxoid cyst 212, 212*f*

N

Naftifine 146
Nail 13, 78, 94, 197
   anatomy 205*f*
   changes 18
   disorders 205
   fungal infections of 144
   involvement of 16*f*
   plate 210*f*, 211*f*
      loss of 210*f*
      thickening of 15*f*
      transverse depression of 209, 210*f*
   psoriasis, severe 21
   spoon-shaped 94
   unit anatomy 205
   white discoloration of 209*f*
Nalfurafine 12
Naltrexone 12
Naproxen 62
   ingestion of 61*f*
Nasolabial folds 35
Necrobiosis lipoidica 73, 73*f*, 201
Necrosis 44*f*
   cutaneous 171
   epidermal 40
Necrotizing fasciitis 103, 104*f*
Neisseria
   gonorrhoeae 111
   meningitidis 109
Neodymium-doped yttrium aluminum garnet 204
Nephritogenic streptococci 96
Neuralgia, postherpetic 124, 125
Neurofibromatosis 4*f*, 89, 90*f*
Neuropathy
   diabetic 75
   peripheral 173
Neurotic excoriation 48, 49*f*
Neutropenia 108
Nikolsky sign 109, 166, 167
Nipple eczema 38
Nodular amyloidosis 80
Nodule 1, 4*f*, 137*f*
   erythematous 187
   metastatic 95
Nonbullous impetigo 98*f*
Non-Hodgkin's lymphoma 84, 85*f*, 187
Nonpalpable purpura 9*f*
Nonsteroidal anti-inflammatory drugs 53, 187
Nutritional disease 67

O

Obesity 70
   acquired 70
   central 203
Obstructive biliary disease 11
Onycholysis 15*f*, 206, 207*f*
Onychomycosis 207
   distal subungual 207, 207*f*
   proximal subungual 207, 208*f*
Onychophagia 45, 45*f*
Onychorrhexis 208
Onychoschizia 208
Onychotilomania 45
Ophthalmia neonatorum 112*f*
Ophthalmology 76
Opioid
   agonists 12
   antagonists 12
Optic gliomas 89
Orchitis 112
Orogenital sex 111
Oropharyngeal candidiasis 155, 157*f*
Oropharynx 111
Otitis media 120
Oxiconazole 146

P

Paclitaxel 201
Pain 12, 111, 208*f*
Palate 122
Palmar erythema 94, 171
Palmoplantar keratoderma 86
   diffuse 86
Palmoplantar pustulosis 18
Pancreatic disease 95
Panniculitis 82, 95
Papular acrodermatitis 132
Papules 1, 21*f*, 69*f*, 121*f*, 122
   erythematous 67, 68*f*, 69*f*, 137*f*, 186*f*, 191
   follicular 22*f*
   keratotic 64, 87*f*
   linear flat-topped 28*f*
   pruritic urticarial 67
   umbilicated 133*f*
   violaceous 23*f*, 27*f*
Papulonodular lesions, multiple 50*f*
Papulopustular rosacea 194
Papulosquamous subacute cutaneous lupus erythematosus 171
Parainfluenza virus 132
Parasitosis, delusions of 45, 51, 51*f*
Paronychia 74*f*
   acute 102*f*, 208
   chronic 102*f*, 209
   pyogenic 102
Parvovirus 55, 132
Patches 1
   hypopigmented 17*f*
Pediculosis capitis 143
Pellagra 78
Pelvic inflammatory disease 112
Pemphigoid gestationis 67
Pemphigus 163
   erythematosus 167, 167*f*
   familial benign chronic 87
   foliaceus 163, 166, 167, 167*f*
   vulgaris 5*f*, 163, 166*f*, 167

Penicillin 55
  allergy 112
Perianal dermatitis 105, 105*f*
Perifollicular abscesses, multiple groups of 100*f*
Petechiae 7, 8*f*, 9*f*
Pethidine 48*f*
Pharyngitis 111
  streptococcal 13
Pharynx 111, 122
Phenolphthalein 62
Phenyl-butazone 55
Phenytoin 55, 198
Phlebotomus 135
Photopheresis 180
Photophobia 120
Photosensitivity 73, 81
Phototherapy 19, 35, 180
Phymatous rosacea 194
Pigmentation 40
Pink macules 121*f*
Pityriasis
  alba 17*f*, 31*f*, 34
  rosea 21
    vesicular 38
  rubra pilaris 22, 23*f*
  versicolor 158, 159*f*
Plantar
  hyperkeratosis 70*f*
  psoriasis 16*f*
Plaques 1, 21*f*, 27*f*, 137*f*, 186*f*
  amyloidosis 80*f*
  erythematous 13*f*, 14*f*, 16*f*
  hypopigmented 47*f*
  large scaling 15*f*
  pruritic evanescent 5*f*
  psoriasis, chronic 14*f*, 18, 20
Plasmapheresis 68, 167
Platelet
  dysfunction 7
  rich plasma 30, 192, 198
Plewig and Kligman classification 194
Plexiform neurofibroma 90*f*
Pneumonia 120
Pneumonitis 124
Podophyllotoxin 132
Poikiloderma 185
Poliovirus 132
Polyarteritis nodosa 95, 171
Polycystic ovarian syndrome 70, 191, 203
Polymerase chain reaction 120, 128
Polymyxin B 11
Porphyria 54, 81
  cutanea tarda 81, 95
Post-kala-azar dermal leishmaniasis 137, 137*f*
Poxvirus 132
Prader–Willi syndrome 70

Prednisolone 67
Prednisone 196
Pregabalin 12, 54
Pregnancy 11, 21, 187
  cholestasis of 68, 69*f*
  ectopic 112
  plaques of 67
  polymorphic eruption of 67
  prurigo of 68
  pustular psoriasis of 67
Proctitis 111
Propranolol 54
Propylthiouracil 198
Prostatitis 112
Prurigo nodularis 11, 49
Pruritus 11, 12, 95, 185
  ani 46
  aquagenic 54
  causes of 11
  chronic 46
  primary generalized 12
  scroti 47
  treatment of 11
  vulvae 47
Pseudomonas 206
  aeruginosa 210
    infection 106
Pseudo-orange appearance 94
Pseudoxanthoma elasticum 82, 91, 91*f*, 94
Psoralen plus ultraviolet A 19, 40
  therapy 54
Psoriasis 3*f*, 6*f*, 11, 13, 15*f*, 17*f*, 21, 47, 211, 211*f*
  arthritis 20
  common sites of 18
  erythrodermic 18, 20
  inverse 18, 105
  pustular 18, 20, 67, 211, 211*f*
Psoriatic nail change 15*f*
Psoriatic plaque 14*f*
  symmetric distribution of 14*f*
Psychogenic excoriation 45, 48
Psychoneurodermatitis 45
Pulsed dye laser 132
Purpura 7, 9*f*
Purulent rectal discharge 111
Pustules 4, 17*f*, 122
  erythematous 191
Pyoderma 63
  gangrenosum 94, 95, 187, 188*f*
  ulcerative 99*f*

Q

Quinacrine 176
Quinidine 28, 62
Quinine 62

R

Radiation
  dermatitis 41, 201
  therapy 44*f*
Radiodermatitis 41
Raindrop
  hypopigmentation 2*f*
  melanosis 64*f*-66*f*
Raynaud phenomenon 171, 177, 177*f*
Rectum 111
Reiter's disease 19
Renal cell carcinoma 187
Renal disorder 176
Respiratory tract infections, 52
Retinoic acid 192
Retinoid 176, 198
  oral 19, 86, 87, 132
  topical 86, 87, 192
Rhinitis 63
Ribonucleic acid 120, 180
Rifampicin 120
Rituximab 168
Rotavirus 132
Rubella 120
Rubeola 120

S

Salicylates 187
Salicylic acid 83, 132
Salivary duct 213*f*
Salmonella 55
Sandflies 135
Sarcoidosis 83, 84, 201
Sarcoptes scabiei hominis 139
Scabies 3*f*, 139, 142*f*
Scale 4
  hair, sensitivity of 198
  psoriasis 18
  ringworm 153
Scaly face 31*f*
Scar 81*f*
  hypertrophic 126*f*, 201
Scarring alopecia 201, 203*f*
Scleredema diabeticorum 73
Scleroderma 177
Sclerodermoid disorders 177
Sclerosis
  progressive systemic 177
  systemic 177, 179*f*
  tuberous 89
Scopolamine 11
SCORTEN scale 60
Scrofuloderma 113, 116*f*
Scrotal tongue 213, 213*f*
Scrotum 3*f*, 47
Secukinumab 20
Seizures 90

Selective serotonin reuptake inhibitors 12, 54
Selenium sulfide 35, 158
Senile purpura 10*f*
Serositis 176
Serotonin-norepinephrine reuptake inhibitors 12
Serum thyroid stimulating hormone 53
Sexually transmitted infection 109
Shagreen patch 90
Silvery white scale 6*f*, 13*f*, 16*f*
Skin 63, 94, 180
   acute autoimmune bullous disease of 163
   atrophy 76*f*
   biopsy 18
   care 35
   chronic autoimmune bullous disease of 163
   chronic inflammatory disease of 13
   darkening of 64
   disease 12
     inflammatory 31
   erosion 61*f*
   findings 72, 77, 94
   fragile 81*f*
   fungal infections of 144
   genetic diseases of 83
   involvement 16*f*
     extent of 96*f*
   lesions 122, 128, 136*f*, 173, 185
   periareolar 39*f*
   sensitivity 20
   tuberculosis of 113
   viral diseases of 120
Slapped cheek disease 122
Slit-skin smear 120
Spectinomycin, intramuscular 112
Sphenoid wing dysplasia 89
Spider angiomas 94
Spironolactone 198, 204
Sporotrichosis 144
Squamous cell carcinoma 28*f*, 64, 65, 66*f*, 86, 87*f*, 92, 149*f*, 162, 183, 195, 214, 214*f*
Stanozolol 54
Staphylococcal scalded skin syndrome 109, 110*f*
Staphylococcus aureus 96
Stasis dermatitis 11, 35, 36, 38, 41, 71*f*
Steatocystoma multiplex 3*f*, 82*f*
Sterile pus formation 5*f*
Steroid, topical 7*f*, 10*f*, 49
Stevens-Johnson syndrome 55, 57
Stomach 20
Streptococcus
   aureus 102
   pyogenes 96, 102
Stress 35, 125
   psychological 198
Striae 76*f*
   distensae 68*f*, 71*f*
   gravidarum 69, 70*f*
   pregnancy-induced 69
Sulconazole 146
Sulfa drugs 62
Sulfamethoxazole 21
Sulfonamide 55, 62
Sun protection factor 194
Superficial disease 35
Sweating 35
Sweet's syndrome 94, 186, 186*f*
Swollen
   eyelids 111
   nail-fold 208*f*
Syphilis 143
   secondary 144*f*
Systemic lupus erythematosus 84, 171, 173, 176, 176*f*

T

Tacrolimus 19, 35
Tazarotene 19, 192
T-cell lymphoma, cutaneous 11
Teeth, X-ray of 53
Telangiectasias, nail-fold 171
Telangiectasis 7
Telogen effluvium 198, 199*f*
Terbinafine 146, 147, 150, 153, 158
Terry classic white nail 94
Testosterone, serum-free 191
Tetanus 132
Tetracycline 61*f*, 62, 196
Thalidomide 11, 12, 49, 176
Thayer-Martin media 111
Thermolysis 204
Thiazide diuretics 28
Thrombocytopenia 21
Thrombocytopenic purpura 120
Thrombophlebitis, migratory 95
Thyroid 76
   disease, autoimmune 199
Tinea
   barbae 153, 154, 154*f*, 155*f*
   corporis 38, 145, 146*f*, 151
   cruris 150, 151*f*
   facialis 151
   faciei 152*f*
   manuum 147, 149*f*
   pedis 147, 148*f*
Tissue
   painful swelling of 102
   progressive calcification of 94
Togavirus 133
Tolnaftate 146
Tongue, geographic 213, 213*f*
Toxic epidermal necrolysis 55, 57, 59, 59*f*
   score of 60
Trachea 122
Traction alopecia, long-standing 201
Transferrin deficiency, congenital 95
Trauma 13, 125
Treponema pallidum 143
Tretinoin, topical 69
Triamcinolone acetonide 195
Trichloroacetic acid 30, 192
Trichotillomania 45, 51, 51*f*, 199, 201*f*
Trimethoprim 21
Tubal scarring 112
Tuberculoid leprosy 116, 117*f*
Tuberculosis 113
   cutaneous 113
   periorificial 113, 116*f*
   verrucosa cutis 113, 114*f*
Tuberculous abscess 101*f*
Tumor
   glomus 212, 212*f*
   necrosis factor 20
Twenty-nail dystrophy 26*f*

U

Ulcer 7, 7*f*, 37*f*, 57, 59, 63, 101*f*, 113, 187
   anesthetic 74*f*
   aphthous 94
   formation, self-induced 48*f*, 51*f*
   infections 74*f*
   leg 71*f*
   oral 19, 176
   peptic 21
Ultrasonography 139
Ultraviolet
   A 194
   B 49
   radiation 125
   therapy 12
Umbilicus 95
United Nations International Children's Emergency Fund 63
Urea 83
Urethra 111
Urethral stricture 112
Urethritis 19
Urinary tract 122
   infection 52
Ursodeoxycholic acid 68
Urticaria 11, 52, 73, 94, 95
   acute 5*f*, 52, 54, 135
   chronic 5*f*, 52
   cold 53
   idiopathic 54
   papular 11
   solar 54
   vasculitis 54, 171

V

Vaccines 132
Vaginal discharge 112*f*
Vaginal swab 53
Valacyclovir 124, 128
Valproic acid 198
Varicella 4*f*, 55, 122, 123*f*, 125
   zoster virus 122
      immunization 124
Vascular disease, peripheral 75*f*
Vascular hyperpigmentation,
    methotrexate induced 62*f*
Vascular laser 194
Vasculitis 53, 94, 95, 171, 177
   pustular 94
Vasculopathy 171
Veins, dilated abdominal 94
Venereal Disease Research Laboratory
   144
   test 53
Verruca vulgaris 129
Verrucous papules 3*f*
Vesicles 4, 43*f*, 44*f*, 59*f*, 61*f*, 69*f*, 122
   bulla 60*f*
Vesicobullae 81*f*
Vesiculobullous lesions 96
Vessel vasculitis 171
Viannia subgenus 135
Virilization, signs of 203
Visceral leishmaniasis 135

Vitamin
   D3 analog 19
   K deficiency 7
Vitiligo 2*f*, 94, 95, 199
von Recklinghausen disease 89
von Zumbusch pattern 18
Vulvar mucosa 103
Vulvitis 157
Vulvodynia, dysesthetic 47
Vulvovaginal candidiasis, chronic 47
Vulvovaginitis 157

W

Warts 129, 130*f*
   flat 129, 132*f*
   oral 132
   palmar 129, 131*f*
   plantar 129, 131*f*
   recalcitrant 132
   treatment of 132
   viral 3*f*
Waxy hyperkeratosis 22*f*
   diffuse 22*f*
Weight loss 198
Wheals 4, 52*f*
White spots, congenital 90
White superficial onychomycosis 207, 207*f*
Whitfield's ointment 106
Wickham's striae 27*f*
Wilson–Turner syndrome 70
Wood's lamp 146
Wound infections 74*f*
Wuchereria bancrofti 137

X

Xanthelasma 78*f*
Xanthomas 78
   eruptive 78*f*
Xeroderma pigmentosum 92, 93*f*
Xerosis 11, 33*f*, 34, 36*f*, 83
X-linked recessive disorder 84

Y

Yeast infection 157
Yellow nail syndrome 211, 211*f*

Z

Ziehl–Neelsen staining 120
Zinc 35
   absorption, autosomal recessive
      genetic disorder of 78
   deficiency 78
      acquired 78
   salt supplementation, intravenous 78
   therapy 79*f*

EU GSPR Authorised Reprsentative
Logos Europe, 9 rue Nicolas Poussin
1700, La Rochelle, France
Phone: +33 (0) 6 67 93 73 78
E-mail: contact@logoseurope.eu

www.ingramcontent.com/pod-product-compliance
Ingram Content Group UK Ltd.
Pitfield, Milton Keynes, MK11 3LW, UK
UKHW051847210426

5322IPUK00019B/284